HANGRY

HANGRY

Simple Steps to Balance Your Hormones and Restore Your Joy

Sarah Fragoso

and

Brooke Kalanick, ND, MS

St. Martin's Press ✿ New York

Mention of specific companies, organizations, or authorities in this book does not imply endorsement by the authors or publisher, nor does mention of specific companies, organizations, or authorities imply that they endorse this book, its authors, or the publisher.

Internet addresses and contact information given in this book were accurate at the time it went to press.

HANGRY. Copyright © 2019 by Sarah Fragoso and Brooke Kalanick. All rights reserved. Printed in the United States of America. For information, address St. Martin's Press, 175 Fifth Avenue, New York, N.Y. 10010.

www.stmartins.com

The Library of Congress Cataloging-in-Publication Data is available upon request.

ISBN 978-1-250-18984-4 (hardcover)
ISBN 978-1-250-18985-1 (ebook)

Our books may be purchased in bulk for promotional, educational, or business use. Please contact your local bookseller or the Macmillan Corporate and Premium Sales Department at 1-800-221-7945, extension 5442, or by email at MacmillanSpecialMarkets@macmillan.com.

First Edition: June 2019

10 9 8 7 6 5 4 3 2 1

To women everywhere who are overwhelmed, exhausted, stressed, frustrated, and tired of all the BS diet and exercise trends, and yet still decided to pick up this book. Thank you. Thank you for trusting in us, and for caring enough about yourself to take yet another step towards finally feeling better. It's our wish that this book will bring you the hope and true healing you have been searching for. You are worth it.

Contents

Acknowledgments

From Sarah:

To my sweet Brooke. I'm so thankful that we tackled this beast of a book together! There's nobody else in the world I'd rather ride on unicorn floaties in Lake George or write life-changing books with. Thank you, for taking on this never-ending project with me and for sticking by me through all the crazy that life has thrown our way! I'm so grateful for you, and I love you.

To John, this book would not have happened without your tireless hours of reading, editing, and input, as well as your unwavering love and support. I am incredibly lucky to have you standing by me.

To Coby, Jaden, and Rowan. From editing to errand running to comedic relief, all of you helped so much with this project. Thank you, for being the most understanding boys a mom who's writing a hormone health book could have; the three of you are my why, and I love you each completely and endlessly.

Sister and Brother, thank you, for being the best, most supportive, loving, and encouraging siblings ever. I love you both to the moon and beyond.

To my tribe of women friends (you all know who you are)—my honorary sisters in this life, the ones I say I love you to because I really mean it, thank you for being powerful, inspiring, warrior women, all authentically who you are.

To Mom. You are still, and forever will be, my inspiration. To Dad. You are right: we are the most blessed family, and I couldn't have made it this far without you.

From Dr. Brooke:

Thank you, Sarah. I can't imagine working this hard on anything with anyone else and I wouldn't want to. You were the missing piece to my work and my life, I love you. I'm also so grateful for your Chico fam: John, Jess, Lynn, America,

Mike, Blaire, Lisa, and Traci—thank you, for everything you do to support our work.

Thank you to the colleagues and friends that teach, inspire, and rally me: Tyna Moore, Jill Coleman, Jade Teta, Jen Comas, Mariza Snyder, Ann Wendell, Karen Smith, and Cass Forsythe. And thank you, Molly Galbraith and Joe Dowdell, for giving me a chance when no one knew who the heck I was.

Thank you to the team that keeps my biz going and talks me off the ledge: Anna, Tomas, Mackenzie, Mariana, and Matt. Thank you, Dorota, for keeping our home together and a special thank-you to my friend, admin, and "Aunt" Sally for everything since day one in NYC, and to Jack for all the Lake George sunsets.

Thank you, Dad, for always supporting me even when my dreams are a little nuts.

Thank you, Margo, Aaron, Noah, Clara, Steve, Sarah, and Noel, for all the '80s dance parties during this crazy, stressful year. You're irreplaceable. Thank you, Carly, for making Brooklyn fun again. Thank you, Taryn and Lorraine, for still loving me even though I never call.

Lastly, Joe and my girls, I love you all so much. Gigi, your spunk embodies #bewhoyouare and all my stress melts away when I kiss your sweet cheeks. Lola, you are the smartest, kindest person I know, and this book would not be possible without you playing with your little sister for days on end as I sat for far too many hours at the computer.

From Sarah and Brooke:

To our Better Everyday Inner Circle Women, our podcast listeners, our online followers, and all the clients we have ever coached or treated—we are forever grateful. Thank you, for your vulnerability and for your trust in us. Without you we couldn't do this work and we are humbled and deeply honored by the support we have received over the years.

To Michael Lang, for taking our pictures and for being so incredibly patient with us. We couldn't imagine working with anyone besides you! You make the hardest part easy!

To our amazing editor, Eileen Rothschild, and the entire kick-ass team at St. Martin's Press, we could tell from that very first phone call that you simply "got" us. Thank you, for turning this book into reality and for your excitement, guidance, and attention.

To our agents Celeste Fine, Sarah Passick, and the rest of the team—you made *Hangry* come to life. We are eternally grateful for your direction, inspiration, and belief in us!

Introduction

We Know What It's Like to Be a Hangry B*tch

> **Hangry B*tch:** A woman who feels hormonally harried and who is frustrated, unfulfilled, tired, and troubled—i.e., overwhelmed and over it.
>
> **Happy Babe:** A woman whose hormones are in harmony, who feels nourished and nurtured and is present and joyful—i.e., finally freakin' fulfilled and healthy.

If you are reading this, you know what it is like to feel like a Hangry B*tch! Ladies, you're tired, you're stressed, you're unhappy. We know this because every other woman feels the same way. Take a look at other women in line at the grocery store, at preschool drop-off, and around your office. Like other women, you've probably spoken with your doctor about how terrible you feel, only to be told (perhaps based on a skimpy panel of tests) that "nothing's wrong" or "it's all in your head" or "you're just getting older" or, perhaps the worst, "every woman I talk to feels this way; it's normal."

It. Is. Not. Normal. We're all worn-out and frazzled and wish we felt different. We commiserate about pesky symptoms like our erratic menstrual cycles (or lack thereof), our breakouts and bloating, our inability to get any restful sleep, and our expanding waistlines, and we frequently answer the daily question "How are you doing?" with "I'm stressed out of my freaking mind!"

We've mistaken common as normal because we're all in the same boat, but just because something is common does not mean that it should be classified as normal. Simply put, we all deserve better.

We wrote this book after years of successfully working with and helping women just like you—but that's not all that makes us experts. We have also been exactly where you are right now, or at least in places that will probably look very similar.

We are your anti-gurus: real women working under real demands with real lives who are in the arena with you. We have both suffered enough to understand what it takes to come back and really live; and after years of work, research, and dedication to women everywhere, together we have developed the Hangry B*tch Reset, a four-week program that takes you from Hangry B*tch to Happy Babe.

Before we introduce you to the Hangry B*tch Reset, we think it's important for you to get to know us a bit better, to give you a glimpse of where we came from and what led us to do the work we do today.

Sarah Fragoso's Story

I grew up watching my mother constantly struggle with her health. When my mom wasn't battling migraines, she alternated between bouts of depression, bloating, and fatigue. Despite what she was up against on a daily basis, my mother was driven. She was always on her game on the home front and in her career as a licensed clinical social worker. My mom did it all, powered through, and, like so many of us, sacrificed her health in the process.

As her symptoms got more significant, she tried everything to be well: she read book after book on natural remedies for her symptoms, juiced her veggies, sprouted her beans and grains, and took mountains of vitamins. Sometimes she felt better, but often she felt worse. She carried the heavy burden of her family's needs, as well as each day carrying home with her the stress of her demanding career.

In 1999, my mom's health took a severe turn for the worse when she was diagnosed with breast cancer, and in 2004 it metastasized and spread to her brain, bones, and lungs. On May 14, 2005, I lost the most influential, powerful, and loving woman in my life.

After losing my mom, I tried desperately to ignore the panic and fear that comes with suffering such a great loss. Instead of confronting my pain, I buried myself in mothering, wife-ing, obtaining my psychology degree, and working, without taking two seconds to breathe or grieve.

Two years later and three months after the birth of my third son, I was a total disaster, battling headaches, candida issues, weight gain, edema, cravings, and constant fatigue—not dissimilar to my mother's story.

In an attempt to do something to turn things around, I joined a local gym that was owned and operated by Robb Wolf, future *New York Times* bestselling author of *The Paleo Solution* and *Wired to Eat*. I was encouraged by Robb to try a Paleo diet and, as I saw the amazing results that unfolded by simply following this food plan and a rigorous exercise regimen, I found myself falling in love with my rescuers: fitness and nutrition. One year after walking into Robb's gym, I was the healthiest version of myself that I had ever been, and I became a trainer at the gym. I leaped into my new career with wild abandon and, to share my newfound passion with the world, started my blog *Everyday Paleo* to document my healthy lifestyle.

My new life, although exciting, was a rinse-and-repeat cycle of total insanity. Although I had lost weight and gained some energy and muscle, my newfound path of pushing harder than I ever had before quickly took over any vitality, vigor, or balance that I thought I had achieved. I was eating healthy and exercising hard, but I once again found myself chronically exhausted and back to being a Hangry B*tch—but this time with more severe repercussions than before. In fact, I had no idea how badly I was crashing until I literally collapsed while coaching a class at the gym on February 11, 2010. The next day at the urgent care clinic my blood pressure was 85/50, which is right above coma, followed closely by death. The doctor checked my heart, ruled out a stroke, and chalked it up to exhaustion and/or "something psychological."

For the next month I literally couldn't get out of bed. My blood pressure stayed chronically low, which made me feel like I was constantly lightheaded or drunk; my kidneys hurt; my joints ached; and I was seriously depressed. At this point, I wasn't just a Hangry B*tch, I actually felt like I was dying, and nobody seemed to know what to do. I was more "fit" than I ever had been in my life, yet I wasn't even able to muster the energy to make breakfast.

I eventually found a local naturopathic doctor who told me that I had "adrenal fatigue," more accurately termed HPA (hypothalamic-pituitary-adrenal) axis dysfunction. There I was, the perfect Paleo dieter who also excelled at training as hard and as often as possible—all in order to hide from my fear and my pain. I had never caught up from countless sleepless nights taking care of kids while finishing my degree, I had never faced the grief of losing my mom, I had never sat with the reality that my life was a total mess and instead continued to distract myself with what felt good at the time but what was actually driving me deeper and deeper into hormonal disarray.

More than all of that, I was taking care of everyone and everything around me—and always putting myself last. My only form of self-care was my punishing workouts. I thought I was doing all I could do to be healthy, but by doing *more*, I most definitely was not doing *better*.

Hitting rock bottom was the beginning of my awakening. After years of revamping everything I thought I knew about fitness; relearning what self-care really means; practicing, researching, and implementing mindfulness practice;

and surrendering to the fact that I simply couldn't do it all, I have made my way back to being able not just to survive, but to thrive.

In 2011 I started my *Everyday Paleo* franchise, which has sold over 275,000 books, and I launched my first podcast, which now has millions of downloads. I loved these opportunities to share my philosophies on life, food, and fitness with devotees and newcomers alike in ways that are practical, family-friendly, and delicious. In 2013 I opened my own gym with my husband, John, and today I am so incredibly grateful to be able to help women who walk the same path as I have. I'm grateful every moment for my health, and I'm honored to share my experiences and truth with women around the world.

Dr. Brooke Kalanick's Story

I am no stranger to stress. I grew up with a mother who modeled overextending herself and repeatedly melted down from the stress. As a single mom working two jobs, she got way too little sleep while constantly trying to keep us in handmade Halloween costumes and making us homemade school treats. This frenzy also kept her from doing much work to heal from her divorce, so the emotional toll rose higher and higher during my most formative years.

As a little girl I didn't understand the strain her behavior caused to her hormones and health; I just saw a frazzled, short-tempered, constantly upset mother, which created a horribly stressful environment for me as I grew up. I didn't realize there was another way; this was the norm in my house. So it's no surprise that I grew up saying yes to everything, constantly overextending myself, pushing myself to get straight As, and trying to be president of everything I could sign up for from middle school to college . . . and handling all of it pretty poorly.

It was business as usual to push myself, melt down, and then cry for days. I repeatedly put the heat on my own health and relationships and continued this pattern well into adulthood. As I slogged through my own divorce at age twenty-four, I left pharmacy school during my last year to pursue a naturopathic medical degree at Bastyr University. During this time, I suffered a miscarriage and a life-threatening infection and, despite these downfalls, somehow allowed myself to miss only four days of class. In an effort to avoid all my emotional pain I threw myself into an insane course load at Bastyr, being one of only three people in my class to tackle not only the rigorous naturopathic medical program and but also, simultaneously, two master's degrees, in acupuncture and Chinese herbal medicine. I was fueled by stress.

As if that wasn't enough, for good measure I threw in a very tumultuous relationship, and to fight my constant dissatisfaction with my body I dieted and exercised hard throughout those five years—often on only three or four hours of sleep. How I decided to live sounds crazy to me now, but at the time it was the only way I knew how to operate.

After school I moved to New York City, where the pressures to "make it" were exacerbated by being surrounded by success. Within nine months I had opened up my own practice in the West Village, and within just a few years I had the chance to co-author a book.

The book I co-authored was a weight loss book, and in addition to running my practice and writing said book, I told myself I had better be in the best shape of my life! All of my internal pressure to look better was also met with external pressure (perceived or real) to look the part, so I threw myself into six days a week of training, often doubling up with two workouts a day, coupled with an incredibly restrictive diet (with far too few carbs for my activity level). Driven by every nasty voice in my head and the fear of being "too fat to be in fat loss," I now had every type of stress breaking me down: psychological, lifestyle, and hormonal.

No surprise that during this time I was miserable—in great shape, but miserable. I was terrified to eat anything "off plan" and missed almost every social engagement, either because I needed to go to the gym again or because I was afraid to have a glass of wine lest I gain ten pounds instantly. My hormones were such a mess that I had horrible insomnia, sleeping only a few hours a night; I began experiencing breakouts like a teenager; and my menstrual cycle had all but disappeared (completely ruining the years of work I'd done to normalize my cycle since I have PCOS, or polycystic ovarian syndrome). I also tore a hamstring thanks to overexercising, and my relationship at this point was in complete shambles. I couldn't have felt more like a hypocrite, as I was falling apart on the other side of my great advice.

Luckily for me, my boyfriend at the time, who is now my husband, stood by me. We were on the brink of a breakup, but instead we started therapy and were able to turn things around. I will never forget what a near miss this was and that it was largely due to my intense and frazzled lifestyle. One of my main jobs during the work we did to salvage our relationship was to learn to rethink my entire way of approaching my life—and my addiction to stress. It's hard to face reality when you have a passion or when you are an incredibly driven person; for me, this insane way of living was all I knew.

By some grace I found myself pregnant, and this launched my stress-addict recovery into hyperdrive. (I know, habits die hard!) I knew something had to change if I was going to have a healthy pregnancy and a healthy baby.

My relationship recovered, we now have two beautiful little girls, my health is intact, my cycle is normal, my skin is glowing, and I owe this all to finding a new way. I owe this all to letting go of constant stress as my badge of honor and heeding my hormonal messages at the first signs that I'm overdoing it. I finally started being my own best friend instead of my own worst enemy, and my desire now is to help other women find this same joy.

The Hangry B*tch Reset Was Born

In 2014, everything we had both worked so hard for finally came together. We met at a conference we both had been asked to attend as guest speakers and realized we could accomplish so much more as a team than we ever could apart.

We started our partnership by first helping each other through a lot of life chaos, and, in the process, we realized that our similar stories and our approach to how we work with women made this partnership the perfect marriage; and that is how we came to create this book and this plan. Our combined experience and expertise have since brought to light that there are thousands of women who think they are doing everything right, or have totally given up hope in their efforts, and they are all on the verge of burnout, if not deep in that cavern already.

Research proves what we've been telling women for years: women who work over forty hours a week (which is the majority of today's women) are more likely to die at a younger age from inflammatory disease ranging from heart disease to cancer than those that don't. This is not a shock to us considering how the women we work with feel and how their health is in tatters. We can no longer ignore that today's women are not happy and thriving; they are barely surviving. Studies like this show us that feeling spread too thin and the symptoms that arise from all this stress is most definitely not in our heads, so what are we supposed to do about this very real phenomenon?

We are not going to give you just another diet or exercise plan that works for a hot minute but later leaves you further metabolically deranged. Instead what we have for you is an adaptable, doable, tangible, and uniquely customizable system that will actually help you feel better, and we promise you a way to sustain the positive outcomes we know you will experience. In other words, we are determined to help you get out of the vicious hormonal cycle of feeling like a Hangry B*tch and instead be a Happy Babe

We are still on our own journeys. Health is fluid; life is always changing, and so are our hormones. Really getting to know who we are as women is empowering, and learning to listen to our own innate cues is step 1, but sometimes we have to fall hard to learn this valuable lesson.

Our goal is to help you before you fall hard, but if you've already landed at rock bottom, that's OK, too—there is hope, and we have it for you.

PART ONE

Why We're All Hangry B*tches

Too Tired to Be Happy

Women today are savvy when it comes to health and wellness. Most have likely read about the stress hormone cortisol, probably know about the "cave-man diet," and have at least heard murmurs that lifting weights is the key to a healthy, lean body. Also apparent is the resurgence of a more natural way of living—even in the city—as more people take to a bit of urban farming, ranging from cultivating a small herb garden on the windowsill to keeping egg-laying chickens in the backyard. Many are also ditching department store skin care for more natural products and drinking out of glass, stainless steel, or ceramic, as collectively we grow weary of so much plastic. Slow cookers have made a comeback, and CrossFit has swept the nation, giving more normalcy to women working out with barbells.

Overall, there has been a positive shift toward a more natural way of living, and while not all of you may be doing these things—or have yet to brew your own kombucha—these practices are not seen as completely "out there" as they were twenty or thirty years ago. But at the same time as we are striving to live more naturally in our homes, most women are still living with the unnatural stresses of filling multiple roles, from mom to employee to entrepreneur to wife to playdate coordinator to everything in between.

We've piled more expectations, more work, and more stress on our plates with each passing year—and all of this in an increasingly toxic and stressful environment rife with chemicals that disrupt our hormones all day, every day. It's no wonder our hormones have gone haywire and our happiness has flown the backyard coop. This has us struggling to manage our obligations, sleep, body weight, and cravings, not to mention losing our joy. Between the two of us, we've worked with thousands of women and have found that nearly all of them are being stretched too thin. From the single working mom to the senior executive to the hustling woman with entrepreneurial dreams to the busy stay-at-home mama, most of us are overwhelmed and oh so very tired.

Women are plagued with this notion that we have to do it all and look good doing it. So we pile dieting and exercise onto an already stressed-out physiology and overwhelmed mind, and of course our metabolism and hormones say "What exactly is your problem, lady?" Then, like an overly emotional teenager (which is what we feel like), they rebel. And just when things are totally starting to fall apart and what we really need to do is slow way, way down, unfortunately what so many of us do is one or more of the following:

- Feel guilty for not being able to handle life and suffer in silence

- Avoid going to the doctor because we don't have time right now and we think we'll have time to take care of ourselves later

- Go to the doctor, only to be told that lab tests look normal enough and "it's all in your head" or "all moms feel that way" or, the worst, "you're just getting older"

- Dig in deeper with diet and exercise and end up doing even more when we need to dial it back

If you've mustered the energy to pick up this book and you're actually still awake and reading this page, you may be thinking, "What am I going to do with a new exercise plan, a new nutrition strategy, time-consuming daily habits like walking and meditating and . . . I can't do this, I need a nap!" Before you drop the book, hang on—we've got your back. We know that adding more to your plate is not the answer. We also know that if you don't put in place some healthier food, exercise, and lifestyle strategies, you're going to sink. So, yes, we are adding some things but we're also throwing you a few life rafts.

We Do Not Expect Perfection. You're going to approach the reset in your own way, whether that's immediately going all in or implementing just the parts that you know you can successfully accomplish right now. We're actually going to say that again: this isn't about perfection. Let that sink in. You're going to do your best and your best will vary depending on whether you're injured, you're sick, your kids are sick, you're up for a promotion, or you're otherwise just having a bad day. It's OK. But we do want you to keep going, no matter what your pace might be. We want you to show up and keep showing up. Our Five Pillars, which you'll learn in chapter 3, will give you a foundation for making the strategies and habits you'll learn become easier and easier, until your new lifestyle feels as familiar as your current one, but with sustainable and real results. While we call this a four-week program, it's really a lifelong program—you can't get rid of us in a month! We're here for you for the long haul. We do, however, want to stress the importance of consistency. No, perfection is not required, but feeling better will happen faster when you start grooving new habits and committing to what works for you (you'll be very familiar with what that means soon). Remember, this is not just another diet you'll most likely fail at; this is a plan that will carry you through the rest of your life!

The Hangry B*tch Reset Covers YOU from Mindset to Meals to Muscles. Most programs will give you a one-size-fits-all diet and workout plan yet neglect mindset and hormones entirely. Others address hormones in relation to diet recommendations but seem to be stuck in thirty-year-old exercise science when it comes to workout advice. Finally, almost all of them miss the importance of mindset and stress management entirely.

What we've created is a customizable program that will work for you instead of you trying to work for it. We'll teach you exactly what you need for your hormones and for *you* to be happier. You'll heal your hormones, gain strength, lower inflammation, and (what we know you want more than anything else) get your mojo back and start living a life that is more joy-centric and less focused on just getting by. We want you to let go of believing that the only way to be healthy is by following a grueling exercise and diet plan. Instead, we want you to embrace self-compassion, love, and trust in order to really be OK for the long haul.

Finally, There's No Test. You may have implemented all of our suggestions at the end of the four-week reset or you may have managed only a few new habits. It's all good, and, test or not, as far as we're concerned you all get an A-plus. You're here, trying to be better for yourself and those you love, and this time around you're going to learn how to stop fighting your hormones and instead be your own best friend. No matter how long it takes, that's a win in our book.

Most of us have been doing it wrong and feeling fatigued and frustrated for a long time. By the time you get to this book, you're likely dealing with multiple hormones out of balance and a chorus of unhelpful voices in your head asking questions like "What's wrong with me?" or "Where do I even start?" or "Is this all in my head?" The truth is, you aren't crazy and you aren't lazy, so all we ask is that you hang in there.

We can already hear you saying the same thing so many other women before you have expressed to us: "But I've tried everything! Nothing works!" We want to be sure you understand that this plan is very different from what's already out there.

The Hangry B*tch Reset is about way more than food. The Paleo movement has done a great job bringing our consciousness back to a more natural way of eating. But your health and even your waistline are about so much more than what you put on your plate. So while we agree that nutrient-dense, low-inflammatory, hormone-happy-making food is the cornerstone of health, it's not all she wrote. Lifestyle, mindset, and stress management are just as important as eating organic or avoiding sugar or any other nutritional strategy.

There is no perfect diet plan out there, including this one. If we handed you another thirty-day diet challenge expecting that you'll all do well on it—both today and ten years from now—we'd be doing more of what hasn't worked for you all along. You need a template to get started, but what you really need is to know how to tweak and adjust that template given your unique set of hormonal issues. This book will teach you how to do just that. You'll be guided on how to think with our Five Pillars and how to eat and exercise with our Five Habits. With these two frameworks you'll have a complete lifestyle plan that's easy to adjust and just as easy to implement.

The same is true of exercise. Many of you might be too tired to do much of anything right now, others of you are doing too much and feeling worse instead of better, and some of you may be finding the time and some semblance of energy to exercise but are getting absolutely nowhere with your results. As with diet, your exercise needs to be grounded on foundations that work for most everyone; however, we will teach you how to customize your exercise regimen for your unique hormone imbalances. You'll find that your workouts will finally make you feel better instead of worse and will also help you get those elusive results you've been chasing after.

The same need for some customization is true of stress management. One technique will work great for your sister and fall flat for you. Your blissed-out girlfriend's mantra may make your skin crawl. Or maybe even the thought of trying to implement stress management makes you even more stressed than you are right now. We'll help you customize this aspect as well by giving you our Twelve Tangible Tools, which are our best stress busters for in-the-moment flip-outs, and you'll hang on to the ones that help and toss the ones that don't. Even better, you'll be living more in the moment and have fewer flip-outs in the long run!

Why Are You So Tired? And Why Does It Matter?

When we speak to worn-out, hormone-harried women, they say that what they hate the most is who they are when they feel this way. They hate that they lack patience with their partners, snap at their kids or coworkers, feel frustrated, frazzled, frantic, and flustered—and the truth is, none of us feel very proud of ourselves when we act like a Hangry B*tch.

Throughout this program we will also be challenging you to give up some time-suckers, overwhelmers, and stuff that can go—even if it doesn't feel like something you can let go of right now. We want you to have a bigger, better, more beautiful life, and sometimes that means you have to create more time and energy for the things that will give that to you. This, of course, will go a long way toward healing your hormones as well.

You'll learn how problems with insulin, cortisol, thyroid hormones, estrogen, and progesterone can lead to your lack of energy, weight gain, and overall not feeling like your best self. However, hormones aren't the only things at play when it comes to your metabolism and great energy. You'll see how much of an impact your environment and everyday products have on your hormones, as well as how to spruce up your intracellular energy makers: your mitochondria. These little furnace-like organelles quite literally turn your food into energy, and they face a host of challenges to properly function in today's woman. Finally, throughout this program, from the diet to the exercise changes to the upgrades in your stress-management habits and personal care products, you'll get a handle on inflammation: the great hormone mess-maker. In sum, you'll tackle hormone optimization and fatigue from every angle.

We know this sounds like a lot, and in some ways it is, but you didn't get here by having just one little thing go wrong. Likely a wave of hormonal disruption is happening in your body that started from one or two things going awry, and now there's cumulative and widespread disruption impacting all of your hormonal systems. But please don't feel overwhelmed; the good news is that you'll learn the best needle movers in food, exercise, sleep, stress management, and supplementation that will give you benefits across a wide range of hormones and physiological systems. Even if you have several hormonal issues to address, we know you don't have the time or energy to waste on an overly complicated plan, so we'll teach you the best habits to employ and the biggest, nastiest things to avoid in order to start feeling better faster.

Ladies, Meet Your Hormones

By the end of this book you'll know your hormones like you know your best girlfriends and you'll understand how they talk to you constantly, giving you feedback about how they are doing with your current nutrition and exercise plan, your stress level, and your joy. While there are about fifty hormones secreted and roaming about your body right now, we'll hone in on the ones that you have the most control over with the habits we'll teach in this book.

Don't feel like you have to fully understand each of these hormones right away; we simply want to introduce you to the big players that we will be working with. They'll become more familiar to you after you take our quiz and begin the actual customization of the reset. Please mark this section, as we will be referring you back here when you start to dig into the details and plan of this book.

Cortisol. Your main stress hormone, cortisol is secreted from the outer part, or cortex, of the adrenal glands in a timed, coordinated fashion. Ideally, cortisol levels are highest around five in the morning and taper off throughout the day, being lowest at bedtime. Cortisol plays a major role in both your immune system and your metabolism. It is essential for dealing with acute inflammation, maintaining blood sugar levels, and even burning fat during a workout. Without its normal rhythm you suffer with low blood sugar, low energy, inflammation, and poor exercise tolerance, as well as a low appetite for protein and often cravings for simple carbs and sugar. With too much of it, you ramp up inflammation and weight gain (especially with elevated insulin or insulin resistance), and have difficulty sleeping, erratic energy, menstrual cycle dysfunction, and a host of disruptions spanning your entire hormonal system.

Adrenaline/Epinephrine. Your other stress hormone, epinephrine (also known as adrenaline) is released mainly through the activation of sympathetic nerves connected to the adrenal glands. This quick-response hormone is released within moments of a stressful event, in contrast to the more timed, coordinated, and ongoing release of cortisol, and its main job is to get you ready to fight or flee. It dilates your pupils to let in more light, shunts blood away from organs like your digestive tract and toward your muscles, and maximizes blood glucose to give your brain and muscles some fuel to put up a good fight. Its related hormone, norepinephrine (aka noradrenaline), has a low-level secretion that is ongoing and is also an important central nervous system neurotransmitter; without it you can have low motivation or depression.

When it comes to fat loss, adrenaline is stimulated by exercise and, together with cortisol, growth hormone, and testosterone, it sparks fat burning. This effect can be blunted when our insulin is elevated or we have low cortisol. Adrenaline receptors have two main types, alpha and beta, and while the alpha receptors increase fat storage (women have more of these in the hips and thighs and they are spurred by estrogen, giving us the classic hourglass figure), the beta receptors increase fat burning.

Aldosterone. Yet another adrenal hormone that is not a stress hormone but does get caught in the stress-related crossfire of HPA axis dysfunction (commonly called adrenal fatigue), aldosterone, along with other hormones (renin and angiotensin), helps regulate blood volume, pH, and electrolyte balance. If you find that you have frequent urination or seem to rapidly pee out all that good water you're drinking, you may benefit from supplementing with electrolytes to support aldosterone while you handle your stressors.

Insulin. Your main storage hormone, insulin shuttles nutrients (namely glucose, amino acid, and fats) out of your bloodstream and into tissues for use or storage. Like cortisol, it's absolutely vital, but with our modern diet and lifestyle it's often out of balance. Insulin's main job is to lower blood sugar, and when it's out of balance you can have increased appetite, lots of sugar and starch cravings (particularly after eating), easy weight gain (especially when cortisol is also imbalanced), fatigue, and depression, as well as possible testosterone excess symptoms such as acne, hair loss, and ovulation problems. When elevated too often, it negatively impacts your metabolism, spurring fat storage and inflammation. Problems or resistance to insulin's message can be mild and simply create imbalances in your ACES (appetite, cravings, energy, and sleep), which you will be introduced to in detail on pages 22–23 or can be more significant, such as in women with PCOS (polycystic ovarian syndrome, a common metabolic and hormonal imbalance), diabetes, or pre-diabetes. Like cortisol, this hormone exerts a huge effect on all other hormones, so the reset really focuses on you tuning this one up.

You release insulin in response to any rise in blood sugar, whether from eating or from stress. Secreted most significantly when eating carbohydrates, insulin is also released when you eat protein (however, protein also releases a hormone, glucagon) and, indirectly, when you eat fat, via the hormones ASP (acylation stimulating protein) and GIP (glucose-dependent insulinotrophic peptide). This is important to note because it's a common misconception that protein and fat are "free foods"—or that carbs are all you have to worry about—when it comes to insulin.

Thyroid Hormones. Made by the thyroid gland, which sits atop your collarbones, thyroid hormones are vital for the metabolism of every single cell in your body. Without adequate stimulation by these key metabolic messengers, cells struggle not only to do their job but also to repair themselves. Because thyroid hormone affects every cell, the symptoms of thyroid problems are widespread but always look like a slowdown: constipation, dry skin that doesn't heal well, brittle fingernails, brain fog, hair loss, depression, irregular menstrual cycles and possibly heavier bleeding, slower reflexes, and of course weight gain. Our modern lifestyle is rife with factors that slow our thyroid glands down, including heavy metals, endocrine disrupters, inflammation, and of course stress. Among the worst offenders for women and thyroid health is chronic dieting.

A further problem is that the vast majority of women with low thyroid function also have an autoimmune attack on the thyroid gland called Hashimoto's disease. This condition creates several unique thyroid- and inflammation-related issues that can make exercise tolerance, fatigue, hair loss, and weight gain big problems for women. We'll cover those specific issues throughout the four weeks of the reset, as this is a rampant problem that leaves women very confused and frustrated—it may be the very reason you feel like a Hangry B*tch!

Glucagon. The often-forgotten hormone of blood sugar, glucagon works with insulin and cortisol to keep your body's energy needs in balance. One of its main jobs is breaking down stored glucose (glycogen) for use, and one of its best tricks is helping stimulate fat burning when insulin is low, such as between meals and (ideally) during a workout. It's also stimulated by eating protein, so this plan will harness its power both with adequate protein and with exercise.

Leptin. This hormone is made by your fat cells and it's basically a fuel gauge. It ideally regulates day-to-day overall hunger by telling your brain you have enough reserves so it's fine not to eat a lot more. Leptin has a significant role in supporting or regulating your thyroid as well. However, because of overeating, especially overeating high-calorie foods, which is so common in our modern world, many women have leptin resistance, and thus the signal to dial down hunger isn't happening. We overeat and don't feel satisfied so we keep overeating. Our plan will help normalize hunger signals by boosting your veggie and protein intake, keeping you full and satisfied without getting overly stuffed and shutting down leptin. By proxy this also supports your thyroid, so it's a win-win!

Ghrelin. Another key hunger hormone, ghrelin provides more of an hour-to-hour signal of "Am I hungry?" in contrast to leptin's overall signal. It can be a tricky thing to know if hunger is true or emotional. Ghrelin is the hormone that signals physical hunger—that is, grumbling in your tummy as opposed to a thought like "Chocolate sounds so yummy right now." Physical hunger goes away when you eat, while emotional cravings persist or even bring on guilt after eating. Physical hunger also builds more slowly (usually three to four hours after not eating), while emotional hunger comes on randomly. Keeping your blood sugar on an even keel can help balance your hormone hunger response, as will avoiding eating to the point you're stuffed. The Hangry B*tch Reset is chock-full of blood sugar balancing tips, and stress-management tools and will help you get to know yourself better so that at the end of the four weeks you will be much more aware of where your appetite and cravings cues are coming from. Also, one of your best tools for balancing ghrelin is sleep, and we'll constantly be reminding you to get more rest.

Adiponectin. An important inflammation-fighting and body fat–regulating hormone, adiponectin, like leptin, is made by your fat cells. The more body fat you have, often the less adiponectin you have, ironically telling your body NOT to burn fat. It seems backward but it's one more way our modern lifestyle, with stress and abundant food, has gotten our ancestral hormonal wires crossed. Adiponectin is also found at lower levels in women with PCOS, which may be part of why this condition can cause frustratingly slow fat loss and why inflammation is elevated in these women. You can boost adiponectin by supplementing with magnesium, as well as by having larger windows of time between meals (i.e., intermittent fasting). We'll help you heal your stress response, give your digestive tract more recovery time, and fine-tune your carbs so that in time you may be able to go longer without eating, further lower inflammation, and spark fat loss, if that's your goal.

Estrogen. Our main metabolic hormone, estrogen is vital for our feminine features (round breasts, full hips, and soft skin), strong bones, and adequate muscle mass; it aids fat burning and metabolism; and of course it has a crucial role in our fertility and menstrual cycle. Estrogen also spurs creativity and bolsters serotonin, helping us feel more like our joyful selves. Low estrogen causes a host of problems associated with "getting older," like osteoporosis and loss of muscle mass, less strong and elastic skin (read: wrinkles), increased fat deposition around the middle due to worsening insulin resistance, and increased inflammation, which will impact all of our hormones negatively. On the flipside, excess estrogen, whether absolute or relative (due to low progesterone), creates an entirely different set of symptoms such as heavier or more frequent periods, tender or painful breasts, bloating, and weight gain (thanks to its effect on those alpha-type epinephrine receptors mentioned previously). This plan will help you harness the power of estrogen as well as give you a host of lifestyle support strategies to minimize estrogen dominance.

Progesterone. Our other feminine hormone, progesterone, together with estrogen, coordinates fertility and a normal menstrual cycle. It is the hormone of temperance. It balances many of estrogen's negative effects as well as buffering some unwanted effects of cortisol. It also is key for a calm outlook and solid sleep as it boosts GABA (our main chill-pill neurotransmitter) and gets converted into one of our most soothing hormones, allopregnenalone. When progesterone is low, we are more stress-sensitive, more agitated, and have more insomnia. We can feel moody and bloated and see added body fat—which doesn't often help our low mood! One of our best tools for keeping our progesterone rockin' solid is managing stress, and this plan is loaded with tools for that.

Testosterone. Typically thought of as a male hormone, testosterone is required by women, too—in just the right amount. Too much, and we throw off our female hormone balance, lose hair on our head and sprout some on our chin and upper lip, break out, gain weight, and retain water, not to mention hinder our metabolic and cardiac health. However, a bit is still needed for women to keep our libido and mood up, keep our bones and muscles healthy, and burn fat during workouts. The best testosterone support habits for women include rest, lifting weights, and not too much stress—and we've got ALL that covered in this plan, as well as some excess testosterone support if needed.

Growth Hormone. The "fountain of youth" hormone, this baby is crucial to you staying lean and healthy. The best way to get more of it is to get enough rest, not overeat (including giving yourself some breaks between meals), and to lift weights. Throughout this plan you'll certainly be focused on sleep and strength training, and in time, as your stress response heals, you'll be able to go a bit longer without eating and reap some growth hormone–boosting benefits there as well.

You with Us? Good . . . but Where Should You Start?

You've got several big hormonal players when it comes to fatigue. These include the mama of energy and metabolism: thyroid hormone; the blood sugar controller insulin; and the stress commander cortisol.

This program will cover cellular energy, inflammation, and other biochemical causes of fatigue so that you can get on top of your exhaustion from all angles.

However, you've got two hormones that profoundly affect your level of fatigue that you have quite a bit of direct control over, although at times it doesn't feel like it. Those are insulin and cortisol. These hormones not only chat at you all day via your ACES (appetite, cravings, energy, and sleep), but they have a widespread effect on all of your other hormones. Again, these two are surprisingly under your control. Each week of this program, you'll dial in your ACES and gain more and more control over all of your hormones, but let's dive in with cortisol because this is one hormone that is way misunderstood.

Cortisol, as you know, is your main stress hormone, and one that's likely become a foe but can most definitely be your friend again. Cortisol gets a bad rap for causing weight gain and inflammation, but it is a life-saving, anti-inflammatory, blood sugar–boosting hormone secreted for a stress response. But the problem is that we Hangry B*tches are calling on it constantly all day, every day. The result is often termed "adrenal fatigue."

If you've ever googled "why am I so tired?" you've likely stumbled across the term "adrenal fatigue," and if you've been treated by a functional medicine provider you've likely spit in a vial or peed on a piece of paper to assess your adrenals and your cortisol rhythm. On the other hand, if you've asked your family doctor about adrenal fatigue, you've likely been told that it doesn't even exist. No matter what you've heard, one thing is for certain: your cortisol rhythm and output are key to regaining your hormonal health, having the stamina to live your life, and feeling a whole lot better—so let's start there.

What Is Adrenal Fatigue?

"Adrenal fatigue" is a bit of a misnomer, as the adrenal glands are not "too tired" to do their job, but rather a woman has lost her ability to adapt and cope with stress. It is truly a brain/body disconnect rather than a problem with the adrenal glands themselves. Adrenal fatigue, or adrenal burnout, is better described as HPA axis dysfunction or a discoordination between the instructions the brain (specifically the hypothalamus and pituitary gland) sends to the adrenal glands. It basically gets harder to keep cortisol output on its normal circadian timing.

> Note: True adrenal insufficiency, known as Addison's disease, is an autoimmune condition where there is an antibody attack on the adrenal cortex or enzymes within the adrenal glands, much like the antibody attack that happens to the thyroid in Hashimoto's disease. This is perhaps true "adrenal fatigue" and not the functional problem we're talking about here. Addison's disease sufferers will ultimately have low cortisol and often need to use cortisol replacement therapy.

From the obvious stress of managing work, busy lifestyles, relationships, and finances to the internal stresses we don't often think about, such as low thyroid hormones, inflammation, chronic infection, and nutrient deficiencies—stress is everywhere. While most often we associate stress with an elevation in stress hormones or high cortisol, what happens in time is that cortisol levels can decline while your other stress hormone, adrenaline, stays high. Cortisol in most women dealing with ongoing stress is high at the wrong times and low at the wrong times, producing a host of symptoms related to this mismatch in brain-adrenal coordination.

When you feel tired, achy, cranky, and have terrible sleep or start gaining weight and have unmanageable cravings it's time to listen up. These symptoms are beacons from your hormones, messages from your metabolism, signaling that you need to make some changes. You will learn to tune in to these symptoms and use them to adjust our plan perfectly to fit your needs.

Are you wondering if cortisol is an issue for you? You will use the Hangry B*tch Hormone Quiz to find out. You'll also discover all the other hormones that might be giving you those signals we mentioned.

You'll get to the full quiz in chapter 7, but below are examples of what your symptoms are telling you about cortisol.

High Cortisol: Fatigued and Frazzled

- Difficulty falling asleep at night, feeling "tired but wired" at bedtime
- Puffy appearance, all over but most often noticeable in the face

- Achy and stiff when waking, with a low appetite in general or cravings for carbs

- Intolerance to exercise, difficulty recovering from workouts and healing from injuries

- Difficulty losing body fat, particularly around the middle

- Cravings for sugary/starchy and fatty foods

Low Cortisol: Wiped Out

- Irritability, lightheadedness, low energy, forgetfulness, shaking, etc. between meals or as the time for the next meal approaches

- Sugar or caffeine cravings, often between meals

- Difficulty sleeping through the night

- Low blood pressure (below 110/70)

- Sensitivity to bright lights and sunlight

- Digestive issues including IBS-like symptoms of alternating constipation and looser stools

- Sluggish fat loss from "fat loss exercise," such as sprints, metcon (metabolic conditioning) or other HIIT (high-intensity internal training)

- Difficulty recovering from exercise, low tolerance to intense exercise particularly

To make this extra confusing, you might have noticed you have symptoms of both low and high cortisol. Huh? For some women, it's clear: they're either wound up or wiped out, meaning their cortisol is too high or too low overall. But what we see most often is women with high cortisol at certain times and low cortisol at other times throughout the day.

These symptoms reveal that your stress mechanism is not as robust and coordinated as it was when you were younger. Remember staying up for days on end during college finals and sleeping in for a few days and feeling as if you were as good as new? Fast-forward to having a newborn baby or vying for a promotion in your thirties and feeling as if you never really recovered from the sleep deficit. Or perhaps in the past you went on an aggressive exercise regimen and dropped weight easily, but that same plan ten years later leaves you achy and exhausted and yields lackluster results. Or you might feel like you have a shorter fuse for any type of stress as time's gone on. These are just a few examples of your stress-coping ability going downhill as HPA axis dysfunction sets in.

As frustrated as you are with this laundry list of symptoms and always feeling like crap, these symptoms will be what you rely on to gauge how you will make adjustments to your diet, exercise, and healthy lifestyle habits within the Hangry B*tch Reset. The main variables that you'll learn to pay attention to several times a day, since they hint to your internal workings of insulin and cortisol, are what we have already referred to as your ACES: appetite, cravings, energy, and sleep.

ACES—Listen Up, These Are Your Hormones Talking

The acronym ACES is the window into your hormone balance. It tells you in real time what you can do differently to feel better.

Appetite. Whether your appetite is high, low, or normal is largely regulated by blood sugar balance and the hormones insulin and cortisol. Your appetite is also impacted by information directly from your gut (via the hormone ghrelin), your brain (via neuropeptide Y among others), and your fat cells themselves (via leptin).

Cravings. Food cravings are largely due to blood sugar swings, and thus the hormones insulin and cortisol are responsible (you'll see this pattern over and over again in this book; thankfully, this plan focuses on these two hormones, which you can largely control). Cravings are also impacted by brain chemistry imbalances, primarily involving serotonin and dopamine. Interestingly, the balance of your brain chemistry itself is largely affected by blood sugar, and thus insulin and cortisol come into play again. Cravings, of course, can also be emotional—not hormonal in origin.

Energy. Your energy level is all about blood sugar balance, which is affected by your stress hormones (cortisol, adrenaline) and your storage hormone (insulin, which stores glucose, fat, and amino acids) and also has a lot to do with thyroid hormone levels and activity (e.g., Do you have enough? Are they in the right form? Are they getting into a cell for activity?). There are also some basic but often overlooked causes of low energy including overt or borderline anemias (lack of B12, folate, B6, or iron), deficiencies in other nutrients such as CoQ10 or carnitine (necessary to metabolize fat as fuel), food sensitivities (which can cause your energy to crash after a meal), and inflammation (which can make you feel weighed down and sluggish). This one is a bit more complicated than variables A and C, but rest assured we're going to address each one of these causes of low energy by the end of the four-week reset.

Sleep. When sleep is off (you can't fall asleep or stay asleep), cortisol is typically involved. Estrogen-progesterone imbalances can also affect sleep because they can hinder optimal levels of serotonin and GABA (gamma-aminobutyric acid), making it harder to calm down and fall asleep.

Understanding your ACES can feel like you've been given a secret hormone-decoder ring. Tuning in to and working with these signals will help you find what you really need to be eating, how you need to exercise, and the care you need to give to lifestyle issues like stress and meditation in order to keep your hormones happy, your energy high, and your jeans size where it feels good to you.

Beyond Adrenal Fatigue

While cortisol is a major player in your hormone landscape, it's far from the only hormone that gets wonky from stress and has you feeling wiped out. In time, as you continue to run yourself ragged, you've likely impacted other hormones such as insulin, thyroid hormone, estrogen, and progesterone. Sometimes these other hormones get out of balance only after cortisol issues arise from ongoing stress, and sometimes they are in trouble for other reasons. For example, insulin resistance can be genetic or part of PCOS (polycystic ovarian syndrome), as well as result from poor diet and lack of exercise. Thyroid issues can be due to genetics, and autoimmune thyroid issues such as Hashimoto's disease are often triggered by some sort of stress, ranging from the hormonal swings of pregnancy to toxic burden, infections, leaky gut, or food sensitivities. Finally, sometimes you can go through normal hormonal changes, like menopause, but this fluctuation in hormones in conjunction with stress might be a recipe for mood and sleep issues, weight gain, and otherwise not feeling like yourself.

Have You Been Told It's All in Your Head?

Every day, there are women in their healthcare providers' offices trying to figure out why they are feeling so bleh, and while HPA axis dysfunction actually DOES start in your head (with the hypothalamus and the pituitary), it's a very real problem. Women these days have brains swirling with to-do lists, obligations, self-defeating thoughts, internal criticisms, and a whole lot of pressure. It can often be hard to tell if you're exhausted because you have too much on your plate or because of your hormones and chemistry. Chances are you are dealing with a bit of both, and one can certainly lead to the other.

When we think of our to-do list, see our email inbox, or glance at the overly booked calendar on our smartphone and realize just how many people we are trying not to let down, most of us instantly feel a wave of tiredness wash over us. The mental defeat we feel just knowing we're set up for failure and the guilt we anticipate from not getting it all done are most definitely exhausting.

All this stress will absolutely drive your internal chemistry and your hormones into disarray. Right now, close your eyes and imagine all the people you're trying to be there for and what that too-lengthy to-do list makes you feel like. There's a rush of cortisol (and adrenaline) as you feel the stress of it. Then there are cravings for all the foods that you know will make you more tired in the long run but will temporarily relieve the stress: the carbs, the starches, the sugar, the wine.

When we give in to these sugary, starchy cravings, we disrupt the next hormone in line: insulin. Remember how key these two hormones are to every other hormone. Not only do insulin and cortisol impact thyroid hormone, estrogen, and progesterone, but the foods we crave when we're stressed often contain highly inflammatory ingredients like gluten, dairy, or processed grains and seed oils. This will hit that thyroid as well as estrogen a little harder.

So it's both the mental aerobics we're doing trying to juggle it all and the hormonal impact that comes with trying to do too much that has us so wiped out. Now our energy is low or erratic, our appetite is low for the things we need, and our cravings are high for the things we'd do better avoiding, and soon all this stress turns our sleep upside down. Soon our digestion is off; we're anxious or depressed; our skin shows our hormonal mess with breakouts, dryness, or rashes; PMS goes on full tilt or our female hormones otherwise rage as other hormones become further unraveled. Now more and more biochemical, hormonal, and life stress just piles on top of each other and we're sadly not our best version of ourselves.

But it doesn't have to be this way! Getting on top of the impact of your mental and emotional stress will come from supporting your hormones with the strategies in this plan as well as learning some key habits and tools to keep that stressed-out, frazzled brain in check—and you *can* go from Hangry B*tch to Happy Babe.

Most women have utterly lost their joy and find themselves asking, "Why am I so unhappy?" This million-dollar question is easier to answer than you may think. We'll dig deep into the questions you need to ask yourself to find out why your joy has all but disappeared. But for now, know that happiness is the goal. So during our four weeks together, whether you drop a pants size or resolve a troublesome lab value such as elevated cholesterol or a high marker of inflammation, we want more than anything for you to rediscover your joy and live your life as your best YOU.

Why have two nutrition and exercise experts gone off the deep end with happiness and joy? Not only does happiness beget good health (in that when we are happier and living in more joy, it's easier to do the things we need to do like eat well and exercise), but lack of joy is a chronic source of stress for women. It's becoming an epidemic and it has to stop. You're simply too important.

2

Stressed-Out B*tches

Let's talk about stress. . . .

"Hum . . . OK, but when does my diet start?"

You might be waiting for the diet and exercise plan, and it is coming—we promise! But first we are going to talk a whole lot about stress, mindset, and how you handle your big, beautiful (and yes, stressful) life. In fact we're going to talk a lot about stress *before* we even talk to you about what to eat or how to exercise or what vitamins to start popping because this is where women (our past selves included!) get it wrong with diet, exercise, and, well, life. For often all the wrong reasons, we chase diet plan after diet plan, trying to lose weight or nudge one certain hormone while neglecting the others, and overexercise or underexercise, rarely getting it quite right, all at the cost of our hormones—and our happiness. Both of us have found ourselves overworked, undernourished, or overeating the wrong things, either exercising like a madwoman or too busy and tired to even try, and what suffered was our hormones, our health, and our sense of self—and we know you have lived this hell, too.

This conversation about stress is important not only because it takes a toll on your mood, your sleep, and your relationships but also because unmanaged stress tends to derail any goals you may have to lose body fat, gain muscle, or fix a hormonal issue. When you neglect to tackle this bear first, you not only end up feeling overwhelmed, wiped out, and without willpower to stick to the plan, but also because, when it comes to the deleterious effects of stress on our hormones, you can't trump the need to manage the mama of stress hormones—cortisol.

So while technically the Hangry B*tch Reset doesn't start until chapter 6, where we'll be walking you through a whole boatload of diet, exercise, and supplement strategies to whip cortisol into shape, we've actually got a few things we will be giving you beforehand that you can start doing to help NOW.

Secret Stressors

Many of the following stressors can be helped by targeted nutrients and supplements. A recap and recommended brands can be found at the end of the section, and more resources, such as our favorite brands, are available in Supplement and Testing Resources on page 382.

Blood Sugar Swings. When you have a lot of carb cravings, when you eat until you're sleepy or find that you're craving that espresso or square of chocolate after meals (or both!), when you get forgetful, irritable, or you are a Hangry B*tch after not eating for a couple hours, or if you can't fall or stay asleep— you have a blood sugar regulation problem and this is stressful! Insulin and cortisol duke it out to right your ship as you swing from high to low all day. You get hangry because you went too long without eating or didn't eat the right stuff in the previous meal and you compensate by overeating some of the wrong stuff at the next meal. OR you overshoot your carb tolerance as cortisol and insulin continue to battle. You can bet that the constant high-to-low cortisol and insulin compensation is stressful as the blood sugar ups and downs continually trigger cortisol! No worries though, we'll get this handled with this program starting on Week 1.

Inadequate Protein. You can be low on protein either from inadequate intake or poor digestion. At a minimum, we recommend 90–100 g of protein per day for a woman, which works out to around 30 g per meal, or 25 g at each of four smaller but similar-size meals. We recommend the four-meals-per-day protocol as a starting place for normalizing hormones, which we will dive into the very first week of the program.

Nutrient Deficiencies. We need adequate nutrients, both macro (carbs, fats, and proteins) as well as micro (such as vitamins and minerals), for everything in your body to function properly from a nerve cell sending an impulse to contract a muscle to your thyroid making thyroid hormones and every and anything in between. Micronutrient deficiencies run rampant even when we eat a decent diet. This can be due to mineral depletion in the animals we eat and the soil that grows the fruits and veggies that feed us, or simply the increased demand for nutrients thanks to our modern lifestyle. Sometimes even when we take in the nutrients we need, gut bacterial imbalance or weak digestive capacity makes us unable to absorb and utilize those nutrients.

The Ripple Effect of Stress Across Your Hormones

Nothing puts the heat on your entire hormone landscape like stress. If you've ever broken out, missed a period, or received a low thyroid diagnosis after a stressful time in your life, you've witnessed this firsthand.

Stress most immediately will get into a tug-of-war with insulin when it comes to blood sugar as cortisol tries to raise it and insulin, in turn, attempts to lower it. You experience wonky appetite and energy and often a spike in sugar cravings. Together, insulin and cortisol will bring on water retention from increased inflammation and often more belly fat, leaving you feeling like "What happened to my body?" Both are vital hormones, but when elevated together, are a recipe for poor sleep, out-of-control cravings, and more body fat. Unfortunately, it doesn't stop there.

Progesterone often is the next domino to fall as stress negatively impacts insulin and leptin (especially if the stress is driven by weight loss), oxidative stress and inflammation increase, or the pituitary signals to your ovaries (FSH, LH) wane as your brain senses it is not a good time to reproduce and you get a late or missed period, worsening PMS, puffiness, and crankiness. Estrogen doesn't get out unscathed either. Like progesterone, it can fall, and your fertility, muscle mass, and libido

And, of course, sometimes we just aren't taking in enough! We recommend 100 g of protein and a pound of veggies a day, so let's all start there. Also, a basic high-quality multivitamin can cover most of your bases. (Note: in certain cases, in order to restore hormone balance and have optimal health, it takes much higher doses than the recommended dietary allowance, which are only high enough to prevent overt disease.)

Zinc. Zinc is key for overall hormonal balance (all hormones, from cortisol to your sex hormones to your thyroid, need it) and for a healthy immune system and beautiful skin. The RDA for zinc is only 8 mg per day, but we suggest a minimum of 30 mg per day for women. While taking too much zinc can hinder absorption of other minerals such as copper, many of us are deficient in zinc. If you've been on the pill, eat a vegetarian diet, have poor digestion, consume alcohol regularly, or for a myriad of other reasons, it's disappear or its metabolism is impacted and this, along with the stress-induced low progesterone, causes estrogen-dominance symptoms of breast swelling or tenderness; more frequent, heavier, or more painful periods; and often increased body fat in the hips and thighs.

All the while, this constant cortisol output is increasing inflammation, which affects every single one of your hormones, perhaps none more so than thyroid hormones. Cortisol's impact on this key metabolic hormone is annoying from start to finish. It will lower your active thyroid hormone levels by hindering conversion of what your thyroid makes, called T4, into what you need, called T3. It also drives loss of this active T3 hormone down an irreversible pathway toward reverse T3, which is inactive. And as you've likely experienced, stress can wreak havoc on your gut, which not only drives more inflammation (mucking up all hormones further) but also hinders gut bacteria, which normally are responsible for forming active T3 hormones known as T3A and T3S (T3 acetate and T3 sulfate).

So stress makes you feel pretty hypothyroid pretty quickly and in a manner not easily diagnosed with standard thyroid testing. Yes, cortisol is not fancy or new on the hormone scene, but it's absolutely vital to have in balance or every single hormone in your body pays the price, and you end up feeling like a stranger in your body with difficult moods, poor energy, cravings and erratic appetite, sleep struggles, and weight gain.

wise to supplement with a bit more zinc. Some multivitamins include 30 mg and you can boost your intake by eating more oysters, lamb, grass-fed beef, eggs, mushrooms, and cashews.

Magnesium. Magnesium is needed for hundreds of biochemical reactions daily; it's known to help us perform in the gym, alleviate our PMS, boost our moods, and have more ease in falling asleep. The RDA for magnesium is only around 300 mg daily for women; however, many women need higher doses to restore their depleted magnesium levels. On a basic blood chemistry panel you want your levels to be 2.0–2.5 mg/dL. There are more sophisticated measures of magnesium stores (i.e., red blood cell magnesium), but this test is easily available from your regular doctor on most standard blood chemistry panels. Note that these serum levels (vs. intracellular levels—for example, your red blood cells) will be the last to change, so if your levels are below 2.0 mg/dL on the

A Quick Note on Protein

Plant based protein sources such as legumes or veggie protein powders (i.e., rice or pea) have a few drawbacks. For example, their amino acid profiles aren't as complete as animal protein; they are lower in amino acids such as leucine, which are key for exercise recovery; and our bodies do not as easily utilize these proteins. Also, while legumes contain protein they are predominantly starch, thus they will trigger insulin, and therefore are better categorized as a high fiber starch rather than a protein source.

As far as digestion goes, it's very common for women to have difficulty digesting protein because of a disruption in the intestines from overgrowth of bad bugs (such as SIBO, or small intestine bacterial overgrowth, candida, dysbiosis), poor output of protease enzymes to digest protein, or low HCL (hydrochloric acid) from the stomach. Digestion can be aided by clearing up the intestinal bacterial balance, taking digestive enzymes, and of course managing stress. The stress response is the sympathetic (fight-or-flight) part of our autonomic nervous system, and digestion (as well as reproduction and regulation of your female hormones) is affected by the calmer, parasympathetic part. When we're constantly under stress and are repeatedly triggering the sympathetic nervous system, the parasympathetic nervous system can't adequately send input to our digestive system for proper enzyme release and digestion. The impact on digestion can be made worse from other common hormone imbalances, such as a low thyroid, and it exacerbates certain hormonal issues already in play, such as low thyroid (vicious cycle!) and estrogen dominance (more on that in a bit).

standard blood testing, your tissues are likely very low in magnesium. This mineral is found in spinach, nuts, and avocados, so be sure to include these in your diet, and there are also various forms of supplemental magnesium available: chelate, oxide, glycine, etc. Magnesium chelate is the type found in nature and is a great supplemental form and easy on the digestion. Oxide and citrate forms tend to cause the most laxative side-effects, and glycinate forms can be the best for anxiety, relaxation, and sleep.

Selenium. An important nutrient for our antioxidant defenses, selenium is key to various aspects of our immune system, and it's part of thyroid hormone

#hangrybitchfix

Did you know that you can support your digestion with a couple of super easy tricks to wake up your vagus nerve? This important nerve is part of your parasympathetic nervous system that stimulates a host of important organs, including your entire digestive tract, and it can get a bit lazy for a variety of reasons. But you can stimulate it to release digestive enzymes and get your gut in gear by quick stress-busters such as taking a few deep breaths before you eat. Breathe in for a count of four and then slowly breathe out for a count of eight. You can also get the vagus to fire into your gut by gargling or gagging (not fun, but incredibly effective) several times per day as well as by singing and belly laughing—much more fun!

activation. While the RDA is very low at 55 mcg, based on the research, we recommend a daily intake of 200 mcg. Brazil nuts are the nutritional stars when it comes to this mineral, just 2–3 per day can give you this 200 mcg dose. You can take too much selenium, so avoid unsupervised doses over 200 mcg from food and supplements combined.

Essential Fatty Acids. These essential fats not only help us modulate our immune system and inflammatory response but also can have a favorable impact on our HPA (hypothalamic-pituitary-adrenal) Axis, helping us adapt better to stress and heal HPA axis dysfunction (commonly called adrenal fatigue). Omega-3 fatty acids get burned up quickly when we're inflamed or under stress. Be sure you're eating twelve to sixteen ounces of cold-water fish (such as salmon or mackerel) or shellfish weekly and supplement with 1 to 2 g of a high-quality fish oil supplement daily. Higher doses are warranted temporarily for elevated inflammation, high cortisol, etc., which we'll cover in later chapters. This is where a supplement's quality really counts! Fish oil can be easily rancid and thus full of oxidized fatty acids, which actually boosts inflammation and oxidative stress, so taking cheap fish oil is worse than not taking any. Also be sure your brand is tested for pesticides and heavy metals.

Poor Oxygen Delivery. With all the fancy energy-boosting and antiaging supplements out there, we can't forget good old oxygen! Talk about the fountain of youth; without sufficient oxygen, you not only feel cold and tired and look pale, but pretty much every tissue in your body is suffering big-time. Among the most common causes of low oxygen to your tissues are deficiencies in iron and key B vitamins (B12, folate, and B6). However, if you need more of these nutrients than diet and a good multivitamin can give you, it's best to get a lab test rather than guess. See the free lab guide available at www.sarahanddrbrooke.com/lab-guide for more information.

Oxidative Stress. We have over one hundred thousand trillion mitochondria and they use over 90 percent of the oxygen we breathe. These are essentially the powerhouse or furnaces of your cells, turning food and oxygen into energy. This is actually where your "metabolism" is happening. They're amazing little things, but they are incredibly sensitive to damage via oxidative stress. This is caused by free radicals, molecules that are missing an electron, which makes them unstable, lonely, and a little desperate—bad combo, right? They bump into neighboring molecules and steal an electron, making them unstable, and now a chain reaction is in place, creating a host of oxidative stress–induced damage. Much of our modern life generates free radicals and thus oxidative stress, including exposure to toxins, infections, allergens, too many bad fats and too few veggies in our diet, blood sugar swings, and alcohol. In addition, even the processes that mitochondria normally perform every day involve oxidation. This is essentially the same process as when metal rusts or an apple turns brown, but it's happening in our tissues, and this manifests as a host of diseases, more rapid aging, decreased exercise tolerance, brain fog, and certainly lower energy. When your mitochondria get damaged and aren't working properly, your metabolism essentially is shutting down. The best thing you can do to keep your mitochondria health is eat a wide variety of brightly colored veggies, which the plan in this book will absolutely help you do! The next best thing is strength training, as it actually makes new, healthy mitochondria. You'll get help on that here, also. Finally, you can take antioxidant supplements; there are several we love, like resveratrol.

Dehydration. Much like oxygen, our internal chemistry needs plenty of water to operate properly. Eliminating this stressor seems so simple: drink more water! Yes, some of us fall short of our hydration needs daily (we suggest two to three liters of water daily, some of which can be sparkling) but many women drink plenty of water yet always find themselves thirsty or they pee out as much as they drink and thus, despite carrying that water bottle all about town, they are still dehydrated. One of the easiest fixes here is to supplement with electrolytes. If you have PCOS, deal with insulin resistance (you may be surprised to find your insulin is struggling even if you have no markers of diabetes or pre-diabetes), work out and thus sweat regularly, or are dealing with any adrenal or cortisol issues, you will be amazed how this one supplement will be a game changer for you. Many women start with over-the-counter electrolytes, but these often fall short on potassium so women don't get the benefits these little gems can give.

Inflammation. Inflammation is the great hormone mess-maker. When you have excessive inflammation in your body, it quickly creates a stress burden on all of your hormonal systems. If you think of a hormone as a key and a receptor as a lock, inflammation is like sticking gum over the keyhole, making it harder for hormones to bind to their specific receptor sites and create an effect inside that cell. Inflammation can interrupt the signaling from the brain all the way to the gland, which in turn alters the entire hormonal cascade, creating widespread disturbance.

If you're experiencing any hormonal deficiency symptoms but show normal hormone levels on your blood work, we recommend that you have your inflammation tested. The great news for you is that the plan in this book will start you on the road to lowering inflammation and healing all of your hormones.

Hormone Imbalances. Stress creates hormonal imbalances and hormonal imbalances are stressful. Not fair, is it? Fair or not, remember that your hormones are highly orchestrated and intricately linked, so when one is off it's a matter of time before others get wonky as well. A great example is perimenopause: as your estrogen and progesterone fall, your brain attempts to signal your ovaries to not give up the fight (via a hormone called FSH, follicle-stimulating hormone), and then the adrenals get stimulated as well to "take over" and increase production of progesterone and DHEA and other adrenal androgens that get peripherally converted to estrogen and testosterone, as they come to your falling female hormone levels' aid. Most women, as we have previously attested to, already struggle with some level of HPA axis dysfunction, making this natural transition even more challenging, since the adrenals are asked to do more than they might be capable of doing. This is why we recommend that every woman going through perimenopause support their adrenals via stress management and supplementation, as the adrenals will be asked to step in for sex hormone production when the ovaries close up shop.

Lack of Joy. Whether you're dealing with overt anxiety or depression or low-level blues because you've simply lost your mojo as you've forgotten to incorporate into your life the activities and parts of you that bring you happiness—well, it is simply stressful to feel this way! Joy is an antidote to the inevitable hard times and pressures of daily living. Without it, all of your hormones and your health are suffering. There's no vitamin or super food for this one—getting your joy back is up to you. Throughout this book you will be tweaking your routine at the gym, upping your game with nutrition, and, most important, finding yourself again. This begins with starting to live from our Five Pillars, which will change the way you look at your entire life and the habits that make up your day. These pillars are what will hold up all the work you do in the gym and in the kitchen in a whole new way; they are the framework for your new, bigger, better life. In addition, we've got daily tools and in-the-moment tricks to help you be less stressed and more joyful. Soon you'll be more in touch with who you really are—what makes YOU happy and mindful enough to know exactly what you need to do to take care of yourself and those you love.

Supplement and Nutrient Suggestions

Multivitamin: Choose a multivitamin that includes 800 mcg methylfolate (not folic acid) and 1000 mcg methylated vitamin B12, offers a wide array of minerals, and does not contain sugar, artificial dyes, or excessive additives.

Zinc: minimum 30 mg per day

Magnesium: 300–1200 mg daily in divided doses

Omega-3 Fatty Acids from Fish Oil: 1–2 g (typically 850 mg EPA and 200 mg DHA per serving) from high-quality fish oil

Selenium: 200 mcg per day

Antioxidant and Anti-Inflammatory Nutrients: We recommend resveratrol (100–400 mg per day) and turmeric (1–3 g per day). Other good choices include boswelia, ginger, and bromelain.

Glutathione: This antioxidant supports good mitochondrial function. Use liposomal glutathione (100–500 mg per day or even more for some women) or n-acetyl cysteine (300 mg one to three times per day; doses range from 600–2400 mg daily). It is recommended to support glutathione with other nutrients such as cordyceps and alpha lipoic acid for better utilization.

Mitochondrial Nutrients: CoQ10 100–200 mg per day, l-carnitine 500 mg twice daily, and a complex of B vitamins, including methylfolate, B12, and other B vitamins

Electrolytes: Brands with additional minerals such as magnesium and vitamin C as well as 100–150 mg of sodium and 150 mg of potassium are optimal.

For more information on testing and labs, and for the names of our favorite products, see Supplement and Testing Resources (page 382) or visit www.sarahand drbrooke.com.

Mindful B*tches

Once considered hippy-dippy, mindfulness and meditation are now so mainstream there's an app for that! Everyone from CEOs to stay-at-home moms has likely been told more than once that they should meditate daily. And if you're on social media, you know #mindset brings up over seven million hits. You know the benefits, you even know all the cool kids are doing it. But do you routinely make time for sitting in uninterrupted silence to meditate? Can you calmly deliver a public speech for work or your community without your stomach being in knots? Are you able to stop mid-losing it with your kids and turn your approach more zen? Do you pause midday and check in on your mindset before you get too stressed? Are you able to approach a trip to the gym with a positive mindset about strength and self-care—or are you slogging it out because you "have to"? And finally, can you sidestep eating a bunch of food that you know doesn't work for you by using a mantra?

If not, you're not alone. Most of us know there's something to this mindset stuff but we either fail to make time for it on a consistent basis or just find the whole thing too intangible to make it part of our lives in any real way. Well, that changes with this program! We believe that how you do what you do matters as much as whether you do it at all. For so many of us, diet and exercise have been a punishment for not being enough in some way or at best just something we have to do because our doctors and personal trainers tell us that we should. No wonder gyms are full on January 1, and come February it's back to the same old crowd! Working out as punishment or some sort of sentence for eating something indulgent is no way to live. Doing those same healthy things with an attitude of self-care, self-love, and nourishment feels completely different and is much more sustainable. Not only do the healthy habits we so often struggle to keep going feel different, this change in mindset keeps us from doing stuff that gets us into hormonal trouble. It's hard to overexercise and undereat when you are able to see that these things are actually an act of self-love. It's harder to complain about cooking when you see it as an act of self-care. Ultimately, it's hard to be a Hangry B*tch when you gain the tools to keep your emotions and cravings under control.

When we change how we think about our life and the hassles, struggles, and rough stuff that come with it, we have one of the most powerful tools to decrease stress: perspective. We will provide you with a framework, which we call the Five Pillars, to help you change the way you think about the million things you feel burdened with accomplishing every day, the frustrations you face with your health, and how hard it can all feel some days. We will also challenge you to give up what is not serving you any longer, whether that's old stories about who you are or what you should be doing or folding your laundry when you know someone else could do it (maybe not perfectly, but still). Our in-the-moment tools will get you out of those tough days when you're worried you may strangle the next person who looks at you wrong or you find yourself staring at the bottom of an empty pint of Ben and Jerry's or a glass of wine wondering what happened to the last five minutes of your life.

We promise you that mindfulness supports more Happy Babe days than Hangry B*tch days, both hormonally and emotionally. What this book offers is the tools to make mindfulness less esoteric and more tangible so you can harness its power and completely transform your life. Again, all this comes before we talk about food or exercise because that's how much it matters. We'll be sharing our best how-tos with mantras and mindset magic, as well as the mama of mindfulness: meditation. Does meditation make you squirmy? Don't worry; you can start with just one little, tiny minute per day.

Meditation: Your New BFF

It's scientifically proven that meditation changes our neural pathways and makes us feel less cranky and more resilient, capable, and happier overall.

As with so many good intentions, it's really very easy to talk about meditating and never actually do it—we get that. Women often tell us they skip meditating even if they make it to the gym, take their vitamins, and stick to their nutrition plan. You may not be able to pinpoint why it's so hard to sit down and be silent, but often that reason is fear. It can be super crazy scary to sit silently with yourself; a lot can come up, and it will, but this is exactly what needs to happen in order to get to a space of peace and less stress—by being able to fully experience your life without distraction and by being present, even for the tough stuff.

There are many ways to meditate: you can listen to a guided meditation such as ours, *Meditation & Mantra Walks with Sarah and Dr. Brooke* (available on iTunes and Google Play). You can use an app like Calm, Buddify, or Headspace. Or do it yourself by following these simple steps:

1. Find a comfortable seated position. (Do not lie down—you will just fall asleep and that's not the point of this practice!) Sit in a chair with your feet planted firmly on the ground, legs uncrossed, hands resting palms-down on your legs or cupped gently in your lap. Or sit cross-legged on a cushion on the floor if this is more comfortable for you. Maintain an upright spine with shoulders pulled back and your gaze forward or slightly down.

2. Set your timer for how long you want to practice.

3. Gently close your eyes and take a few deep, cleansing breaths. Breathe in through your nose, filling your belly and lungs completely with air, and then slowly exhale every drop through your mouth.

4. Now breathe normally through your nose, focusing on your breathing. Notice where you feel your breath: in your belly, in your chest, flowing across the top of your lip, in your nostrils. Just notice. Don't judge, react, or contemplate.

5. Let thoughts come and let them go. Don't go chasing after your thoughts and do not feel like you are doing anything wrong when they come. Notice your thoughts, and notice if there's a pattern with what comes up, and then gently let them go while you keep returning your focus to your breath. If you find yourself caught up with your thoughts, your to-do list, your last argument with your spouse, it's OK—stop judging or worrying that you are "messing up" your meditation. Just gently continue to refocus on where you feel your breath. This is a safe and sacred place, a time just for you, and an exercise to be practiced just like anything else. The point is not to be a perfect meditator. The point is to allow yourself space to just be, to be present, to see how you are able to observe your thoughts rather than being gripped and controlled by them. Meditation is learning that you can always come back to the present; it's a practice that helps you "wake up" to the moment and not let the chaos in your head dominate every second of your life.

6. As you are meditating, you might notice tension in certain places in your body. That's OK. Observe what you feel, breathe into that tension, and if you can, let it go and then return the focus once again to your breath. If you feel like you're going to lose your mind, or if the position you are in is truly painful, it's OK to move a little, but try to stay focused on the moment, on your intention, and on your breathing.

7. When the time is up, allow a few seconds to open your eyes and come back to the room, to observe how you feel in that moment, to notice your body, your emotions, and your mood. Avoid jumping up and rushing on to the next thing.

If your meditation pillow has an indent of your booty from a regular practice, we're only asking that you add one more minute to your time there. If you're new to meditation entirely or only practice sporadically, you'll simply start with one minute per day. Feel free to increase that as you're ready, but throughout the four weeks of the reset, we'll be asking you to add just one more minute per week. You can do that; we know you can.

Here's how: set a clear-cut plan for yourself. Make space for just one minute a day to start, or add one more minute to your current practice. For busy people (duh, that's you), the morning is usually the best time, before life gets crazy. Wake up, go pee, drink some water, meditate. Just do it. Commit. You got this. Do not look at your phone, your email, or anything else that will pull you away from your intention.

Finding that joy and peace you crave is just around the corner; we promise. Oh, and when you have that overall sense of well-being, those other things like lifting weights and eating veggies become so much easier.

Tired B*tches Need to Sleep

Sleep, glorious sleep. The hormone reset switch. The Happy Babe–making magic. The metabolic healing balm. Sleep is the nutrient most of us are not getting enough of and an absolute nonnegotiable when it comes to healing your hormones, losing body fat, keeping your lean muscle, and not acting like a Hangry B*tch.

We know you feel like you have way too many things to do to get in bed and get your rest, or that you must get up crazy early to get a few more things done before your day starts. Or you've had some personal trainer tell you that you weren't committed enough if you didn't make it to the gym by 5 A.M. every day regardless of how wiped out and exhausted you are. If your trainer is still telling you this #noexcuses type of garbage, send them our way; we want to politely flick them in the forehead for you.

Nothing, truly nothing, is worth losing sleep over. Yet we know sleep is complicated for women. Even if we're not pressuring ourselves to rally on too little rest, many of us have trouble getting ourselves into bed on time, falling asleep easily, or staying asleep once we get there. These are all problems we want to solve, like, yesterday. We've got some hormone-specific strategies you can use in the weeks to come, but for now let's ensure you're doing the basics.

Commit to a Consistent Bedtime. If your circadian rhythm is out of whack, the best way to start to repair it is with consistency in your sleep cycle. Aim to go to bed within fifteen minutes of the same time every day—yes, on weekends, too. By that same token, aim to wake within fifteen minutes of the same time every day as well. For any new mamas reading this, obviously you can't commit to this with little ones waking you periodically throughout the night. For you, the advice is slightly different: rest whenever you can and keep as much consistency as possible, knowing it won't be perfect. This phase will pass in time; such is a mama's life.

Step Away from the iPad. Turning off electronics (including the TV, computer, and smartphone, iPad, or tablet) by 8 P.M. can feel like abandoning our first-born for some of us, but it's crucial that we help nudge hormone balance by using our normal light and dark cues. Melatonin, your sleep hormone, can't be triggered while there's still light coming into your eyeballs. If there's no way to avoid working on a device, at the very least use a blue light–blocking app such as NightShift on your phone or computer. Or try amber glasses such as those made by Uvex or Solar Shield: while not really a fashion statement, when worn in the evening they help block blue light and nudge your melatonin along.

Keep It Cool, Dark, and Comfy. Light is a powerful hormonal cue that is all out of sync these days thanks to artificial light, swing shifts, and stress. If you have a hard time falling asleep or currently depend on taking melatonin to doze off, consider switching to low-light lamps rather than bright overheads, or even go full-on candlelight as soon as you get home from work. It's mellow and lovely. If this doesn't work for your entire family, at least try candlelight in the bathroom and bedroom to keep your bedtime ritual relaxed. Keeping the lights low stimulates more melatonin and less cortisol. Blackout shades may be the best money you'll ever spend, as they will help keep your room completely dark. In the morning, expose yourself to daylight as soon as possible to stimulate your CAR (cortisol awakening response) by pulling open those shades or, better yet, getting outside.

Furthermore, temps much above 65 degrees Fahrenheit are not conducive for good sleep, so keep it cool as well. And if you haven't already, invest in a good mattress and ensure that your bedding is comfortable.

Get to Bed and Let It Go. So many women we work with have trouble just getting their bodies into their bed at a decent time. To heal your hormones, you need seven to eight hours of restful sleep. This starts with knowing what time you have to get up and how long it takes you to fall asleep, and requires being responsible enough to do the math and get yourself in bed at a time that allows you those seven to eight hours. Are there people who thrive on less sleep? Yes, of course; however, they likely don't have any hormonal issues that would ever lead them to pick up a book called *Hangry*. So in short, it's imperative that you commit to getting your beauty sleep and hormone-helping rest.

But what about all that STUFF you have to do? It will be there for you tomorrow. And trust us: the world won't actually end if you go to bed with an incomplete to-do list. We wanted to be sure, so we committed to this ourselves, and you're all still here, so it turns out the world does keep turning. Make your to-do list for tomorrow and let it go. And before bedtime, avoid anything that gets you riled up—whether that's talking to an irksome person on the phone, exercising intensely, or even reading a gripping novel. You need to guard your chill zone and protect your calm. If you currently get far less than eight hours of rest, you'll simply start by bumping up your bedtime by fifteen minutes every week during the program and continue that until you are there. Please feel free to start now! No need to wait for the program to get rolling; get more rest tonight if you can.

Sleep is a complicated hormonal and biochemical mix that many women struggle with, especially as we age. It is also negatively impacted by our habits; for example, when we drink alcohol and when we're not managing our stress. We will offer some hormone-specific strategies in the chapters to come so you can get better sleep, but we've got a few tips here for you to start with beyond the basic sleep-hygiene advice we mentioned above. Here's what we suggest you do if you're having issues with winding down.

Start a Nighttime Sleep Ritual. Try taking a warm bath with Epsom salts; the bath is relaxing, and the magnesium from the Epsom salts is great for muscle recovery and helping your nervous system calm down. Bedtime is a great time to get your thoughts out of your brain and onto paper, which is why before-bed journaling can be a great wind-down tool. Or you can read a comforting (but not stimulating) book. Things that are best left out of your nighttime ritual include intense conversation, TV shows, or Internet surfing that may get you all excited or upset. And if your current ritual includes the all-too-common "winedown" to fall asleep, yet you know wine actually disrupts your sleep later on in the night, let that go—at least for now. We're going to ask you in Week 1 to avoid the alcohol, for a while anyway; think how much less terrible that advice will be if you're well rested.

Support Your Sleep with Herbs. Bedtime teas are one of our favorite sleep supporters and can easily replace a glass of wine if you are one who enjoys sitting and sipping on something at the end of the day. There are a variety of sleep-supporting tea products out there that we love, including Tazo Calm and Yogi Bedtime Tea for example.

If you try the suggested teas and find they are somewhat helpful but do not offer quite enough support to get you soundly snoozing, consider using the same herbs found in the teas, such as chamomile, passionflower, valerian, and lemon balm, in capsule form instead in doses of 100–300 mg each. You can try these on their own or, in addition to any of the following sleep-supportive nutrients: 3 g glycine (one hour before bedtime), 200 mg L-theanine or 300–600 mg magnesium glycinate at bedtime. Or get several of these easily in one product such as our sleep supplement blend called calm+sleep at www.sarahanddrbrooke.com.

#hangrybitchfix

If you like the idea of a bedtime tea but have had lackluster results, the key is to make it strong. This is herbal medicine, so you need a dose high enough to create an effect. You can use three to five tea bags to make a cup of calming tea. Happy Babes need their sleep, and this is an easy and nourishing way to help you get your z's.

Rethink the Wine. Wine contains biogenic amines like histamine and tyramine that can be stimulating well into the night, making it difficult to stay asleep and hard to fall back asleep once you wake up. This is especially important for women over forty who are experiencing hormonal changes as it can make this effect even worse. Furthermore, the enzymes that metabolize these amines can be sluggish (due to lifestyle or genetics), causing them to build up in your brain and nervous system. These amines are stimulating in their own right and potentially cause the release of cortisol directly, and we have already covered why we want to keep this important stress hormone in check.

Can't I Just Take Melatonin?

While melatonin is sold freely over the counter, don't forget this is a hormone and thus a powerful messenger to your body. When you take melatonin, your body can't gauge how much melatonin it needs to make on its own, so it slows its production, which causes the natural rhythm of this hormone to get out of whack. Melatonin is ideal for travel-related sleep disruption, especially across time zones, but it's meant to be taken for just three days or so, not daily.

When you do take melatonin daily, this is a problem because melatonin and cortisol regulate each other. These two hormones have opposite rhythms and timing of release (cortisol release is high in the morning and lower at night, and melatonin release is the opposite). As melatonin release down regulates due to daily supplementation, it causes cortisol abnormalities followed by both stress and blood sugar issues and affects thyroid, female hormones, fat loss, immune system, etc. over time.

If you've been taking melatonin for years, you may not be able to sleep without it. If you try and just can't manage, that's a sign that your own melatonin production and rhythms are disrupted, and we can assume you'll have some cortisol and blood sugar issues because of it. In this case, you may need to stay on melatonin long-term to be able to sleep because not sleeping is worse than taking melatonin!

The best ways to ensure good melatonin release is to decrease blue light exposure in the evening and to have good cortisol timing and release. We will explain later on how to specifically address any cortisol issues (high or low) as your body makes melatonin by trying to coordinate with cortisol's rhythm.

Be sure you are not low on vitamin B6 or iron; both are key nutrients in serotonin (melatonin's precursor) and melatonin production. Look for a multivitamin with at least 50 mg of B6 and know that taking hormonal birth control or hormone replacement will quickly deplete B6, so in this case you may need more. To determine if you are deficient in iron, you need to do a couple of blood tests. See Supplement and Testing Resources or www.sarahanddrbrooke.com/lab-guide for more information.

We will cover cortisol in more detail in Week 2, but in this scenario, you may also be struggling to metabolize tyramine, histamine, or your own uppers, dopamine and epinephrine.

The enzymes you're dealing with here are MAOA (monoamine oxidase A) and COMT (catechol-O-methyltransferase). MAOA metabolizes dopamine, norepinephrine, and serotonin. COMT helps you process catechols (such as those in green tea, coffee, and chocolate) and estrogens, as well as dopamine, norepinephrine, and epinephrine. When these enzymes are running slow, several stimulating neurotransmitters can accumulate and you can feel a little amped-up, which is no good at bedtime.

To Support MAOA and COMT

Avoid taking supplements with quercetin, rhodiola, or ECGC (green tea) later in the day.

Increase riboflavin by including lamb, liver, salmon, and eggs in your diet, or consider taking 100 mg riboflavin one or two times per day.

Consider avoiding cured or fermented foods, including aged cheese and meats (a cheese plate with a glass of wine can be a sleep nightmare for women!), sauerkraut, and kombucha. And avoid high-tyramine and high-histamine fruits, including avocado, strawberries, and bananas, in the evening.

Avoid taking calcium and iron supplements in the evening, as they will slow COMT, but do take 100–400 mg magnesium in the evening. Magnesium supports metabolism of these upper-type neurotransmitters, reduces anxiety, and helps you sleep. Magnesium glycinate is our favorite form because the glycine also supports calm and sleep.

And of course stay away from caffeine in the afternoon or evening and avoid excess intake overall. Caffeine will slow MAOA directly and it will stimulate adrenaline, which needs to be processed by MAOA and COMT. And that's not all, coffee and tea contain catechols, which also have to be metabolized, putting an even bigger burden on COMT. All of this is to say that coffee, tea, and other sources of caffeine can leave you unable to wind down for multiple reasons.

Finally, Talk Yourself Down. Sometimes we just need to purposefully quiet the chatter in our minds. Try the following mantras and deep breathing to help you get into a safe place for sleep:

- I am safe, I am OK, I can sleep.

- Deep peace, deep sleep.

- Sleep can heal. I can sleep.

- Everything is OK.

#hangrybitchfix

The mantra "Everything is OK" will work in pretty much any situation where you feel stress, and while it may not feel true, you can trust that it is. No matter the outcome, it's somehow going to be OK, even if we can't see quite how yet. If saying "Everything is OK" feels like BS when you're in the thick of it and you don't believe it one bit, try "Everything is going to be OK."

Now you have a much broader understanding of the multiple stressors that can impact your sense of well-being and your hormones, and you're on your way to addressing stressors like lack of sleep, lack of calm, and biochemistry imbalances. Before we get to the details of the plan, we want to first introduce you to a foundation to rest all your healthy habits on because for so many women, the gym, the food, the vitamins, and finding a minute to meditate can easily contribute to MORE stress. In the next chapter we'll share our Five Pillars, the big-picture ideas that will provide support as you commit to doing more for yourself. We know what you've experienced time and time again: trying to employ other exercise and nutrition plans without a solid foundation, only to see your best efforts crumble like a house of cards. Our Five Pillars are what we are the most passionate about sharing with you. Of course, the diet and exercise plan is coming, but first let's build your foundation.

The Five Pillars That Take You from Hangry B*tch to Happy Babe

Self-care, thank goodness, has become a common topic these days on wellness blogs and social media, and most of us now realize how important it is. However, the practices we might think of as self-care—getting manicures, taking bubble baths with a fancy new soap, having dinner with friends, getting a massage—may feel good for a bit and create some distraction but do not offer any lasting effects of inner peace and satisfaction. We're here to tell you that finding your joy is not about manicures and massages. As nice as those things are (and we still want you to do them if they are something you love to do), they are not *real* self-care.

Self-care is not what you do but how you do it. It's how you live your life day to day, how you talk to yourself, and how you view yourself in the world, especially when times are tough. Getting out for a girls' night or going for some pampering is totally fine! Even encouraged, if that's what makes you feel like *you*, but these are watered-down versions of the kind of deep self-care that will change your life. What will change everything for you is tuning up how you speak to yourself, especially in a moment of stress, upset, failure, or frustration, what you choose to give your time to each day; and how much value you place on your overall peace and happiness.

That tape in your head—the one when you say you should've done more, should've done better, or ask, "What's wrong with me?"—has been playing for a very long time and it won't be easy to shut it off. But you can change the tape to a new one by making different choices daily. Instead of beating yourself up, start to give yourself the benefit of the doubt, choose grace over guilt, and trust that your best is simply your best even if you had hoped for better. This is a practice that you will hone over time, supported by tangible tools that we will be teaching you throughout the program. Before we get to the daily tools, we need to talk about the framework for a life where you are kind, compassionate, and less of a Hangry B*tch. This framework is our pride and joy: the Five Pillars. These tenets give you five simple anchors to make intangible, "fluffy" ideas like self-love and self-care more concrete and actionable.

This chapter will give you an overview of these five fundamental ideas and you'll actually start working on the first pillar right now. During the four weeks of the program, you'll be given more tools so you can implement all of these on a bigger scale one week, and one pillar, at a time.

The Hangry B*tches Five Pillars

1. Find and commit to what works for you

2. Opt out of overwhelm

3. Full-engagement living

4. Be your best friend

5. Be who you are

Living from these Five Pillars makes what you do with diet and exercise more effective. In fact, without them you will never have lasting success with your health—or your happiness, which, let's face it, is the ultimate goal anyway, right? Losing weight or transforming your body in some way doesn't inherently bring you joy, turn on your inner light, or improve your health. Your life is about so much more than that (it's why we wrote this book, actually!). These fundamental pillars will give you a solid base to build your health upon in a way that nourishes and sustains you.

As you continue to read the first section of this book before embarking on the four-week program, we want you to wrap your head around the first pillar, finding and committing to what works for you, because this sets the Hangry B*tch Reset apart from your average "thirty-day-challenge-follow-it-to-the-letter-or-else-type diet."

Pillar #1: Find and Commit to What Works for You

Everything you're told about health and fitness is pretty black-and-white: do this, don't do that. All gurus and experts—let's give them the benefit of the doubt—are well-meaning and believe in their way of doing it. Unfortunately, this dogmatic approach has left us with so many "rules" and hard-and-fast dos and don'ts when it comes to food and exercise and even lifestyle that we feel like failures when we follow the rules and still remain stuck.

This book is all about finding what works for you given your unique goals, priorities, and current set of hormonal imbalances. Throughout it, we are going to give you our best diet, exercise, and lifestyle strategies, based on research and also what our practical experience has shown us works best for women with wonky hormones, fatigue, and sluggish metabolisms. However, we promise to not be dogmatic. We will provide you with the necessary tools so you can evaluate how our advice is working for you. You will be able to rely on your results as well as your symptoms to assess if your hormones are diggin' a particular strategy. In other words, you'll be able to customize everything in this book uniquely for you, rather than just following our rote plan. If all is well after following your path on the Hangry B*tch Reset, that's great; keep doing it. However, if your hormonal cues based on your ACES (appetite, cravings, energy, and sleep, which we will focus on in Week 2) are still off, then we know that particular strategy isn't working for you. Instead of telling you that you aren't trying hard enough or that you aren't doing it right, we'll guide you to make adjustments that will work better for you.

Sometimes it's easy; you swap out your current breakfast for a new option and voilà! You're doing great. Sometimes giving up a certain food or style of workout gives such obvious, instant results it's easy to let it go and embrace the change. Other times it's harder, comes with more emotional backlash, or is just way more complicated and takes more detective work. But we ask that you commit to doing that challenging work because, ladies, off-the-shelf plans, as you know, just don't work for all of us! It is part of why you're so frustrated and it's exactly why we created this plan. The "how to know what works for you" is coming, but right now we want you to start thinking about what it will be like when you DO find exactly what works for you. Knowing what you need to do but not being able to do it—well, that's the biggest frustration of all.

Most of us have been here in one way or another: knowing that there IS something that works for us but we just plain don't want to do whatever that thing is. Maybe being gluten-free makes you feel great but you just don't want to "live that way forever." Or maybe your symptoms are resolved when you eschew sugar and stay away from wine but you feel restricted and rail against this. Or maybe you just don't want to lift weights, because it's boring or because you have no idea where to begin. Or, on the flipside, maybe you are incredibly, very, super-duper reluctant to give up some form of exercise, be it long runs, spin class, or daily, intense CrossFit metcons, because you love the rush you get from it. We get it; we both love exercise and hated stepping away from intense workouts even though our hormones and injuries were clearly telling us to. And yes, we both want to drink wine all day most days, too, but that just doesn't work for us either! Like you, we have had to commit to what works for us and we get it: some things are simply harder than others.

Throughout the Hangry B*tch Reset, you'll be given insight into what works for your unique biochemistry and hormonal issues. Your job is to treat yourself with the love and care you deserve by not doing things that hurt your body or your hormones. Making peace with your diet can be harder than making peace with exercise, but don't worry: we have lots of ways to help you make this potentially tough transition, including a little food relationship counseling. So often we see women derail their best efforts with their commitment to do what works for them because it's just so tough to sort out their food issues. We get it; we too have struggled with this very real problem, which is why we want you to start thinking about your relationship with food before we even jump into our diet suggestions. Your first food-relationship counseling session starts now!

Achieving a healthy relationship with food can look exactly like what it takes to have a healthy relationship with anyone—but this "food relationship" is really about your relationship with yourself. At the end of the day, food is just food; it's how we feel about ourselves that dictates whether we use food as a tool or as a weapon (one that might make us feel better initially but often worse in the end). As with any healthy relationship, a good relationship with food involves the following elements.

Trust

- You were likely never taught to have any sort of trust in your food, or you've likely lost faith that food is healing or even nourishing because every diet you've ever tried has probably felt miserable or has produced less than stellar results. You might typically think of food as the enemy or as comfort or celebration or maybe just as essential, but we want you to consider your relationship with food in a spiritual, meaningful, and trustworthy sense.

- In order to regain food trust, it can be incredibly helpful to get in touch with your habits around where your food comes from. For example, if you decide to be more aware of small aspects such as doing some of your shopping at your local farmers' markets, getting to know the hardworking people who grow your vegetables, or seeking out opportunities to buy your meat from local grass-fed and pasture-raised sources, it will help you feel more in touch and appreciative of your food rather than distant and uncertain.

- This kind of trust-building relationship will help you see the bigger picture and help cultivate a sense of responsibility around how you obtain the food that nourishes you; and this alone is helpful in committing to what works for you. If you can't find all or even some of your food from local farmers, just the simple act of growing your own small window box herb garden is quite often enough for women to feel more trustworthy around and in touch with the spiritual healing nature of food. Getting closer to the source provides a positive connection to your food vs. how you might feel about the typical packaged diet fare that often only comes with feelings of frustration or discontent.

- We also want to encourage you to think about what it would feel like to eat food that doesn't hurt you. Just like in any other relationship, you must trust that the food that is right for your body will not cause pain or discomfort, emotionally or physically. Once that has been established, you can feel free to enjoy it, rather than always anticipating how bad you're going to feel after you eat something. Once you've gained trust in your commitment to what works for you, you can break up with the food that harms you, and simply relax and enjoy the food that loves you back!

- Finally, we encourage you to really examine why you might be going back to the foods that you know don't work for you. It can be very challenging, but you'll need to address why you use food for comfort. For example, did you have trust issues in past relationships that made you turn to food to fill an emotional void? This is tough, but it must be considered and addressed.

Acceptance

- After establishing trust, we encourage you to accept where you are with your new and more positive relationship with yourself and the food you know works for and nourishes your body. Just because your relationship is getting better doesn't mean it's always comfortable; it may feel strange until you're used to it.

- We want you to know that there is no good food or bad food, but there is food that works for you and food that doesn't, and accepting this new fact is an important first step in healing your food relationship. Just as some toxic people aren't necessarily bad people—they just don't work for you—and the same goes for food. Some people might be able to hang out with that same person (or eat that food) and be fine, but you cannot and that's OK, too. It's about honoring and accepting what does and does not work.

- We ask you to accept that every food relationship is and can be different. No two relationships are the same, but if you figure out what works for you, that's all that matters. As with human relationships, we all communicate a bit differently, feel a bit differently, and behave a bit differently around food. Your body might respond to a food differently than other people you might know and that is OK because you are discovering what works for you!

- If certain foods are fighting against you, making you sick, exhausted, and hangry, even though your taste buds might love them it's not a good idea to keep coming back for more. We ask you instead to work on accepting that there is a lot of food that you do enjoy that will completely and unconditionally love you back.

Respect

- If you don't respect yourself, it's almost impossible to respect the relationship—you must heal your relationship with yourself before you can truly have a healthy mindset about food, which is why our program has such a focus on mindset, meditation, stress reduction, and self-love and compassion.

- We ask you to consider respecting yourself as you would your own child, spouse, lover, or friend. You are amazing at respecting and taking care of everyone else in your life, and it's time that you respect your own body enough to give it what it needs! It helps if you can decide if a particular food is worth your respect and be OK with it if sometimes that changes. Relationships are fluid. If something works for a while and then stops working later, it's OK to have enough respect for yourself to address that reality and make a change.

- It's important in healing your relationship with food to learn to respect food that doesn't hurt you. This is pretty straightforward: only food that loves, heals, and respects YOU should be deserving of your respect.

- As you move forward through this program, we want you to respect the journey, the challenges, and the times that you are not perfect because there is no perfect. No relationship is perfect; this is a journey to doing better, feeling better, and living life to its fullest. Remember, the challenges that you face are offering you the opportunity to learn and grow.

Safety

- You should feel safe in any relationship, including your relationship with food, and nourishing foods that you know work for you can and should provide a sense of safety, both physically and emotionally. Remember that your body is your safe house and treat it as such.

- We want to encourage you to feel safe and reassured in your choices through education. Remember that animals feed but humans EAT—you need to make your own choices by learning what is safe and what is not instead of blindly following the pack.

- As in any relationship, if you realize that you are in a situation with your food where you do not feel safe, make changes! You might need to really examine what this means for you, including changing your routine, whether that means finding new places to shop and eat out to finding new ways to cope, and to start new habits that make you feel comforted and cared for that have nothing to do with food. We will give you several tools throughout the program that will give you a safe and positive way to cope with the struggles often associated with any sort of change. Know that no matter what you choose, it should feel nourishing and uplifting.

Commitment

- Committing to a bad diet is like committing to a bad relationship. It never ends well. We ask you to make the conscious decision to change your perspective and, instead of committing to yet another "diet" that's doomed to fail, commit to your health by gaining a better understanding of your body's needs rather than trying to work toward a weight-loss goal. We suggest that you change your ideas around why you are trying to make these changes and that feeling better should be your first commitment rather than aesthetic goals; the rest will come after you achieve health.

- In any relationship, commitment is about who you are, rather than whom you are with. Even if that person is "perfect" for you, the relationship won't work unless you are psychologically healthy enough to make a commitment—and the same is true with food.

- This is also your invitation to assess before you commit—just because it worked for your best friend doesn't mean it will work for you. We will give you the knowledge to learn how your body works; this is why you are reading this book, to learn how you operate and how to stop being so exhausted that you can't find time to commit to your health. Your time is now!

Realistic Expectations

- Food should not fill a void. As with a human relationship, food should complement your already healthy self! Food does not fix everything, and this is why we have more than one pillar of health. Our plan is comprehensive because we know you can't just address one area with the expectation of a magical fix. Your life will start to feel full when you have enough energy to be joyful again, and good eating habits will just be a by-product of your joy rather than what brings you joy.

- We do want you to expect that you will have to play detective. We are not offering a magic solution, and some things, such as committing to the foods that work for you, are not always figured out overnight. This is why as you work through the Hangry B*tch Reset you'll see that what we prescribe is not a one-size-fits-all approach. We do not want to set you up for failure, so we are giving you the tools to know what needs to be changed with your plan based on your unique needs. This is something that all relationships should be built upon: the realistic expectation that life (and hormones) are always changing and that, in order to be successful with your food relationship, you must adapt according to what your body needs. We also want you to NEVER give up, because there is always better.

Satisfaction

- You'll know you've found a healthy relationship with food when you feel satisfied with your choices and are no longer anxious or unsure about what to eat, when to eat, and how much to eat. When food stops being at the forefront of every thought, then you are living a satisfied coexistence with food rather than constantly battling the food demons. Feeling satisfied with your food will give you so much freedom, and we can't wait to offer you the tools to get you there!

Once you take our Hangry B*tch Hormone Quiz (starting on page 127) and gain more insight on your unique hormonal issues, your journey to finding what works for you will really begin.

Pillar #2: Opt Out of Overwhelm

There can be no joy or optimal health when there's utter overwhelm. This is one of the biggest problems we hear about from women trying to make healthier choices.

"How do I do it all?"

"Where will I find the time?"

"But I don't know how!"

"I don't have the support (or the resources or the money) to do this!"

And finally, "What's wrong with me that I can't make it happen?"

Nothing's wrong with you—and you're not alone. Feeling harried and overwhelmed is unfortunately the female condition. We know just finding the time to read this book was a challenge for most of you and that our plan will require more of your time and mental energy. We get that, and we want to help you succeed because we also know that getting your haywire hormones in check and following the Hangry B*tch Reset isn't the only thing on your plate!

Overwhelm kills results—as well as happiness—but it doesn't have to be that way. Overwhelm is a choice and we're going to teach you how to choose instead to #optoutofoverwhelm. Here are two ways that you can choose to opt out: getting good at saying no and living in gratitude:

Get Good at Saying No

Saying no is hard for most of us, and it is really, *really* hard for some women. Whether you're a people pleaser or feel obligated more often than not, the reluctance to say no can drastically increase your stress and decrease your time. Saying no is a skill, one you'll have to practice until it feels easy for you.

What most of us can't do in the moment is assess how important this thing is we're being asked to do—to us. To the person asking it, it's super important! It's easy to get infected by their urgency or excitement or desperation and say yes . . . when you know you shouldn't or just don't even want to. What you have to learn to do is assess how important it is for YOU, right there on the spot. This takes time and practice and you'll mess it up a few times, but here's how to start practicing your NO.

If you are a constant "yes" girl, get in the habit of always asking for at least an hour before you give an answer. Maybe it's not possible to take a week to think it over, but most of the time an hour is reasonable. This gives you a window to assess how important this is for you, how it fits in with your schedule, and the value it has for you and for those you care about.

If you already feel stressed, be willing to say no to something if you say yes to something else. For example, if you are asked to be on a new committee at work or school, right away decide what you can delegate, stop doing, or put on hold before the words "sure I will" can even escape your lips. You have to make room for new obligations instead of piling them onto your plate with all the old ones.

Practice with stuff that doesn't matter. When you are seemingly unable to say no to just about everyone, practice saying no in situations where the stakes are low and there's less emotional charge for you. For example, practice saying no when you're asked if you'd like something at a restaurant. Yes, it sounds weird, but saying no to "would you like fries with that" is practice for saying no to the bigger things that really count. When asked at the post office if you'd also like to buy some stamps and you don't need stamps, practice your firm but polite no. You may be saying no to these smaller things already, but get really present when you do say it. Really feel how it feels to say no and witness how the world doesn't end. Observe that the cashier at the post office doesn't tell you that you're a horrible friend, mother, or community member for passing on their offer for stamps. The reality is that with most high-stakes situations this won't happen either.

Finally, you will inevitably find yourself in the situation where you say yes when you really meant no. Or you say yes and quickly feel yourself drowning in the stress of adding one more thing to your plate, so now what? You are allowed to change your mind. Crazy, right? We know no one has ever let you in on this little secret, but you are 100 percent within your right to say, "You know what, I said yes but I am realizing now that I shouldn't have. I'm sorry for that and I can give you (three days/one week/ten phone calls/whatever) in order to help get this obligation transferred to someone else."

This brings us to what follows on the heels of saying no: disappointing people. Oh man, is this hard! But as long as you are kind, courteous, and as helpful as you are able to be without wrecking yourself, you don't need to feel bad. Whatever upset is present on someone else's part has more to do with them than with you. Now, we never want to leave anyone in a lurch, but most of the time you can help find someone else to do it, do a smaller percentage of the work, or simply say no and skip the hand wringing as it's your job to take care of yourself.

Finally, when you really aren't certain if saying no was the right thing to do, think about whether what you are saying no to will feel important when you are on your deathbed. Morbid, we know, but this trick really works! We are certain you'll want to think about time well spent with the people you love, how you filled your big beautiful life with moments that really mattered, and how you were able to care for yourself first so that you could really show up as your authentic, healthy self for those who truly did need you, like your children or other loved ones. So if someone is upset at you for saying no, simply hand him or her a copy of this book and let yourself off the hook.

Live in Gratitude

It's easy to feel good when things are good, but there will be times when all you want is something other than what you've got. It's during these inevitable times that it's important to still find and appreciate the good in what you do have, even though it mostly feels like you want a vacation from it all! Living from this place, whether you are faced with something good or bad, is a powerful tool in opting out of overwhelm, but it takes practice.

To cultivate more gratitude in your life, we want you to start each morning by thinking about what you are grateful for and giving thanks for what you have. Each morning, in your head or out loud (or write it on paper, typically called a Gratitude Journal), simply say, "I'm so grateful for A, B, and C!" This is a wonderful way to start your day with gratitude, rather than contemplating all the crap you have to do. The crap will still be there, but a simple reminder to yourself of the abundance in your wonderful world will set the tone for a joy-filled day. Even showing gratitude for the things you really aren't all that grateful for will help keep you open to whatever positive lesson will come from said thing. For example, if you are dreading grocery shopping because you simply don't love doing it, instead give thanks for your ability to be able to afford the food you are about to get, or the empowerment you now have knowing that you are shopping for food that will help you feel better.

No matter how bad things get, you can always find at least one thing to be grateful for. In the darkest of times, we can still find one glimmer of good that opens our eyes to one more thing we're grateful for, and one more, and on from there. There is always, *always* a silver lining, a meaning, and a reason for everything that happens—good or bad. This is why we so strongly believe in this daily gratitude list and practice; however, gratitude is much bigger than this exercise. Living in gratitude is a full-immersion experience in "I could just break into utter joyful tears right now because I am so grateful." Start with the exercise each morning and continue to look for opportunities to feel submerged in the feeling of wanting what you have right now so much more than getting what you want in the future. In other words, living in a state of gratitude can look like letting go of always wanting more and instead deciding that what you have right now is enough.

We live most of our lives wishing and hoping for better health, a better body, a more fulfilling career, and more money. We may plan to do really noble things with this stuff we want, but, even so, it keeps us in a state of longing and desire for an imaginary future. Wanting what you have now—not just appreciating it but desiring it—that's gratitude. That is living with the experience that you're taken care of, you're gracious, and you're 100 percent OK. That is life-changing, and will open you up to allow space for even more abundance.

Will you be moved to tears of gratitude today by what feels like a messed-up metabolism, frustrating hormone issues, health issues, finances, or troubled relationships? No, probably not. However, as you continue to practice not only the morning gratitude routine but also start to approach your entire life with gratitude, life will truly change. You'll be more content and at peace than you've ever imagined possible (talk about cortisol lowering!). And this doesn't mean you love having no energy, a nonexistent sex drive, breakouts, or pants that don't fit and it doesn't mean you give up your dreams. It means that you don't desire them any more than what you already have. It means you want more for yourself without hating where you are now. When we marinate in gratitude for what we've got, it brings us more of what we want—not to get too quantum science-y on you, but it's true. And let's say the worst happens: you don't get what you want . . . aren't you happier being at peace with what you already have? Of course you are.

In the end, it's really hard for anger, resentment, judgment, and shame to live in gratitude. Gratitude is a bad-mood buzzkill, and we understand it's challenging to remember to find something to be grateful for when you feel like you are falling apart, but we promise that if you keep flexing the gratitude muscle it simply makes life easier, allowing you to opt out of overwhelm and opt into joy instead.

Pillar #3: Full-Engagement Living

Taking the number-three spot on the Five Pillars list is fully engaging with our lives and with the people that matter to us. In our overly busy and often stressful lives, we often end up living in the future ("I'll be happy if . . ." "It will be OK when . . ."), which means we are unable to be truly present.

This pillar focuses on having a different experience of everyday life, one that is not about distraction from discomfort but about absolute connection to what's going on, no matter what the experience might be. We want you to really connect with the people you love: really listen, really stop and look into your lover's eyes, really get down to eye level with your kiddos. At least once a day, just "be" with your people in the most engaging ways possible. This will draw you smack into the present moment and will be a strong reminder of what is most important. If you simply decide to make this type of connection a priority, all the other things we are asking you to do, such as learning to say no, will become easier. Full-engagement living is self-care at its finest. It's learning to really tune in to what is happening in your world rather than constantly distracting yourself from it.

We also want to encourage you to get away from today's primary distraction: the phone. You can be available for phone calls or texts should you need to, but in order to avoid the distraction of social media and the internet, set aside times every day when you keep your phone out of reach, like up on a high shelf or in a closet with the door closed. Make the conscious choice to be present in your real life and not your digital one every single day. You will feel so much intense joy in these moments—we promise your mind will be blown. For those of you who have children, it's especially important to model for them what full-engagement living looks like. We are raising a generation that doesn't even understand what a real conversation looks like and our kids *need* us to be connected to them.

The next aspect of full-engagement living is learning to be OK with discomfort. Happiness is not a constant state, although we are shown through everything from TV to social media that, no matter what, we are always supposed to wear a smile and walk around being really friggin' happy, well dressed, and put together. Well, that's simply not achievable. Happiness, like all other emotions, happens in moments rather than being constant. And of course, not all moments are happy! But all moments are worth fully experiencing as often as possible, and when you really tap into what brings you joy, what it means to you to be happy, you will feel an overall sense of well-being, peace, and contentment, even when crap gets crazy. Learning to be OK even with the bad will help you feel less exhausted because frustration, anger, sadness, and stress are all draining—especially when you expend so much energy fighting against those very real and normal emotions.

Go ahead and let yourself feel your "bad" emotions, because none are really bad—all emotions are parts of our human experience. Instead of shopping, eating, drinking, gossiping, or exercising to avoid an uncomfortable feeling, we ask you to just sit with it for a moment and breathe through it rather than fight it. As you practice this tool you might find that you have to work through some really uncomfortable stuff that you would rather distract yourself from. This is why meditation is so important: it's the practice of being observant rather than reactionary. Meditation is the door to full-engagement living, which is why this practice is so strongly recommended throughout our plan. Sitting with those uncomfortable feelings that come up when we meditate and subsequently in life is what we like to call "putting your toe in the hot water." It can be shocking or even a bit painful at first, but just as getting into a hot tub can initially feel uncomfortable, as you immerse yourself and relax you get more and more used to it, and it actually feels pretty darn great.

As you start to let yourself sit with your uncomfortable emotions, you may find that you need to cry or say out loud what you are experiencing, and you should. Write it down if you need to or, even better, phone a friend or talk to a counselor about some of the stuff that might come up. Most important, don't shut down, and don't close your heart. Stay open by letting those feelings come through you until they begin to dissipate. It's easier to do this by remembering that you are not defined by any one emotion. Bad feelings like hurt, resentment, or jealousy or good feelings like happiness, joy, and excitement will all come up, but these feelings aren't you. You will feel more content and be able to stay more present when you honor all of your emotions and let them be a part of who you are instead of a definition of who you are.

Full-engagement living enhances the beauty of life, and just as we ask you to breathe through the scary, tough stuff, we want you to breathe through all the wonderful stuff that comes up, too. Soak in the good moments, really relish them, explore them, and be open and OK with how good life can feel. Fully engage in them; be a part of each moment in its entirety before you move on to the next "have-to" on your list. Sometimes we shut down during moments of joy because we are distracted by thinking that those moments will be over soon and that there may be worse moments around the corner. Rather than miss out on good times by worrying about possible impending bad times, remind yourself that all you have is right now, and just be there, present and engaged.

Like the other pillars, this one takes time to master, so just keep trying to be more engaged, more comfortable in your discomfort, and more aware of your distractions. During Week 2, we'll practice becoming more engaged in our lives by doing something that can't be undone. It can feel endlessly defeating that much of what we do all day is undone in an instant: laundry, dishes, answering emails. Almost as soon as it's done, it's getting dirty, messy, undone, or piling up again. We'll be helping you do something every day that can't be undone: write, draw, express your love, perform a random act of kindness, dance in the kitchen, make a memory, or have a real conversation with someone who values you and whom you value as well. Create memories and moments that last—something that *will* matter to you on your deathbed.

If all you take away from this book are the lessons we are hoping to instill with this pillar, we feel like our work has been done. This is a bold statement for a nutrition and exercise book, but that's how much we want you to dive into full-engagement living, because at the end of the day, that's what life is really all about.

Pillar #4: Be Your Best Friend

As you navigate the choices you make each day, from high-level career decisions to parenting or caregiving choices to diet and exercise options, you need to be your own best friend. Of course we all love our friends, but the friend you really need is yourself. Unfortunately, however, most of us have spent our lives being our own worst enemy and nastiest critic rather than our biggest cheerleader. We punish ourselves with diets and exercise and set unrealistic standards that we lose sleep and sanity trying to uphold—all because our inner critic is cracking the whip.

While this voice feels as real as the pages of this book you hold in your hands, it's only one option, and you will be able to find and develop a positive voice you can truly rely on. You can continue to listen to this Nasty B*tch (let's be honest; she is a real piece of work) or you can tune in to the encouraging cheerleader, the best friend who always seems to look at you with love and

Nasty B*tch and Best Friend Go on a Diet

There's perhaps no area of a woman's life where distinguishing between these two internal voices is more of a challenge than body image and weight loss. Look, there are a thousand crazy-ass things we could tell you to do to lose weight. Much of it would further your hormonal mess and most all of it would be unsustainable. Some of the more intense, restrictive, and hard-core programs may work initially (we know, it feels really good at first to see "progress"), but maintaining them would make you miserable. In the end, as enticing as they are, all restrictive diets fail, even the "good" ones like Paleo, and all aggressive exercise regimens have a shelf life.

When it comes to weight loss, you have to answer some fundamental questions and pay particular attention to which inner voice you're hearing as you answer:

- Will achieving a particular goal (size 6, X number of pounds, etc.) give you a bigger, better life? Get honest about what this goal means to you, and decide whether reaching it will truly make you happy or is it just something you think you need to do to be more worthy, lovable, or accepted.

- Does this goal feel good to you? Simple but profound question. If it lights you up, great. Then go for it in a loving, nourishing way that honors your hormones first.

- Is your goal the right one? What we mean by this is, would five or even ten pounds short of your goal actually be your sweet spot, where you could feel you were living the life you wanted and not feel overly restricted in terms of gym time and diet?

kindness. Think about how different life would be if, after a tough day, your best friend voice chimed in with, "It's hard to see now but you are beyond lovable and worthy and I want to help you feel better. We got this." Instead, what we usually hear is, "OMG you are such a loser! On top of screwing this up like you do everything else, you are never going to be happy. Oh, and you look fat

- Do you really want to lose weight? So many women respond to this with "Of course I do—that's why I'm here! Are you sure you two are experts at this stuff?" However, upon further investigation, we find they have zero interest in doing the things they need to do to lose weight. They've thought for so long that weight loss is a mandate, a must-do, just part of being a woman. The truth is, some health parameters may improve with weight loss, your jean size may change, and you may even feel more confident, but you and only you can decide if losing weight is something you want to do. If it is, again, go about it in a loving, nourishing way. If it's not, let yourself off the hook about it and spend your energy elsewhere. And either way, know that you're lovable and worthy of joy and happiness now.

The point of these questions is to get really honest about what losing weight means to you—and what you're willing to do to get there. Many women are shocked when they are told they don't actually have to lose a pound. They are surprised to hear that strength, confidence, and better hormone balance are also options on the menu when it comes to health and fitness. If they choose to lose weight, women must go at it in a way that honors and even heals their hormones and creates more happiness, because being smaller but miserable is no way to live.

All of this matters. It's not just about the diet—because stress management and good-quality sleep are paramount for your health—and absolute necessities when it comes to success with weight loss and sustainability. These key elements need to be addressed before you can even think of how many carbs to eat or how many deadlifts to do, and there's not much that's more stressful to the average woman than dieting. What we do and how we do it when it comes to most weight loss advice is part of the problem, not the solution, for women to be healthy and happy.

today." Both voices are present in your head but the nasty one chimes in faster than you can say "better go on a juice cleanse." So you've got to be on your toes.

When you are just starting to let your best friend voice take the reins, your task is simply to constantly check in with yourself to see who's running the show up there. Women always ask, "Well, how the heck do I know?" You start to listen to the tone of your internal dialogue. Just observe—don't try to shush Nasty B*tch; she just gets louder. Instead, listen to her and get to really know what she sounds like.

Often, what you'll hear is basically your BS. It's all the haggard old stories about how you don't measure up, aren't good enough, and are somehow unworthy of love or happiness. The voice spewing these stories is usually rude and mean, but your inner Nasty B*tch can also be sneaky. When she's downright critical it's fairly easy to spot, but sometimes she's a "frenemy," masquerading as a friend and persuading you to do something not in your best interest, which might sound like this:

"You worked so hard today, you deserve that glass of wine or that entire cake."

"You are awesome; eff that new diet. You don't need to worry about gluten and those achy joints you get when you eat pizza; that's all in your head. Screw those girls that wrote that dumb *Hangry* book; what do they know?"

"Indulge now and you can work it off at the gym tomorrow! YOLO, right?"

"This whole healthy (or weight-loss) thing is so unfair! You should be able to eat like so-and-so and be fine. Your genes suck so bad! It's not fair that you have to try so hard! You hate this. Why bother?"

Your frenemy voice is great at making a lot of justifications and feeling entitled. Your best friend voice, on the other hand, is kind but not above telling you the truth if it's helpful. She is practical, nurturing, and a real cheerleader. She won't pressure you to drink wine if she knows you're trying to cut back. She will suggest a nap instead of a workout if you are sick or low on sleep. She will appreciate your hard work even when things don't pan out. Your job, starting now, is to constantly check in with whose advice you're taking. In Week 3 we'll help you get better at heeding your best friend voice and telling the Nasty B*tch voice to simmer down.

Again, this takes a LOT of practice. For so long you've done things that keep you at war with yourself. You've fought your hormones and metabolism like they were the enemy instead of being on their side. It might not have seemed like it as you battled fatigue and extra pounds, but your hormones are constantly trying to keep you going, so you have to rally and decide to be on their team. They want to be besties with you again, and life will be so much better when you are. So moving forward from here, instead of listening to the Nasty B*tch saying "my stupid body just won't ever cooperate; how's this going to be any different?" channel that best friend voice and say "I trust my body. It's doing the best it can—it always has and it always will—and if I support and love myself I know I can heal."

Pillar #5: Be Who You Are

When we're tired, cranky, stressed out, and maxed out we tend to forget who we are. Part of being healthy is living from a place of authenticity, being gentle and kind to ourselves, and doing things just for us. It's not being selfish; it's living "self-first" and it's essential! If you aren't nurturing yourself, there's no way you can be fully present and available for the important people in your life. When we lose who we are, we end up carrying around a lot of pent-up anger, resentment, and bitterness, which creates more unwanted stress. Part of living life as a Happy Babe, rather than as a Hangry B*tch, is focusing on finding what brings you joy. But how do you do that? It's simpler than you'd think: it starts with making a commitment to be exactly who you are.

We are painfully aware that many of you have lost touch with who you are and what brings you joy because you've taken care of the kids, the career, and the laundry for so long that taking care of yourself seems as foreign as fluently speaking Sanskrit. The time to reconnect to YOU is now.

Start by making a list of things that you love or used to love to do or have always wanted to do, like dance lessons, playing the guitar, knitting, reading, mountain climbing, writing, singing, traveling, cooking, art, or any creative pursuit—things that are purely fun and focused on bringing you closer to your authentic self and how you want to be in the world.

You may be tempted to add things like working out and eating healthier to your list, but that's not what this list is about. Your list has to be made up of things (or even just one thing) that make you smile or laugh out loud with joy. They could be things that push you just a smidge out of your comfort zone or that get you fired up inside. Remember your high school drama days, when you played the lead role in the school play and felt like you were Julia Roberts in *Pretty Woman,* and you never wanted to do anything else in your entire life but that? Yeah, that sort of thing is what we are talking about. However, your list doesn't have to be extravagant. It just needs to include things that make you feel more alive.

After you've figured out what activities might bring you closer to being your authentic self, the next step is to make time for one of them. You may have to take time from something else, but do it. This is that important. Schedule a time for this activity and stick to it! This is your task before you start the rest of the program and it doesn't have to take hours every week. Even fifteen minutes of playing the piano can bring you more joy. The point is that you're expressing who you are and having fun! That's it.

This is a biggie and you may not figure it all out in a week or maybe even a year! We'll practice this pillar in Week 4. But for now, it's important to make time to do things that you love because, let's face it, there's nothing more stressful (to you and your hormones) than not being who you are.

What a Hangry B*tch Should Eat

When it comes to what you should eat in order to move toward feeling more like a Happy Babe and less like a Hangry B*tch, we think the best approach is to find the diet that works best for you. But how do you know what that is? Well, it won't be the same for all of you, which is what makes this program unique. We'll show you how to customize your meals—both the timing and the content—to work with your own hormones, but first you need a template that you can customize.

The basic Paleo dietary template is a fantastic starting point for women and has a solid reputation for being the catalyst that can help to clear up, or significantly improve, a lot of health issues and hormonal imbalances. Paleo avoids grains, soy, and legumes, as well as dairy, highly processed foods, and sugar, all of which can cause inflammation and blood sugar swings, and much of which is not tolerated well by many women.

The core tenets of a Paleo diet stem from the concept of eating in a manner closer to our hunter-gatherer ancestors and opting for more natural, unprocessed choices. This diet provides an upgrade in nutrition quality for most women compared to what they are currently eating, as the Paleo menu is rich with these nutrient-dense foods:

High-Quality Protein. In addition to wild-caught fish and game, recommended meat sources include grass-fed beef, pasture-raised pigs, and free-range poultry. Animals ideally should be raised without added antibiotics or hormones and fed an organic diet. This makes for less-inflammatory protein

Um, Excuse Me, Is Your Gut Leaking?

Your gut normally allows only very small molecules to cross from the intestines into your bloodstream through small openings called tight junctions, and this is how you absorb nutrients from your food and supplements. This regulated permeability by your intestinal cells is vital for health, but it can get disrupted when the protein zonulin is released, damaging those tight junctions. Certain foods, such as gluten for some people, as well as infections, stress, and aging can cause the release of zonulin and thus create a hyperpermeable, or "leaky," gut.

Now we've got a mess. Toxins, microbes, and undigested food can escape your intestines and hitch a ride in the bloodstream to the rest of your body, putting an increased burden on both your liver and immune system. Your immune system sees these molecules as it would any infection or invader and mounts an attack, leaving you with a range of symptoms that can include headache, joint pain, water retention and puffiness, stuffy nose, rashes or breakouts, or any other signs of inflammation.

Gluten is a common cause of leaky gut, but other inflammatory foods, such as dairy and alcohol, are possible culprits as well. Gut infections such as SIBO (small intestine bacterial overgrowth), candida, and intestinal bacteria and parasites, as well as medications including ibuprofen (Motrin, Advil, etc.), antibiotics, steroids, acid-blocking medications, and environmental toxins such as pesticides, BPA in plastics, heavy metals, and our old friend stress all can create leaky gut and hyperpermeability.

Wondering if you have leaky gut? You may if you have any of the following:

- Digestive symptoms such as gas, bloating, diarrhea, or IBS
- Skin issues including eczema, acne, or rosacea
- Autoimmune issues including Hashimoto's disease, lupus, rheumatoid arthritis, celiac disease, or psoriasis
- Seasonal allergies or asthma
- Mood issues such as depression, brain fog, anxiety, or difficulty concentrating

Yikes, right? Well, the great news is that your gut and liver are very adaptive and can heal. We tell you exactly how later on in this chapter on pages 69-71.

sources and fewer hormone disruptors, and addressing both of these aspects is absolutely key for women.

Vegetables and Fruits (organic is preferred). Getting plenty of fruits and vegetables bolsters our antioxidant, phytonutrient, and fiber intake, normalizing hormones such as insulin and estrogen and improving overall health and digestion. Ideally all produce is organic, to avoid pesticides, such as glyphosate, which has been linked to cancer, endocrine disruption, leaky gut, and more.

Healthy Fats. Extra virgin olive oil, coconut, avocados, nuts, and seeds support our fat-soluble vitamin needs, including vitamins D, A, and E. Healthy fats also support female hormone balance, aid in feeling satisfied from meals, and normalize inflammation, which improves all health parameters. Remember, inflammation is the hormone mess-maker!

The Paleo diet does not include the following:

Grains. Paleo dieters are told to avoid grains largely because they are typically processed into tasty treats in combination with sugar and fats like cookies, breads, bagels, and doughnuts, which wreak havoc on our health because of the crazy carbohydrate load. However, there are other compelling reasons to avoid grains as well. Grains contain lectins, which attach to receptors in the intestinal lumen and are transported through the intestinal lining and into our bodies intact. These lectins can be treated like "invaders" much like other bacteria, or viruses, leading to a host of problems like joint pain, inflammation, autoimmune issues, and cancer. Damage to the gut lining also inhibits nutrient absorption. Phytates in grains will bind to essential nutrients such as magnesium, zinc, iron, calcium, and vitamins A, D, and K and prevent or greatly inhibit their absorption. Finally, gluten, whose components gliadin and glutenin are highly inflammatory for some people, is found in grains such as wheat, barley, rye, and some oats. Due to food processing and technology, our modern gluten is very different from what our grandparents ate and is more problematic for many people well beyond celiac disease.

Dairy. After our toddler years, most humans produce only a small amount of lactase, the small-intestine enzyme that digests lactose (the sugar found in milk), which is one reason dairy causes so much gas, bloating, and tummy trouble. Furthermore, it is very common for people to have sensitivities to casein and whey, the proteins found in dairy, which can cause gastrointestinal problems as well as headaches, congestion, fatigue, and behavior/mood issues.

Legumes. Beans, lentils, and other legumes make the no-no list on Paleo because they contain a few troublesome components, including phytic acid, which can bind nutrients in the gut, hindering their absorption (basically, you get less good stuff from your good meal). They also have saponins and protease inhibitors, which both contribute to leaky gut. Furthermore, the oligosaccharides in legumes make them a high-FODMAP food, which means they can be difficult to digest and cause a lot of bloating, especially if you have any underlying gut imbalances such as SIBO or IBS, which are both very common these days! Finally, legumes, like many other plants, contain lectins, which can also contribute to inflammation and leaky gut in many people. So, while in theory legumes are a great high-fiber food with a decent amount of protein, with all the nutritional chemistry factored in they are less than ideal for most. Cooking them properly can improve their digestibility, so although legumes are eschewed on Paleo, as you work with the Hangry B*tch Reset Diet, you might find that they do work for you as a high-fiber carb source down the road.

Soy. This highly genetically modified legume has all of the same issues as other legumes, but in addition it is a very common food sensitivity, creating symptoms ranging from headaches to bloating to stuffy nose. Soy also is a potent phytoestrogen that could help or hinder a woman's hormone balance. As well, soy in high amounts could possibly hinder thyroid function.

Sugar and High-Fructose Corn Syrup. These processed sweeteners are to be avoided for obvious reasons, especially high-fructose corn syrup, which is processed by the liver and can lead to nonalcoholic fatty liver disease (NAFLD).

Vegetable Oils. These modern-day highly processed oils, including canola, soybean, corn, peanut, sunflower and safflower oils, are almost always rancid and extremely high in linoleic acid, which can increase systemic inflammation, which, as you will learn in this book, worsens all hormone function across the board.

By simply removing some of the most offensive foods and replacing them with foods that are considered low-allergen, less glycemic, more nutrient-dense, and not prone to causing inflammation, a lot of women achieve great results from a Paleo diet, including improved digestion, hormone rebalancing, fewer aches and pains, and weight loss.

By adopting a Paleo diet filled with higher-quality foods boasting more nutritional value, most people feel so much better and can overcome a host of digestive, hormonal, and other health issues but, unfortunately, simply "going Paleo" doesn't solve all problems for all women—it can even create a few! Much of that is due to women's unique hormonal landscape.

How to Fix Your Digestion

Bloating after eating or bloating that gets worse as the day goes on, tummy aches, skin issues, headaches, fatigue after eating, constipation, diarrhea, or increasing sensitivity to more foods—all of these symptoms indicate a need to fix your digestion in order to fix your hormones. The seat of health or the seat of inflammation, the gut is a major player in your hormone balance and unfortunately it's easily damaged from stress, eating foods that don't work for you, or taking medications such as antacids, acid blockers, steroids, or antibiotics.

The first step in fixing your digestion is removing foods that are aggravating your gut or causing inflammation. While you can be sensitive to or agitated by literally anything, the Hangry B*tch Reset Diet will remove the biggest offenders. If you eat certain proteins every day (we're talking eggs for breakfast every day or chicken at almost every lunch), swap them out for other protein sources, even if you don't think they're causing major digestive issues, as a disrupted gut is prone to developing sensitivities to things you eat regularly. While sensitivity can happen with any food we eat routinely, such as nuts, veggies, and fruits, the reaction is to proteins within those foods. Thus the biggest offenders tend to be our go-to, eat-on-the-reg protein sources. Instead of trying to figure out what foods to avoid through trial and error, you can instead get food sensitivity testing done through Cyrex Labs (www.cyrexlabs.com, see Supplement and Testing Resources on page 382 for more info). This is absolutely the ONLY food testing we recommend, as the various other tests on the market, while less expensive, are highly inaccurate. If you choose not to do food sensitivity testing, you'll simply follow our plan and then systematically reintroduce foods when you're ready.

Next, this is the time to nurture your gut with some good nutrients and clean up your microbiome, meaning the bacteria that live in your intestines, and help your hormones and health. Here are the nutrients and supplements that can help:

Supplemental digestive enzymes can be life changing for women with low digestive enzyme output. Your supplement should contain a wide range of enzymes including protease, lipase, and amylase, as well as HCL (hydrochloric acid) and possibly ox bile. Take them with meals (we recommend taking them about five bites into a meal so that they aren't sitting on the top or bottom of your food). We suggest starting with a moderate amount of HCL, as you may have a delicate gut after years of disruption. Start with 200 mg and go up to 600 mg if needed. If you get any burning or discomfort, simply back off by at least 200 mg. If you find that even this low dose of HCL gives you issues, choose a digestive enzyme that doesn't contain any HCL.

Probiotics are the good guys, but these beneficial bacteria can cause an uptick in bloating if you have issues such as SIBO or significant dysbiosis (microbiome disruption), so we suggest during this initial phase of healing you switch to saccharomyces (a beneficial strain of yeast) for at least two weeks, then add probiotic products with *lactobaccillis* and *bifidobacterium* for another two to four weeks. Then, if tolerated, soil-based or spore forms of probiotics can be a good move (consider Prescript Assist or Megaspore). Note that these can be difficult for some to tolerate, so if you find that these don't work for you, opt instead for a more traditional probiotic with a variety of strains and at least 25 billion to 100 billion units per day and work with a functional medicine provider to get your gut bacteria in better balance.

Next up is repairing the lining of the intestines so that you have both less inflammation and less food reactions. L-glutamine is an amino acid that is fuel to your enterocytes (intestinal cells), helping them regrow and repair. Healing doses are in the range of 3–10 g two times per day for at least a month. Other helpful herbs include slippery elm (which contains soothing mucilage and stimulates your gut nervous system to secrete more mucus as well as helpful antioxidants), DGL (deglycyrrhizinated licorice, which also supports healing the stomach and intestinal lining), and marshmallow root (another mucilaginous herb that soothes an inflamed gut and protects the digestive tract lining). Bone broth and collagen supplements are also amazing gut healers, as are nutrients such as zinc and vitamin A. Typically all of these herbs and nutrients are used together in a combination formula, but if you choose just one, start with l-glutamine.

Finally, because the good guys have been out of balance, likely some bad guys (bacteria, yeast, parasites) have taken up residence. You can test to see what specifically may be lurking in your intestines through Genova Diagnostics Comprehensive Stool Analysis (www.gdx.net) or the GI Map test (www.diagnosticsolutionslab.com) or you can take a general approach and hit the most likely offenders such as candida, *H.Pylori,*

Blastocysitis homini, and *yersinia enterocolitica.* Antimicrobial herbs can be taken for four to six weeks with all of the supplemental support mentioned above and should be broad spectrum. You can include caprylic acid, berberine, artemsia (wormwood), bearberry, and black walnut. Certain infections such as SIBO and candida can be harder to clear, so if this regimen doesn't clear your symptoms we suggest you find a functional medicine doctor to help you get the rest of the way.

For our full gut-healing protocol and suggested products, see page 385 of the Supplement and Testing Resources, or visit www.sarahanddr brooke.com for more info.

From Grog to Greek Goddess

When you take to Google and start checking out Paleo blogs, you'll notice that many of them are more suited to men. There are exceptions, of course, but when women try to use advice suited for a caveMAN, we are bound to run into some problems, as women have some specific considerations to make when they go Paleo. You need to think less loincloth-clad Grog and more ancient Greek goddess—and we're about to show you why.

While most of the hormones we'll help you dial in with this program are not unique to women, the interplay between them is highly intricate and nuanced for women as compared to men. Because of this reality, we need to approach the Paleo template for women a bit differently, and although our plan has its roots there, Paleo leaves some serious holes when it comes to women's hormones that this plan will shore up.

Women, Paleo, and Carb Confusion

Many women on a Paleo diet fall into the undercarbing camp, replacing their usual breads, pasta, and cereals with plenty of protein but not enough starchy carbs or even fruit. This practice can cause your energy to tank and can also ramp up cravings, as well as aggravate cortisol (and, by proxy, estrogen and progesterone) and hinder thyroid function. Signs that undercarbing is affecting you include an erratic menstrual cycle, worsening PMS, insomnia, fatigue, brain fog, and even weight gain. Talk about feeling like a Hangry B*tch.

Other women will fall in the opposite camp and simply swap out their old comfort foods with "replicas," like Paleo pancakes for breakfast made with bananas and almond meal and topped with maple syrup or treats chock full of honey or coconut sugar. These food choices end up putting some serious heat on their blood sugar and insulin. Still others simply overdo Paleo-friendly carbs like sweet potatoes, eating them with abandon because "they're Paleo," with those same consequences. Without understanding how their hormones respond to excess carbohydrates (whether gluten- and grain-free or not), women often find themselves gaining weight, see rising blood glucose numbers on test results, feel lower-energy, experience more cravings, and notice an increase in appetite. The Hangry B*tch Reset, however, will help you find your unique carb tolerance—the carb types and amounts that work best for you—and you will avoid this entire carb conundrum and start achieving Happy Babe status.

One final point of carb confusion, and something that is often overlooked when it comes to carbs, is how your hormones respond when those carbs come served with a lot of fat. A popular Paleo example might be a breakfast of bacon, eggs, and sweet potato hash cooked in ghee or duck fat. However, this is not just a Paleo problem—it can be any high-fat and high-carb combo, like a doughnut, cheesecake, steak frites, a cheeseburger and a big thick bun (gluten-free or not!), or pizza with sausage and cheese. The issue is the exaggerated insulin response that can happen when we eat carbs and fat together. Yes, you read that right: our supposed hormonally neutral dietary fat actually has some insulin-triggering effects, especially when combined with carbohydrates. This combo can worsen insulin-resistance issues, increase your appetite and cravings, and set in motion a cascade of hormonal events that trigger fat storage and hinder fat burning. Thankfully, we've got that covered! You'll become more aware of your specific hormonal issues by taking our quiz, you'll be able to check in on how your hormones respond in real time to what you eat and how you exercise with your ACES, you'll find your unique carb tolerance, and you'll learn exactly what you can do to optimize functioning of all of your hormones.

Fat Frenzy Free-for-All

It might sound like we hate dietary fat, but we don't—not at all! It's key to the absorption of fat-soluble vitamins and it makes food taste better! We are not advocating a low-fat diet, but there are a couple of issues with dietary fat as it relates to hormones that we need to address (even though our advice may ruffle the feathers of a few of our pro-Paleo colleagues). It's easy to eat excess fat on a Paleo diet, and the consequences can be a much bigger deal than a few extra calories.

The primary issue is something called persistent organic pollutants, or POPs. These chemical by-products, such as pesticides, plastic residues, and various chemical solvents, are lipophilic, or fat-soluble, so they build up in our own body fat and the fat of the animals we eat. These endocrine-disrupting (or hormone-whacking-out) chemicals are in our air and our water, on our produce, and, yes, in our meat. Organic products and grass-fed and free-range animal products contain lower levels, but these little buggers are incredibly ubiquitous. Even the healthiest meats (from animals not treated with antibiotics or hormones) are still subject to environmental exposure, and the fat in them can bring a big POP load. And of course that load is bigger when we eat a lot of animal fat—again, as the Paleo diet tends to advocate.

Our advice is not to avoid animal protein, because we believe it is key for a woman's metabolic balance. Nor do we recommend eliminating animal fat altogether or returning to the fat phobia so popular thirty-five years ago. What we are saying is that if this is all brand new to you, don't worry; we've made sure our plan is optimal for women's hormones. And if you have dabbled with Paleo and the skies didn't part with angels singing or if Paleo seemed to make any of your hormonal issues worse, this POPs issue may be why, as they can create issues for a woman's hormone balance via several different mechanisms.

Research has demonstrated that POPs can damage the beta cells of the pancreas, which makes our important hormone, insulin. With dysfunction in the beta cells, we are more at risk for elevated blood sugars, insulin resistance, and even type 2 diabetes. You'll soon learn a whole lot more about insulin resistance and hyperinsulinemia and how it may be playing into your increased appetite, low energy, sugar cravings, and weight gain, but for now know that heeding fat quality will help this important hormone.

POPs are known to decrease thyroid hormones via various routes, including decreasing thyroid hormone production in the gland itself, decreasing conversion of T4 into the active thyroid hormone T3, and increasing the breakdown of T3. Lack of thyroid hormone leaves us feeling brain-dead, tired, cold, constipated, and depressed and can cause hair loss, make losing weight difficult, and make finishing a workout—or even a walk—almost impossible.

Some POPs actually have estrogenic activity of their own and compete with our own estrogen for receptors, creating a wide range of estrogen and progesterone imbalances as well as estrogen dominance symptoms. Many women notice an improvement in PMS-related symptoms such as a heavier flow, cramping, and breast tenderness by simply taking the animal fat down a touch.

Finally, when we embark on a new diet, such as the Paleo diet, and lose some body fat, whatever POPs we have in our own body fat will get released from their safe storage into our bloodstream and wreak havoc again. Obviously, the more exposure we have from pesticides, our water supply, low-quality animal products, and plastics (which is inevitable in our modern world) to these POPs that are so resistant to breakdown, the more POPs we will have in our own body fat. So when they get dumped into our system as a result of our own fat loss, we can suffer those estrogen-related symptoms, feel sluggish in general, or have our fat loss plateau because of their thyroid and hormonal impact.

The other consideration is that a diet high in conventional red meat has been linked to estrogen-related conditions such as breast cancer and endometriosis. The correlation is likely at least partly due to the POP effect we just covered, but we also have to remember that even those grass-fed, non-antibiotic-and-hormone-treated cows have their own estrogen metabolism, some of which occurs in their own body fat, which we, of course, eat. A diet high in red meat also has a funky effect on our gut microbiome, causing higher levels of beta glucuronidase, which is made by bad gut bacteria. An excess of beta glucoronidase hinders our ability to metabolize estrogen and thus it can recirculate, leading to estrogen-dominant or estrogen-progesterone imbalance symptoms.

Paleo Is a Plant-Based Diet—Or at Least It Should Be

Vegetables—remember those? With all the anti-grain and pro-bacon talk that abounds in the Paleo-sphere we forget about veggies! We've both been guilty of looking back at a day full of adequate protein but only one little salad, and we know you can relate. It happens! But every single one of your hormones (but especially insulin and estrogen) will benefit in some way from a higher-vegetable diet with all its fiber, phytochemicals, and antioxidants. Because of this, The Hangry B*tch Reset recommends that you eat a pound of veggies a day. We want you to see mostly veggies when you look down at your hormonally balanced plate!

Calorie Overload

We are thankfully past the days of thinking of our bodies like a calculator, where the only thing that matters is calories in and calories out. Most of you now know that your metabolic math is more complex and what plays the bigger role in how you "burn" energy from your food is actually how effectively a calorie gets utilized, what hormones are triggered in the process, and what your existing hormonal balance is like. This will, however, be different; particularly what hormones get triggered, be it from a calorie that comes from a

Paleo Pop-Tart vs. a grass-fed steak, for example. Calories are not the end-all be-all of nutrition, but they do still matter and they can still add up. Although we're thrilled that strict calorie counting is no longer the only parameter to tend to anymore, years of dieting have still left us thinking of food as good or bad, on plan or off plan. With this philosophy of good food equals green light on calorie consumption, we frequently see women who are following a Paleo

The Evolution of Everyday Paleo

Hi, Sarah here! When I started the blog *Everyday Paleo* and wrote my first few books I was "all in." Thanks to a Paleo diet coupled with intense work-outs, I turned my health around quickly, shed a few pounds that were lingering after the birth of my third son, and was soon in the best shape of my life. Eating Paleo and exercising literally changed my life and it worked really, really well—until it didn't. Thanks to piling on the stress like the frenzied woman that I can be, and the hormonal changes inevitable with getting older, I found myself a few years after my Paleo switch to be an exhausted mess, and I realized that I needed to make some changes.

I have always been a veggie pusher but I loved loved LOVED my ani-mal fat. Can you say bacon and eggs for breakfast every single morning for six years straight, plus cooking in duck fat, beef tallow, and leftover bacon grease? Well, besides the exorbitant amount of stress I wasn't tending to, I was also dumping a good amount of POPs into my daily diet, and my estrogen started to talk to me in a big way. Especially after losing my mom to breast cancer, the last thing I wanted to see on my test results was an inability to detox excess estrogen. Thanks to working closely with the amazing Dr. Brooke and reeducating myself on what my female body really needed, I was able to turn my hormonal disarray around.

Yes, I still love bacon. Yes, I still think animal fat can be a part of every-one's healthy diet to some extent. But no, I don't think bathing in it, rub-bing it daily on your body as a lotion, or eating it at every single meal is the best idea for most women, myself included. As I continue to work with women around the globe, some who are Paleo diehards and some who aren't, I see women turn a corner when they adopt a more Mediterranean Paleo approach. I'm still grateful that Paleo exists, but the reality is that Paleo and Paleo alone doesn't work well for everyone, myself included.

diet consuming very high-calorie foods too frequently or just large quantities of food in general. Don't start panicking, the Hangry B*tch Reset Diet contains absolutely no calorie counting, but we see this scenario so often we had to point it out. Consider this: you're home from work after a long day; maybe the kids are going a little crazy and it's been too long since your last meal so you're downright hangry. While you're hurriedly prepping dinner, you munch on a handful of nuts and scarf a package of uncured turkey pepperoni. Then you eat your dinner in a rush—too quickly to catch any of your hormonal cues that you are getting full—unknowingly having already consumed a little over 700 calories worth of Paleo-friendly appetizers plus your whole plate of food. Yes, they all might have been "good food choices" but eaten-while-hangry-too-quickly "good food" can still wreak havoc on your hormones and simply add up.

What we've found from working with thousands of women collectively is that when your hormones are balanced and you follow your hormonal cues, counting calories is not necessary to maintain or to even lose weight. But when you forget the basics, are too rushed to be mindful while eating, and/or you adopt the mindset that foods are "good" or "bad" because they fit into a certain diet dogma or "unique approach" it's easy to overdo it, especially with foods that are higher in calories. This not only can bring with it some weight gain but also can be a stress on your insulin, which can quickly create other hormonal imbalances.

#hangrybitchfix

One of the most mentally freeing and hormonally liberating things you can do is to stop thinking of food as good or bad, friend or foe, on plan or off plan and instead as food that works for you or food that doesn't work for you. This eliminates the guilt you feel from eating something deemed bad, and makes it easier to eat more foods that work for you. As you recognize the connection to how food makes you feel and how your hormones behave, it lessens the emotional pull toward certain foods. This small but significant mental shift can change your entire relationship with food, especially those foods you feel you have no control over, and this mindset shift will help you become and stay a Happy Babe.

Finally, in the shift toward recognizing the importance of hormones involvement in metabolism after the last twenty years, some of us have forgotten that calories still do matter. It's easy for some women to just plain overshoot what they need in a day when consuming a high-fat diet. While fat is typically very satiating (which is one of its metabolic benefits), when hormone signals are deranged because of stress, sometimes that satiety signal isn't as clear and we can easily miss it.

So What Are We Talking About Here?

We are talking about harnessing the best of the Paleo diet by eating more whole foods and fewer processed ones, keeping sugar low, caffeine minimal (especially if you have adrenal issues), and alcohol intake reasonable (or avoiding it altogether if it hinders your sleep, throws off your estrogen balance, or causes weight gain). We want you to avoid eating too many or too few carbs and instead find your sweet spot—your own unique carb tolerance, or UCT. We are advocating eating a pound of organic veggies each day. We want you to opt for high-quality, humanely raised animal protein with as few contaminants as possible, keeping fattier cuts of meat to one or two times per week, especially if you have insulin, thyroid, or estrogen issues. Finally, we encourage you to keep your diet full of plant-based fats from coconuts, avocados, nuts, and olives, all the while honoring your unique female hormonal balance.

Aside from the coconut, this Paleo diet now looks a lot like the Mediterranean diet, doesn't it? As one of the most well-researched diets when it comes to cardiovascular health and lowering inflammation, the Mediterranean diet certainly gets a lot of things right. However, if you're thinking this means all-you-can-eat pasta, we do hold true to the Paleo philosophy that it's still wise to let the grains go, at least until you're better balanced and can see which of them, if any, do in fact work for you and your UCT.

What we can borrow from the Mediterranean diet is the emphasis on olive oil, leaner meats, and loads of phytonutrient-rich veggies, thus giving the Paleo diet a much-needed makeover. This makes our hormone-healing nutrition plan the perfect combo of the best of what low-inflammatory, hormone-happy-making eating has to offer. Not to mention beautiful and deliciously healthy—just like an ancient Greek goddess.

But Wow, Eating This Way Sounds like a Lot of Work

One of the most common complaints we hear when we preach the real food lifestyle is, "I don't have the time or energy to cook. Chop, dice, roast, sauté . . .

What Your Hangry B*tch Reset Diet Will Look Like

We have already established that we all need a customizable approach to nutrition, but without a guideline, how do you know where to begin? When hormones go haywire, they send you mixed messages, and who hasn't felt like their body is telling them to eat chocolate for breakfast? During Week 1 we'll give you a starting point and then help you tune in to what your hormones are actually telling you, as well as when they may be lying to you, so that you can discover the elusive "what works for you" magic.

To recap, the basic template of the Hangry B*tch Reset Diet is a Paleo-Mediterranean hybrid, with an emphasis on lean proteins, plenty of fibrous nutrient-dense veggies at every meal, and healthy fats from plant sources such as olives, avocados, and coconuts. During your first week on the reset you will tune up a few key metabolic hormones and step away from nutritional habits, like grazing all day or skipping meals, that may not be working for you. At the very least you'll give your metabolism a jolt in the right direction, as your metabolic set point tends to get stuck when you've been doing the same thing for a long time, be that intermittent fasting or small frequent meals. After Week 1 you'll be armed with your quiz results, and you will learn to adjust this template in various ways from carb type and amount, and how often to eat, etc., for your unique hormonal issues.

I'm tired just thinking about it!" We hear you. Please know you aren't alone, as most women feel this way, at least from time to time. Part of the foundation of this plan is mindset and how we do what we do, which is why meditation, mantras, and the Five Pillars are all such important parts of this book. Yes, we have some time-saving tips and favorite kitchen gadgets that make cooking easier, and we live in the real world with you so we know you can't possibly cook three times a day, which is why we offer recipes in this book that will easily and deliciously transition from dinner to breakfast and then on to lunch. That said, you *will* spend some time cooking! Rather than suffering through it, you can use this time as a meditation and an act of REAL self-care.

Meditation doesn't always have to look like sitting in the lotus position with your eyes closed. We can find a little place of peace even in the mundane, and decide to choose joy, acceptance, and connection even with day-to-day tasks like preparing meals.

First, set your intention. When you're shopping for or preparing food, reframe a negative thought such as "This is more than I can handle" or "I can't even cook" or "I don't have time for this crap" to something like "I choose to nourish my body with food that heals me and doesn't hurt me" or "I'm making these changes so I can live my bigger, better life." Or even something simple like, "Cooking is fun" or "I'm an awesome cook."

Once your intention or intentions have been set, take a few deep breaths and really start to focus on what you are doing with the perspective of connectivity and total presence. When you pick up a piece of fruit or a vegetable, for example, really notice it—the feel of it in your hand, the color, the shape, texture, and even the smell.

While you are preparing your meal, listen to the sound of the knife as it cuts through the food, notice how your hands work, see how the food looks spread out on your cutting board, hear the sizzle it makes in the pan, smell the aroma as it's cooking in your oven or slow cooker. In other words, get totally involved with what you are doing rather than letting a gazillion thoughts or distractions pull you away from the moment.

If you are feeling like everything is in total chaos and you really need to just feed yourself but life is spinning out of control, take three deep breaths in through your nose, and exhale out through your mouth. Decide that everything else can wait, because it can. There is never anything as urgent as caring

#hangrybitchfix

If the distractions around you include kiddos driving you crazy while you're trying to cook, the best way to handle the stress of keeping them busy while you're making a meal is to involve them in the process. This might mean a slight kitchen overhaul, setting them up with small cutting boards and their own bowls, or simply giving them age-appropriate things to do like setting the table or folding napkins. Kids love being a part of what you are doing, and when you decide to make it fun, they will decide to make it fun, too.

for yourself should be. You can turn on some music that you love or light a candle to set the mood if that helps, and just be with the task at hand. Decide that all you have to do right now is to simply be immersed in the process of making your own beautiful food. Even if it's a quick two-minute lettuce wrap, dive into the moment and enjoy the fact that you are creating food that will help you feel better and will give you the nourishment your body is craving.

You might find that shopping at your local farmers' market and getting to know your food producers helps you feel more connected and excited to prepare your food. You might decide that a subscription service that delivers organic veggies to your door is a worthwhile time-saving, stress-busting tactic that helps you feel good about the extra time you will now be spending in the kitchen. Look at different ways you can get more connected to your food source and we promise you'll start to appreciate the process as you continue to reframe and get present to why you are taking the time to feed yourself well.

Getting It Right with Exercise

Exercise—this subject one way or another has created a lot of confusion over the years, leaving us frustrated at best and hormonally wrecked at worst. Whether from self-inflicted beat-downs at the gym thanks to our Nasty B*tch voice or from following a myriad of advice that has driven our hormones haywire, exercise for women tends to be too much or too little and often punishing in spirit. So many of us have found ourselves working out for all the wrong reasons and have ignored our hearts or our hormones as they begged us to do it differently. If this describes you, it's not your fault: you've been sold a bill of goods that for a woman to have any worth she needs to be skinnier, smaller, or otherwise fit the expectation of what a woman's body "should" look like. This inevitably will drive us to do all the wrong things for our hormones and psyche when it comes to diet and exercise!

If your goal has been to lose weight you've likely been advised to "just go exercise more." If you've discovered high-intensity training and metabolic conditioning, you've probably been told that feeling like you want to puke by the time you leave the gym or that having arms so shaky you can barely steer your car out of the parking lot are signs that you did it right. On the other hand, if you've been diagnosed with adrenal issues, a low thyroid, or autoimmunity, you've probably been told the opposite: that you can only walk or do yoga and anything else will ruin you. Unfortunately, as well-meaning as they may be, these approaches are ALL wrong.

The Hangry B*tch Reset will turn all this bad advice on its head by showing you how the right style of training is actually an act of real self-love and the truest form of self-care. With our Five Pillars and this book's commitment to helping you quiet that nasty voice in your head, we'll be tackling the spirit in which we want you to exercise. If it's not a healthy relationship right now, we promise it will be by the time this program is over. How and why you exercise is as important as what you do in the gym—remember #nourishnotpunish—but your attitude isn't the only thing we need to fine-tune. Before we get into how we want you to exercise, let's address how you might be currently missing the mark and clear up some common confusion and myths around the big topics like cardio and lifting weights. Let's first talk about a few ways you might be getting things wrong with your current routine.

Forgoing Weights for the Stairmaster. If you were around forty years ago, you remember the aerobics craze. It was all the exercise we thought we needed. As of late, many fitness gurus have flat-out said cardio will kill you. The truth is somewhere in the middle, especially for women with weak adrenals or low thyroid function. Cardio is not something to be scared of, just something that shouldn't be overdone. Cardio is also not the only form of exercise you need by any stretch of the imagination; in fact, that forty minutes of steady state cardio on a machine at your gym should be on the bottom of your exercise to-do list in our opinion, especially if you're struggling with cortisol or thyroid balance. Steady state cardio or fat-blasting sprints may or may not have a place in your exercise routine, and in Week 3 of the program we will help you determine what form of cardio is right for you. For now, we're encouraging walking as your only cardio. As part of our Five Habits, which you will soon be very familiar with, we want you to walk at a leisurely pace, outside if possible, for forty-five to sixty minutes at least five times per week.

Not Getting Your Lean, Longevity Hormones in the Game with Heavier Weights. From our experience, many women typically avoid lifting heavy weights because of one of the following three reasons: they are afraid of getting injured, they are concerned they might bulk up, or they follow popular strength training programs that have them convinced they should be lifting tiny pink dumbbells or only using resistance bands to achieve a "lean body." If you step back and think about it, your purse, your bag of groceries, and definitely your toddler are all heavier than a set of five-pound dumbbells. Our program will show you how to lift enough weight to trigger the hormones you're after, gain strength to help you in your day-to-day life, and stay safe while doing it. We will also address the fear of bulking up, which is harder to do than it seems and can be avoided by adjusting your diet to tap into fat loss.

Overdoing It Entirely. Many women are really just overdoing it in life and then follow it up by also overdoing it in the gym. Although the kind of stress that is produced with exercise is beneficial, too much stress in the gym can be very detrimental over time. The truth of the matter is, your body might not be able to handle the huge amount of stress piled on by spin classes, CrossFit, or other super intense styles of training. It's possible to tolerate this higher-volume or higher-intensity training for a while and even be addicted to the adrenaline rush that follows a crazy-hard workout, but if you picked up this book, we know one of two things: your exercise efforts are no longer giving you the results you want OR you are feeling so crappy that you know something's gotta give. Still, if you love to exercise, we know how hard it is to step away from this style of training. You may worry what will happen to your strength, ability, mental state, or body composition if you cut back. Well, if it was working, we'd be all for it! We know that intense training sessions are indeed more effective at torching body fat, but if your hormonal system can't handle what you are dishing out, you won't be getting those promised results. And when it becomes too stressful, your hormone balance and your health start to fall apart—from your period to your gut health to your sleep, it all begins to unravel. You can also overdo it with lower-intensity exercises such as long-distance cardio like running or distance cycling, which trigger stress hormones but not the fat-burning, advantageous hormones (like growth hormone and testosterone). Because of this women who do this type of exercise typically don't get optimal results with losing fat, building lean muscle, or optimizing hormonal health.

To determine whether you are overtraining, look for these four warning signs, which have the acronym **RAMP**:

Reluctance to train: You start to feel overwhelmed or otherwise upset when you think about your next workout because you are struggling to get through your workouts and/or are unable to recover from them.

Achiness or extreme soreness: Your joints ache and your muscles or tendons feel overly sore, even when you take a day or two off from training.

Moodiness: You experience an increase in anxiety or depression.

Puffiness: Your face, hands, feet, or belly are swollen or puffy; this is a sure sign of inflammation. Other signs include getting sick more frequently or chronic or increased rate of injury.

Clearing Up Cardio Confusion

Traditional forms of cardio, like jogging, biking, or working on a cardio machine for thirty to forty-five minutes, offer some clear benefits such as exercising your heart and lungs, boosting serotonin and thus your mood, and burning some fat while you are exercising. The downside is that traditional cardio doesn't tend to continue burning fat after your workout is over. It also triggers cortisol but will not trigger your lean, rejuvenating hormones like growth hormone.

On the other hand, more intense cardio such as sprint work and high-intensity intervals (bursts of intense exercise no longer than sixty seconds followed by a short period of rest and repeated for a session of no more than ten to twenty minutes total) can be great for fat loss. Also in the same camp as these short cardio sessions would be higher-intensity strength training or metabolic conditioning done while using weights, performed in the same short-duration fashion. This type of metabolic conditioning also gets the heart rate up and will produce some of the same benefits of heavy lifting but with the perks of high-intensity cardio. Unlike longer-duration (i.e., "more traditional" cardio), these shorter intense workouts trigger growth hormone and testosterone as well as cortisol, and they produce similar effects to weight training in general.

High-intensity intervals and sprint work also create a great after-burn effect, where you can burn more calories throughout the day (especially if you eat the right diet). Many people also find these sessions fun and less boring than other forms of cardio, and because they are short, they save time as well.

Although high-intensity interval training has some huge advantages over traditional cardio, it's important to understand that this style of training can often turn into too much of a good thing. Many women who have adopted this kind of training find that it initially provides great results but eventually leaves them feeling run-down and achy; sleeping worse; and experiencing lowered mood, increased anxiety, and cravings that are all over the map. The takeaway is that if this type of workout is no longer giving you the same results it once did, then it's a sure sign you're overdoing it.

As you can now see, cardio has many faces, from slogging it out on a cardio machine, running a 5K race, or taking an hourlong boot camp, spin, or CrossFit class to doing quick bursts of activity like sprinting or a metabolic weight-training session. However, it's also one of the quickest ways we can wreak havoc on our hormones when we overdo it. While short burst and metabolic conditioning save time and offer hormonal perks when it comes to fat loss, many women are dealing with hormonal issues that make this type of training not only less effective than it looks on paper but also prone to promoting further hormonal and metabolic disarray. Exercise is a stress, no doubt, so the more stressed you already are and the more hormone issues you have, the more sensitive you'll be to that stress. And in order to harness the power of exercise for healing your metabolism, you need to be strategic about exactly what stressors you place on your physiology.

Cardio and metabolic training is the first thing we're going to pull back on in the Hangry B*tch Reset, but that doesn't necessarily mean you have to pull back from it forever. If you want, you can return to this style of training when you're more able to reap its benefits.

What we really want to drive home here is that cardio isn't the be-all and end-all of exercise and yet it's not going to kill you, either. Training the cardiovascular system is important, but it's even more important to understand from a hormonal perspective how to tweak your cardio sessions to work for you and not against you. In the end, maybe that will be a mix of traditional cardio and sprint work or maybe you'll simply incorporate some cardio into your strength training sessions, and hopefully it's in a way that gets you results, keeps your hormones happy, and includes activities you love doing. We don't expect after reading this section on cardio that you'll know what exactly YOUR body needs right now as far as cardio is concerned. However, we hope we cleared up the confusion and helped you opt out of glorifying or vilifying it and that you are clear on what's coming with your plan. There will be weights, walking, and, if necessary or desired, a cardio plan that's perfect for you.

Laying to Rest the Fears of Lifting Heavy

Strength training is when you put a demand on your body that causes it to adapt. If you are under heavy load, your body will have to figure out how to sustain the environment you are in by adapting to the exercise by putting on muscle mass. As we age and our hormones change, our metabolism starts to slow down. As estrogen and progesterone drop (which can start as early as thirty and certainly by age thirty-five), we become better at storing fat but worse at maintaining muscle mass and more sensitive to all stressors. This has a host of unfortunate side effects including weaker bones, more body fat (especially around the middle), more inflammation, and muscle loss. This is not a great combo by any means. Luckily, heavier strength training slows this all down. With all that magic mojo, why are women wary of weights?

Many women have a kneejerk fear of getting bigger if they lift more than a few pounds. This is one of the most common ideas about strength training, but we assure you it's more myth than reality. While you will put on some muscle with this program, remember that it's calorie-burning, hormone-magic-making muscle. Most women actually struggle to put on muscle mass in any significant amount; it truly is much harder to look like a ripped bodybuilder than you imagine! We are in awe of the amount of work competitive female bodybuilders are required to do. When you see a female bodybuilder, know that her muscles are the result of a meticulous diet and hours upon hours of time spent daily in the gym—this doesn't accidentally happen to everyday exercisers. What many women do experience when they first start lifting heavier is that they lay down some muscle under their body fat and they see themselves get a bit bigger at first. This is where the panic sets in! But we assure you this is more of an issue with not yet figuring out your diet and sorting your hormones to shed some body fat; you're not gaining massive amounts of muscle. We will talk about this more in the program so you'll know exactly what to do to optimize fat loss if you want to. We're confident that you'll feel a lot better and hope that you'll embrace this slight shift in your body composition.

The exception to this is women with insulin resistance: they really do put on muscle more easily. They also put on body fat more easily and have a more difficult time taking it off. You'll know if you're in this group when you take the quiz in chapter 7 and we'll help you get the results you want throughout this program and improve your insulin sensitivity. One thing is for sure: it is absolutely vital to lift weights for you to have that nice amount of lean muscle. Muscle is your depot for excess glucose, which you struggle with if you have insulin issues, so a little bit more muscle will be key to resolving your insulin issues, maintaining a healthy body composition, lowering inflammation, and preventing diabetes.

Another fear associated with lifting heavy weights is getting hurt, and this is a legitimate fear—if you don't have proper instruction. This book will clearly show you the right technique for safe lifting, and you can find video instruction at www.sarahanddrbrooke.com. Perhaps the most important thing to know besides proper form is that "heavy" is completely relative. For some women, heavy means simply their body weight; for others, a barbell with a few plates is heavy. What we mean by "heavy" is that it needs to be challenging for you based on your current level of fitness, and we will guide you so you know what that level is.

You'll be amazed at your progression and the myriad benefits associated with a legitimate strength training program.

So put out of your mind that strength training means tiny weights with high reps, and remember you have to pick up things that are heavy every single day: kids, groceries, pets, laundry, suitcases, and the list goes on and on. You need to be strong and you need to know how to gain that strength in a smart and safe way. The last thing you want to do is injure yourself by simply living your life, so learning proper technique in the gym and adapting that technique to your daily environment is not only empowering but also essential!

We can't tell you how many times women have told us how amazing it feels to be strong and capable in their own bodies and how many women have overcome feelings of powerlessness, fear, and inadequacy simply by implementing a program of heavy lifting. We are obviously big fans of strength training for all its benefits, both mental and metabolic. It is truly awesome, and even if it's scary and maybe right now doesn't sound like a lot of fun, you can't ignore the scientifically proven benefits of incorporating strength training into your life. We promise, the effects it will have on your hormones will override any of your concerns and you will grow to crave it—and that's the kind of craving we want you to have!

Hopefully we have cleared up some confusion and dispelled some common myths when it comes to exercise, but there are still a couple more areas of concern to highlight, and it's mostly all about mindset.

The reality is that exercise, particularly lifting weights, is so important to our hormonal health and longevity that we have to find a way to do it—but, most important we need to do it right, and for the right reasons. When we're not doing enough exercise, either because we're too busy, we hate the gym, we don't know what to do when we get there, or we're just too tired to even consider it, we aren't creating a favorable environment for fat loss, longevity, or health.

Let's start by addressing the problem of not having enough time. Look, we totally hear you, and unfortunately this program does not create more than twenty-four hours in a day. (We're working on that, so stay tuned. . . .) However, beginning to live the Five Pillars will create less stress, more ease, and thus more space and time for you to get in the hormone- and health-helping exercise in this plan. We've also made our Hangry B*tch Fitness Plan both manageable and customizable, so that you can do just enough to get results, but not so much that you're wrecking yourself or wasting your time. We also prioritize what will give you the most bang for your buck: lifting weights and walking.

What's that? You don't like the gym or lifting weights? We wish there was a "get out of the gym free" card, but when it comes to being capable now and as you age—normalizing hormones and lowering inflammation, not to mention achieving a healthy body—you need to exercise. More specifically: you need to lift weights. If you just can't fathom going to a gym, we will give you tips on how to outfit a home gym. You could also consider hiring a trainer, which is a great way to keep you accountable. (See How to Outfit a Home Gym, on page 309, and How to Interview a Personal Trainer, on page 312, for tips on setting up a home gym and on finding a trainer who will work with the templates we suggest for you based on your hormonal profile.) Bottom line is, you need to lift weights, and we will do everything in our power to make sure that you love it and give you the mindset tools to make your new habit stick!

Why It's All About Those Weights

One of the determining factors for being able to care for ourselves in our later years is being able to move independently. So if nothing else gets you lifting weights, focus on capability, strength, agility, and autonomy. You need to be strong enough, especially as you age, to get down on the floor and up again easily. A marker of declining health is when you get to the point where you can't get up or down from the floor without using your upper extremities for assistance, so holy guacamole, at the very least, let's be motivated to be strong enough to get ourselves up from a fall or up and down off the toilet as we age! Weight training is essential for living a long and healthy life, and it provides a ton of benefits along the way.

Strength training is also your way to a better metabolism. Guess what burns most of your calories? Muscle. Strength training will stimulate the release of lean hormones such as glucagon, anti-aging hormones like growth hormone, and immune regulators called myokines, which lower inflammation. However, in order to stimulate this anti-aging, anti-inflammatory, strengthening, lean-body-producing hormonal soup, you have to challenge the muscle. You have to create enough stress to trigger these hormones. This means you have to lift heavy—whatever heavy is for you.

This may mean squatting with a loaded bar across your back or it may mean squatting down to and back up out of a chair, but you might also be somewhere in the middle. The most important thing is to start at the appropriate place for your fitness level. We want you lifting weights safely and effectively. You might be ready to start lifting now or you might need a foundation laid first based on your abilities, limitations, and fitness level before you can employ all of our strength training suggestions. Either way, in time you'll be lifting and·triggering the magic hormone mix of body change and longevity without running yourself into the ground in the process.

Our approach to fitness and training is focused on healing your hormones and body first while incorporating strength training and conditioning at a level that is right for you. We want you to do the stuff you love but not at the expense of your health.

Not Your Average Fitness Plan

By now we are sure you're catching on that the Hangry B*tch Reset is decidedly NOT a one-size-fits-all workout and diet plan. You may be using our strength-training template by Week 3 or you might still be doing one of our base workouts. There are no extra points for finishing this program on time, and the most important thing is that you are taking the appropriate steps to get the promised benefits and to avoid injury. So, with that being said, where you are is exactly where you need to be.

Our Hangry B*tch Fitness Plan has three workout templates in total, but to begin with we're going to give you two of our templates to choose from as a starting point. If you have a bad back, neck, or hips, or are postpartum and have not healed your core and pelvic floor, you'll start with our HB Core+ Floor Recovery Template. If you are not injured but haven't been training regularly OR have been only doing high-intensity or metabolic conditioning, you'll do the HB Hormone Reset Template for two weeks and then we'll introduce you to our third workout: the totally customizable HB Strength Training Template that you'll adjust based on your hormones. You'll get all this in Week 1 and Week 3 of the program. For now, know that your hormone fairy godmothers (that's us!) will be delivering the perfect exercise plan designed just for you!

There are infinite ways to exercise, but for difficult fat loss and hormonal trouble, we've found the Hangry B*tch Fitness Plan to be the most effective. Our three workouts within the plan honor the best about metabolic training, work multiple energy systems within a muscle cell to avoid overtraining, work with rather than against your hormones, and avoid the bad stress that so easily occurs with weak adrenals, autoimmunity (such as Hashimoto's disease), and hypothyroidism.

Weights and Walking: The Hormone Happy Makers

We've sold you on weights by this point—we hope! But what about walking? Like many women, you may be wondering, "Isn't it just, well, too easy?"

Take a minute and look down. We all got 'em: two legs that move us around from place to place all day, every day. Unfortunately, we don't use our amaz-

Exercising Post-Pregnancy

If you have been pregnant, even if it's been a long time since you've had a baby, we can almost guarantee that you need to do some sort of rehab to heal your pelvic floor and your core. The pelvic floor is a group of involuntary and voluntary stabilizing muscles that do things like keep us from peeing when we are jumping, walking, or running. When we are pregnant and then give birth, these muscles have to do a lot of moving, stretching, and sometimes even tearing.

Unfortunately, in the United States we do not routinely recommend women get adequate physical therapy or rehab after giving birth. If we were exercisers before becoming pregnant, we typically dive back into the gym doing heavy squats, jumping rope, or running and resign ourselves to pee leaks as "normal." We may even ignore the discomfort of a prolapse or work around the weakening of our abdominal wall due to the ever-so-common diastasis recti (abdominal muscle separation).

This post-partum neglect of women's core and pelvic floor healing is almost criminal because these issues do not resolve on their own. And although strength training is awesome, we also need to incorporate specific rehab and physical therapy to heal, strengthen, and repair our precious pelvic floors and cores. This is why, even after you get through your minimum three weeks of core and floor work, you'll continue to see most of these exercises in your warm up. Do not ignore our plea for proper pelvic position during your lifts as well because, believe it or not, even women who have not had babies often experience pelvic floor dysfunction later in life (or even earlier in life) because we neglect to strengthen this area! This is important work, so please don't skip it; your floor and core will thank you. We promise.

ing legs like we used to and often we end up sitting for long periods of time in unnatural positions that lead to a lot of unfortunate consequences. Research now correlates too much sitting with some similarly horrific consequences as smoking, hence the phrase "sitting is the new smoking." Here's the deal: from an evolutionary and scientific standpoint, we are intended to walk, a lot. We are bipeds, as in meant to move on two feet, but our modern lifestyle and even our gyms with their plethora of machines have us not doing nearly enough bipedal movement.

Walking is a movement that our bodies understand. It's low-impact, easy to do, and, like everything else we prescribe in this book, something that will make your hormones happy, no matter where you are in your health journey. Basically, walking is an amazing habit when it comes to regulating cortisol; it is helpful whether you're crazy from high stress or burned the heck out. Unless you are extremely frail, you should be able to do our recommended forty-five-to-sixty-minute walks five times a week once you get to Week 1. If it's not something you can tolerate right now, we'll also show you how to adjust that recommendation.

But still you may be wondering if it's really that important to just walk. We know that spending an hour in the gym doesn't undo the negative hormonal and metabolic consequences of sitting all day. The simple truth is that we have to make a conscious effort to get up often throughout the day and move around, as well as make time to walk, and walk often, in order to keep our hormones happy.

Research done with patients that have high inflammation who started walking regularly throughout the day—you guessed it—shows that they improved all markers of health and lowered inflammation. Walking is so important that even if it's the only habit you take away from this book, your hormones would be happier and healthier from this one simple activity so we just can't stress it enough! We will offer strategies to make walking something you look forward to and, just like with strength training, once you start, you'll feel so much better that you just won't want to stop!

What About ALL Those Other Types of Exercise?

Coming along with us on this plan may mean giving up your favorite boot camp, Zumba, or spin class and that may feel really scary for you! But please trust us that the Hangry B*tch Fitness Plan is the full-meal deal; we've got you covered from the weights to the walks and everything in between. Yet, we know that some of you have a favorite form of exercise and that you are getting sweaty palms right now thinking of giving it up. We hear you . . . but here's the deal: you need to heal, and we know you are tired of not getting results.

Certain activities are going to drive hormonal derangement in a way that won't allow healing. We can understand and have empathy for you missing your spin class, but we can't change the physiology of the situation. Within the four-week reset, we'll guide you through which exercises you can do in addition—not in place of—the Hangry B*tch Fitness Plan, which ones you may have to let go of for now, and how to keep some of them in at a lower volume. This will be a fitness plan that feels just right and totally doable for you, even if you've never stepped foot into a gym. You'll have the exact tools, resources, and guidance you need, and the resulting confidence to know you're doing the right thing for your hormones and health.

What Do I Do If Walking Is Not an Option?

Restorative movement such as walking is important, but we understand that walking simply might not be possible for you due to mobility issues, injury, safety, or weather. If that's the case, there are still options for you to get in some of this healing, Happy Babe–making movement. We are huge fans of restorative yoga, which is much different than other yoga classes. Restorative yoga places an emphasis on being in a pose that is not challenging, grueling, or strenuous but is more focused on proper breathing and position. Each pose is intended to relax the body and re-lease tension, and you're encouraged to rest and find a comfortable po-sition versus pushing past what feels good. It's just enough movement to yield some of the same benefits as a gentle stroll and it's easily modified for those whose mobility is compromised.

Another fantastic option is swimming—not swimming laps as a long-duration cardio exercise, but swimming at a level similar to walking, with the added buffer from impact thanks to the water. Gently swimming for thirty-plus minutes at a pace that won't make you out of breath while doing so is a wonderful restorative movement when you are unable to walk.

Finally, if you can't walk outside due to safety or bad weather, opt for an indoor treadmill, if possible.

First, though, we have one more overlooked part of exercise, and that's breathing. If you thought the walking came out of left field, then you probably haven't read about, talked about, or heard anyone sing the praises of proper breathing. That's about to change—and set a much-needed foundation for your training and stress reduction.

Better Breathing and Better Posture

Two things that many people overlook when it comes to exercise and move-ment are breathing along with rib and pelvic position. Rib position, what the??!! Who knew that was so important? Well it is! We will teach you how to practice key positioning and breath work before, during, and after your workouts.

Several factors including pregnancy, sitting too long, or not handling our stress will result in poor posture for most of us. We tend to hold tension in our upper back, which in turn causes us to elevate our shoulders and hold them tensely and tightly up around our ears. From prolonged sitting, pregnancy, or even wearing high heels, our ribs tend to be flared from lower back hyperexten-sion, and thus we walk around with an exaggerated anterior pelvic tilt (where your back is arched and your abdomen is protruded).

As for breathing, we tend to be "mouth breathers," constantly taking shal-low breaths through our mouths and into only our upper lungs as if we are in a state of panic—never fully taking advantage of the great gift of oxygen and further increasing neck and upper back tension. On top of this, many of us are borderline or overtly deficient in oxygen-delivering nutrients like iron and B12. We're hungry for this super nutrient—and it's free and always available! Forget turmeric and chia seeds: oxygen is your super food!

Poor posture combined with shallow breathing is a recipe for mobility is-sues in our lower and upper back as well as in our shoulders—not to mention hip flexors and hamstrings. It also results in a core that lacks proper stabil-ity. Getting posture and breathing on track is important to keep you safe and injury-free for progressing to heavier weights and more advanced exercises in the gym as well as for picking up things in your everyday life.

We will teach you how to incorporate specific breathing techniques into your warm ups to bring you into better alignment before you lift. These tech-niques will activate and strengthen your core prior to putting your body under load, enabling you to bring your lower ribs into the "down position," creating a neutral spine and a more natural and safe postural position. These techniques will also help you open your upper thoracic spine, release your shoulders from your ears, and bring your awareness to where you SHOULD be breathing.

We will also show you how to breathe and brace during your lifts to create your own "weight lifting belt" so that you can decrease your chance of injury and lift heavier weights without compromising position or technique. Finally, before you leave the gym or weight room, your program will include restorative breathing techniques (like a mini meditation) that will bring you back to baseline, ready to reenter the world in a calmer and happier state.

Be a Happy Babe in the Gym

There will be no more punishing workouts. No more slogging it out in the gym, hating your body. No more time looking in the mirrors that abound at every fitness facility, criticizing your thighs or triceps or that little bubble of flesh almost all of us have to some degree between our armpit and breasts especially after we shove them into a bra. No more heading to the gym because you're "not enough," "not lovable," or other such unkind motivations. Walking is an act of real self-care, gaining strength is a true act of self-love, and everything we teach you in this book is about being more of the *you* that's already more than enough.

The Five Pillars, the meditations, and the mantras will all help you quiet that critical voice in your head and we think the following tenets are more supportive than your best sports bra:

- You can want more for yourself or work toward a body you feel more at home in without hating the one you have now. We call this acceptance without resignation.

#hangrybitchfix

The gym environment can be ripe for triggering negative self-talk and body image struggles, as often our whole purpose of working out is to fix our feelings of inadequacy. This motivation is not only ineffective but also causes us to do crazy crap like aggressive workouts we're not ready for physically or hormonally, which make us miserable at the gym. This is particularly the case when exercise is part of a fat-loss goal, but there is a way to do it right. Happy Babes go to the gym because of self-love, not self-loathing, and our perspective around our why in the weight room matters way more than making sure our workout plan is perfect. #nourishnotpunish

- You can respect your body without being 100 percent happy with how it looks to you. This is neutral; it lives between feeling great about your body and feeling terrible. Appreciate what your body can do as you start to appreciate how it looks as well.

- You can exercise as an act of self-love instead of self-loathing.

- You can focus on strength over fat loss—or let it at least be an added bonus.

- You can decide if you want to lose a single pound *or not*. Weight loss is a choice for a woman, not a mandate.

- Regardless of where you are with your health, fitness, or body composition, you are absolutely worthy of love, respect, and kindness just as you are right now.

You're Ready to Rock!

OK, you have gotten the big (very big) picture about stress and your hormones; you've been given the secret hormone decoder ring we call ACES and can now listen up when your hormones are talking to you; we've shown you the overview of how you'll be eating and exercising on the four-week reset (and beyond!); you've begun implementing the Five Pillars; and now we are ready to get this hormone-balancing party started! In the next chapter you'll begin the Hangry B*tch Reset and start to synthesize all of the elements that we've taught you, as well as customize this entire program for your unique issues. We know that can feel a little daunting, and you may be wondering how you'll know if it's working.

There are several ways to measure progress with this plan: fat loss, ACES in balance (normal appetite, minimal or managed cravings, consistent energy, great sleep), improved lab test results, or more "no" answers on our Hangry B*tch Hormone Quiz (you'll take that during Week 1). Assessing your level of joy or how much you are living by the Five Pillars can seem a bit more difficult, which is why we've got a tool that you can use daily (or at least weekly) to check in and see how you're faring, called the Hangry B*tch Scale. If you score less than 5, you are doing great and all this stress management, perspective shifting, and mindset choosing is working as you start to feel more consistently like a Happy Babe. If you score above 5, well, you still probably feel a bit like a Hangry B*tch. No worries though, because every tool you need is here in this book, so if you have a high score today, you can lower it as soon as tomorrow.

Simply recommit to practicing the tools in this book and trust that, no matter how you feel right now, the very next moment is a chance to feel better.

The Hangry B*tch Scale

Score yourself from 0 to 3 on each item below, 0 meaning you are 100 percent rocking it in this area and 3 meaning it's a disaster. Aim each day to keep your Hangry B*tch score less than 5. If your score is less than 5 you know your hormones are happy, your mindset is right, and you are engaging in REAL self-care (i.e., living by the Five Pillars). If your score is over 5, assess each area and use the tools we've given you thus far (and know that every week we'll give you more tools) to feel better!

ACES Are Balanced. Your appetite is not too high or low, your cravings are minimal and well managed, your energy is even and adequate, it's easy for you to fall asleep and stay asleep.

Tolerating Exercise Well, Not Under- or Overtraining. You are not feeling that energy is depleted after exercise or showing any signs of RAMP (reluctance to train, aches and soreness, moodiness, and puffiness; see page 83).

Feeling Positive and Peaceful Overall. You are using meditation and mantras, choosing a positive perspective more often than not (listening to best friend voice), experiencing little to no stress, anxiety, and overwhelm.

Able to Stay Present in Your Life. You are using meditation, mantras, and third pillar tools for full-engagement living, and you are feeling little to no distraction from the present moment.

Being Who You Are. You are confidently speaking your truth, engaging in activities solely because they bring you joy and help you feel more like yourself.

#hangrybitchfix

Know that you are as worthy of love and happiness if you score a fifteen or a two. But also know that frequent check-ins will help you get the results you want from this program and will keep you taking those small steps toward better health, happier hormones, more energy, and more moments of pure joy.

PART TWO

The Four-Week Hangry B*tch Reset

- Heal Your Hormones
- Hone Your Joy

and

- Find What Works for YOU

Week 1

The Hangry B*tch Reset

Time for the nitty-gritty. Your mindset is primed, your self-care flame is fanned, and you're ready to get started with the Hangry B*tch Reset. This is very exciting because the first week of your four-week journey truly kicks off the rest of your life! Remember, although this is a four-week plan, it does not by any means end in a month. The tools you'll learn in this plan along with learning to tune in to your hormone talk will serve you for the rest of your life, no matter what comes your way—high stress, a new diagnosis, pregnancy, perimenopause, or anything else. Right now, what's most important is that this plan will take you from feeling like a Hangry B*tch to a well-rested, less-stressed, digestion-humming-like-a-dream, hormonally balanced Happy Babe.

This first week is a recalibration: an opportunity to speed up if you're going too slow or to slow down if you're going too fast. Wherever you might be, you will land in the middle this week as you hit the hormonal reset button and bring an end to over- or underdoing it with food, stress, rest, and exercise.

Think of this week as laying the foundation for what's next: customizing the plan for your unique hormonal issues. For one week you will follow our Five Habits template exactly as is. This template uses a super simple "5-4-3-2-1" framework to help make your initial diet, exercise, and lifestyle changes manageable. At the end of the week (or the end of this chapter), you'll take a quiz that will help you determine how to customize the Five Habits specifically for your unique issues in the weeks to come.

Most diets are focused on a specific goal, such as lowering cholesterol or losing body fat. The goal of our plan is to make your hormones super-duper happy, and since those other goals are typically the by-product of happy hormones it will be a win-win no matter what you bring to the table. Unfortunately, many diets sacrifice hormonal balance and health for their end goal. As you have likely experienced, when we mess up our hormones for the sake of weight loss or a short-term fix, not only is it impossible to stick with whatever plan you might be on at the moment, but the next plan gets harder to follow and is usually less effective as well. What you will hear us preach from the mountaintops is that no diet or exercise plan, and especially no weight-loss plan, should ever sacrifice hormonal balance and health. It's just plain not worth it.

Before we get to the Five Habits, it's important to remember that your hormones will dictate the exact tweaks you'll be making to our template in the upcoming weeks. How do you know if your hormones are happy? Lab tests are of course super helpful, but there are a couple of challenges with this approach. First, you have to get them from a provider, which can take days to weeks, and certain hormones need to be checked on certain days. For example, your progesterone should be tested on day 19 of your menstrual cycle, so you may have to wait a month for the right day to test.

Second, not all lab tests are created equal. Take your stress hormone cortisol for example—standard tests typically only measure morning cortisol, which is inadequate for assessing the normal timed output of cortisol that should actually be checked four times throughout the day. Furthermore, much of the testing in the conventional medical model is great for ruling out major pathology like kidney failure, discovering an infection, or giving a clear diagnosis such as diabetes, but most providers typically dismiss the borderline test results because they are not pathological, but this does not mean your results are optimal. Everything in the middle unfortunately gets overlooked because there's no overt disease present even though you may be feeling downright terrible.

Finally, modern medicine also tends to be too myopic in evaluating the intricate web of female hormone issues. If hypothyroidism is diagnosed, your doctor may start thyroid medication without also evaluating your immune system (that is, checking for Hashimoto's disease, the autoimmune cause of upwards of 90 percent of cases of low thyroid function in the Western world), the impact of stress on the thyroid, and the interplay of estrogen and testosterone on free, active thyroid hormone levels. When we miss the landscape as a whole by focusing on just one hormone in our complicated system, we miss feeling as good as we possibly can, getting the results we want, and lowering our risk for disease.

Testing is a great tool when used properly, so if you go that route make sure you are getting the full scope of information that you need by working with a provider who can help you utilize it. You can get any manner of tests, from hormones to DNA, directly from the internet, but remember the information you get from these tests will only be as good as the interpretation of it. For a great guide to lab testing, visit www.sarahanddrbrooke.com/lab-guide or see the Supplement and Testing Resources on page 382 for more info.

Before you run out for a lab test, what if you could learn today, in real time, how your hormones are doing? We have a secret to tell you . . . your hormones are talking to you right now, and we want to apologize that no one has ever taught you how to listen. That's about to change, as it's high time you start to tune in to your hormone talk so you can start to uncover the elusive "what works for you." Your hormones speak to you via signals such as your appetite (what you want to eat and when you're hungry), your energy level, and your sleep pattern. When you understand what these signals mean and how you can adjust to them in real time, you'll be more empowered to take control of your health than ever before. Many of these signals are driven largely by insulin and cortisol, which are among your most important (and easiest to control) metabolic hormones, but other hormones such as estrogen and thyroid send you signals as well.

The fact that your body is actually talking to you may sound almost like science fiction. However, it is more straightforward than you think, and using the acronym ACES, as well as tools like a glucometer, will help you tune right in.

ACES—Listen Up, These Are Your Hormones Talking

The ACES acronym we introduced in chapter 1 is the window into your hormone balance. It stands for appetite, cravings, energy, and sleep and tells you in real time what you can do differently to feel better and get better results. For this week you will simply tune in to your ACES and get clear on the signals your hormones are sending, both immediately after eating and then in the span between meals. During Week 2, after you've taken the Hangry B*tch Hormone Quiz on pages 128–32, chapter 7, you will learn what adjustments to make to balance your ACES, starting with digging into which carbs work for you, which ones don't, when they work best, and how much you need or don't need. During Week 2, we will help you find your unique carb tolerance, or UCT, as well as a few other ACES-balancing tips.

Once you wrap up Week 1 of the Hangry B*tch Reset and are tuned in to your ACES, you will then adjust each of the elements of our Five Habits template. It's super simple and designed to keep your to-do list very short: walk, work out, drink water, eat good food, rest, be positive, and engage in real self-care. And it's all laid out in the easy-to-remember format of 5-4-3-2-1—to feel and look your best. This template also allows you to start where you are and then to customize it for your current hormonal state, as well as anytime down the line when your ACES or lab testing indicate your plan is no longer working for you.

All right, let's dig in, because it's reset time.

The Hangry B*tch to Happy Babe Five Habits

This week you'll follow the Five Habits as laid out below, and in the coming weeks you'll get to work on adjustments that will take you from hormone reset to customized hormone plan. Just think: **5-4-3-2-1**.

5 walks per week plus 5 minutes of breathing work per day

4 meals per day

3 strength training sessions per week

2 liters (or more) of water per day

1 daily commitment to rest, recovery, and real-self care

5-4-3-2-1 5 Walks per Week Plus 5 Minutes of Breathing Work per Day

Walk This Way

Walking is the great hormone normalizer. This low-grade cardio exercise is best thought of as restorative exercise—or movement our bodies were meant to do every day.

While we recommend you stand at least as much as you sit each day, we also encourage taking a walk five times per week for forty-five to sixty minutes. Even the most hormonally wiped-out women will usually be able to do this walking recommendation. However, if walking for forty-five to sixty minutes is too much for your body to handle, do your best to get five more minutes of walking than you're getting currently, and with subsequent walks continue to increase your time every couple of days or every week until you are able to walk the recommended forty-five to sixty minutes per day. If you experience increased achiness or fatigue as you add minutes, dial it back and walk less until you figure out your walking tolerance. Remember, it's OK to push yourself, just not to the point of pain or exhaustion. Your body will let you know if you are doing too much. Remember, this is not about pushing past your limits but restoring your hormones and health, so increase slowly and continue to check in with yourself.

Ideally you should walk outside for the added benefit of fresh air and some sunlight and vitamin D, but walking inside will do in a pinch. This is also a great time to work on your mindset and reduce stress; think of it as a moving meditation. While you are welcome to walk in silence, listen to a podcast (like ours!) or book on tape, or chat with a friend, this time can also be spent focused on your mantra, which we will be covering later in this chapter.

Five walks per week is often the absolute game changer when you're stuck in your progress with a tough hormonal issue like a low thyroid or PCOS and especially menopause. While it is a bit of a time commitment, we promise that in a week you'll be craving that long walk—really.

And to answer your next question: if splitting up your walking time—say walking twenty minutes now and twenty minutes later—is the best you can do, then do it. However, our recommendation for one steady walk of about an hour a day still stands. It's a profoundly effective part of your plan that ideally you'll do just as prescribed.

Just Breathe

We also recommend you do five minutes of breathing work daily, which can be easily incorporated after your walks. Restorative breathing helps you learn how to breathe deeply and tap into your parasympathetic nervous system. You will also practice restorative breathing after your workouts, which is a wonderful way to start tapping into a few minutes of zen after you move.

Here's how to practice restorative breathing: Lie down on your back with your feet up on a chair or bench so that your low back is supported. Place your arms down by your sides with your palms facing up for receiving or palms facing down if you feel like you need some grounding. Your shoulders should be pulled down away from your ears, letting any tension in your neck and shoulders go. If you can't keep your neck in neutral when lying on your back, it's OK to lay your head on a pillow. Close your eyes and let your tongue rest gently on the roof of your mouth. Start breathing deeply through your nostrils down into your belly using a slow count of 3–4 on the inhale; make sure you are sending that air down into your chest and belly, not up into your shoulders. After you inhale, exhale fully also through your nostrils to a count of 8–10. Do a set of 5–8 breaths or, even better, commit to staying put for at least five minutes. Make sure you breathe through your nostrils the entire time as this will train you to breathe more evenly throughout the day and through your nose rather than shallow breaths through your mouth that keep you in a constant state of fight or flight. Remember that amazing nutrient we mentioned in chapter 5, oxygen? If you start to feel out of breath or anxious from not breathing through your mouth, stop and take a few breaths in and out through your mouth and then return to nasal breathing. This is a learned exercise that can be quite challenging, but it's incredibly important. See www.sarahanddrbrooke.com for a video demonstration.

As a bonus, restorative breathing can truly be done anywhere. As you continue this practice post-walk and/or post-workout, you'll start to become more aware of when you are taking shallow breaths and "mouth breathing" throughout your day. You can tap into restorative breathing wherever you are. We love doing some nasal restorative breathing while walking, while driving, and when sitting at our computers. Do the same inhale and exhale as described, but of course if you are walking or driving, keep your eyes open!

5-4-3-2-1 4 Meals per Day

Welcome to the Hangry B*tch Reset Diet. You'll be eating four meals per day, all roughly the same size—with a focus on 25 g of protein per meal and plenty of veggies; shooting for one pound of vegetables per day, be sure to get some at every meal—yes, breakfast too! The reason we recommend four meals a day is because this is the best way to honor the biggest hormone issues you'll face when it comes to your hangry metabolism: insulin and cortisol.

As you jump on the Hangry B*tch Reset Diet, we know you are probably wondering about the carbs. In Week 2 we will help you find your own carbohydrate magic, but for this week as we help you reset, we want you to eat a moderate amount of our allowed starches/sugars for your carbs (e.g., sweet potatoes, squashes, fruit) to help you avoid either over- or undercarbing. With a couple of your meals each day, include ¼ to ⅓ cup or 4–6 bites of the recommended carbohydrates, and pay attention to how your body responds (i.e., the hormone messages of ACES: appetite, cravings, energy, and sleep).

You may find that this small amount of carbs a couple of times a day works remarkably well or you may find it to be too much or too little. You probably won't know completely what works for you during this week, but you will start to see how each of the ACES changes based on the amount and timing of your carb consumption.

This week is all about tuning your ACES antenna and decoding the previously "secret" hormone talk that you're experiencing all day. Then, after you take the quiz and dig into the carb nitty-gritty to come, you'll be armed with the info you need to fine-tune exactly what works for you when it comes to the crafty carbs that seem to have us all so nutritionally confused!

Depending on your hormone imbalances, you may need to structure your meal schedule differently, which you'll learn how to do in Week 2. But during this first week of the Hangry B*tch Reset, you will break the habit of either grazing all day or skipping meals entirely and adopt the habit of eating four meals a day. As with the smaller servings of carbs, this may or may not work for you long term, but for now it will stop some bad habits, tune you in to your ACES, and shake up your metabolism a bit, which almost always produces favorable results.

Your meals should consist of real food choices, meaning no more prepackaged or processed foods. To keep it simple, avoid eating food with labels. This might sound daunting, but we have made it extremely easy for you by including quick and easy recipes (found in the Hangry B*tch Food Fix on page 314) that are totally doable and easily customizable, even when you're feeling your worst. Even better, most of our recipes are easy to make in large batches, so you can take advantage of leftovers and repurpose them for other meals. Remember, what you eat has a profound impact on how you feel, and until you make this important change, things simply won't get better.

#hangrybitchfix

If you have a known autoimmunity issue such as Hashimoto's disease, we would like you to consider a trial elimination of certain foods beyond what we have already asked you to avoid in order to see if you notice any improvement of your symptoms. Still follow the Hangry B*tch Reset Diet but also eliminate the following: nightshade vegetables, including all varieties of peppers (bell, poblano, jalapeño, etc.) and pepper-based spices (cayenne, paprika, chili powder, etc.), eggplant, tomatoes, and white potatoes (not sweet potatoes). Eggs also should be avoided during this elimination period as well as nuts and seeds. For those with autoimmunity, the above list of foods can often cause a flare-up and increase symptoms, especially if gut health is already compromised. The good news is that after you have healed, you may be able to add several of these foods back into your diet!

The Hangry B*tch Reset Food Guide

When possible, organic is always preferable for vegetables and fruits. When it comes to protein, grass-fed/pasture-raised meat is preferable, as are eggs from pasture-raised hens and wild-caught seafood.

k recap of what you'll be eating this week:

a day, roughly the same size, all of which will include

25 g of lean animal-based protein

1 large handful of veggies (aim for 1 lb of fibrous vegetables a day)

¼ to ⅓ cup or 4–6 bites of the recommended carbohydrates twice a day

Fats from recommended sources—approximately 1–2 tablespoons per meal

Here is a list of our recommended foods:

Proteins

Beef

Buffalo or bison

Eggs and egg whites

Fish such as bass, cod, and salmon, fresh or canned (limit fish high in mercury such as swordfish and tuna to one serving per week)

Game (venison, elk, boar, etc.)

Jerky from bison, turkey, or lean grass-fed beef (gluten- and sugar-free)

Lamb (higher in fat; limit to one time per week)

Lunch meats (minimally processed, nitrate- and gluten-free)

Pork, lean (chops, tenderloin)

Poultry and chicken or turkey sausages (without gluten/sugar)

Shellfish (shrimp, crab, scallops, lobster, etc., avoid fake crab and lobster)

Fibrous Vegetables

Artichokes	Bamboo shoots
Arugula	Bean sprouts
Asparagus	Beet greens

Bell peppers

Broccoli

Cabbage

Carrots

Cauliflower

Celery

Collard greens

Dandelion greens

Eggplant

Endive

Fennel

Green beans

Hearts of palm

Herbs, fresh (such as chives, cilantro, basil, mint, dill)

Jicama

Kale

Kohlrabi

Mushrooms

Onions

Radicchio

Radishes

Shallots

Snap beans

Snap peas

Snow peas

Spaghetti squash

Spinach

Summer Squash

Swiss chard

Turnip greens

Carbohydrates (Starches/Sugars)

Starchy Vegetables

Beets

Parsnips

Plantains

Potatoes

Sweet potatoes

Turnips

Winter Squash (such as acorn, butternut, delicata, and pumpkin)

Yams

Lowest-Sugar Fruits—optimal

Apples

Berries (blueberries, raspberries, blackberries, etc.)

Pears

Tomatoes

Higher-Sugar Fruits—allowed but watch for blood sugar symptoms and adjust according to your ACES

Apricots

Bananas

Grapefruit

Grapes

Kiwi

Mangos

Melons (honeydew, cantaloupe, watermelon)

Nectarines

Oranges

Papayas

Passion Fruit

Peaches

Persimmons

Pineapple

Plums

Pomegranates

Tangerines

Fats

Avocado oil

Avocados

Coconut oil

Coconut meat (fresh or unsweetened shredded)

Coconut milk

Ghee

Macadamia nut oil (in salad dressing)

Nut butters, natural (almond, cashew, etc.)

Nuts, raw (such as almonds, Brazil nuts, cashews, hazelnuts, pecans, pine nuts, pistachios, and walnuts; avoid peanuts)

Olive oil, extra virgin

Olives (fresh, canned, or jarred)

Seeds, raw (pumpkin seeds, sunflower seeds, etc.)

Walnut oil (in salad dressing)

Miscellaneous Allowed Foods

Bars: Epic Bars, Perfect Keto Bars, and Primal Kitchen Bars

Mustard (natural, no artificial colors or sugar added; read labels for modified food starch)

Salsa (no-sugar-added varieties; avoid if eliminating nightshades)

Spices, dry (watch for hidden gluten such as in certain mustard powder or curry powder)

Sweeteners (stevia, erythritol, xylitol, monk fruit, or Truvia)

Tahini (sesame seed paste)

Tea, organic (black, green, or herbal)

Vinegar (balsamic, cider, plum, red wine, white balsamic, white wine, etc.)

On the Hangry B*tch Reset, Here's What Your Day's Meals Might Look Like:

Breakfast: Fabulous Frittata (page 322)

Lunch: Arugula Chicken Salad with HB Ranch Dressing (page 331)

Third meal: Two-Minute Lettuce Wraps (page 332)

Dinner: Spanish Meatballs (page 356), Root Veggies and/or Winter Squash (page 347), and Zesty Cabbage Slaw (page 335)

What You **Won't** Be Eating During the Hangry B*tch Reset

Don't eat crap. We need to be blunt. If you want to stop being a Hangry B*tch, you must focus on real food choices. However, there are several real foods, like grain and dairy products, that aren't included among our food basics. Below is a more complete list of what you'll be skipping and why.

Processed/Packaged Foods. Particularly those with hydrogenated oils, modified food starch, added sugar, gluten derivatives, or soy. It is very tough to keep this diet as low-inflammation as it needs to be when utilizing packaged foods. If you do use them, read the labels to make sure they don't contain any of the ingredients listed above.

Sugar (in all its forms). Including table sugar, Sucanat, raw sugar, maple syrup, agave nectar, and honey. Opt instead for small amounts of raw stevia, xylitol, or monk fruit instead.

Legumes. Including lentils, soybeans, kidney beans, black beans, and peanuts. These are common reactive foods for those with PCOS and autoimmunity such as Hashimoto's disease.

All Grains. Including processed grains such as those in baked goods and cereals as well as whole grains. Grains to avoid include wheat, corn, oats, rye, barley, rice, millet, sorghum, quinoa, amaranth, and buckwheat (these last three are technically seeds but for our purposes they count as grains). Do your best to avoid all traces of gluten as well.

Processed Meats. Such as hot dogs, most sausages, most bacon, preserved meat, and most lunch meats. (Applegate Farms, Diestel Farms, and Butcher Box meats are exceptions, as they are both gluten-free and minimally processed, or look for other natural brands that meet the same high standards.)

Fattier Cuts of Meat. Such as ribs and highly marbled steaks such as T-bone. In general, for red meat stick with leaner cuts of grass-fed beef and bison.

Alcohol. Yes, we know this one is tough, but as we have already mentioned, it's worth it to heal!

Here is a list of other foods you'll want to avoid, some that might be obvious and some that might have been previously thought of as healthier options.

Butter spray substitutes, margarine, and other vegetable oil spreads (such as Smart Balance or Country Crock)

Trans fats and hydrogenated fats

Corn, safflower, sunflower, canola, peanut, or other processed seed oils

Coffee creamers (contain dairy and often sugar; opt instead for Nutpods almond and coconut milk creamers)

Conventional mayonnaise (Opt for avocado oil–based mayo, or make your own; see page 375.)

Sugar-laden condiments such as barbecue sauce, ketchup, relish (many also contain gluten)

Energy bars and protein bars (most have too many carbs to keep blood sugar in check; most also have rice, dairy, or soy.)

Ice cream, gelato, frozen yogurt (fat-free or otherwise)

Rice- or soy-based frozen desserts

Popcorn, chips, and pretzels. Commercially prepared salad dressings (many contain loads of sugar, low-quality fats, preservatives, and gluten. Homemade is better; see pages 377–79.)

Already a Grain-Free Devotee?

If you've been following a low-carb, keto, dairy-free, grain-free, gluten-free, or other Paleo-type diet for some time, chances are you aren't always 100 percent strict. We'll ask that during Week 1 of the Hangry B*tch Reset you get on board with our guidelines 100 percent as this will set the stage for the customized recommendations to come.

We can also bet that if you've been specifically following a Paleo or keto diet for a bit, you're not afraid of fat. We wouldn't be surprised if you've been eating your fair share of bacon, full-fat red meat, egg yolks, duck fat, ghee, and sausage. All totally cool in theory, but it is common for women to overshoot their fat intake on a Paleo diet, and for reasons we have already touched on and that we'll cover more in detail next week, a diet high in animal fat can wreak havoc on estrogen balance. Thus, during the Hangry B*tch Reset we want you to swap out fattier meats for leaner meats—eat more chicken, turkey, lean pork, fish, shellfish, and bison and limit bacon, steak, and other fatty meats to one or two servings per week. Aim to get your fats mostly from plant-based sources like extra virgin olive oil, coconut oil, and avocados and their oil.

You also need to ensure you're eating enough veggies. It's common for Paleo dieters to end up skimping on vegetable consumption, and this plan, while not vegetarian is meant to be plant-based. What we mean by that is that vegetables are a cornerstone of each meal, the thing you want the most of on your plate each time you eat. You should try to eat five or six handfuls of veggies per day, or a total of one pound per day. This alone favorably impacts all your hormones, from insulin to cortisol to estrogen.

If you're a devotee of the Paleo/primal camp that advises three meals a day, or if you've been dabbling in intermittent fasting, you're going to need to dial it back or dial it up and eat four meals a day for this first week. In order to truly reset your hormones and make higher-level adjustments in later weeks, this is a must. Pay attention to what shifts with your ACES so you can learn from this four-meal-a-day experiment, and then we will help you tweak this recommendation to what optimally works for you in Week 2—chances are it's somewhere between what you're doing now and this template.

5-4-3-2-1 3 Strength Training Sessions per Week

During this week you'll start on the Hangry B*tch Fitness Plan and will be given two of our three templates to choose from.

If you have had a baby and haven't sufficiently healed your core and pelvic floor or if you have low back or hip and/or pelvic pain, we want you to do the HB Core+Floor Recovery Template for three weeks before you begin the HB Hormone Reset Template. If you fall in this camp, you might think that starting here puts you a bit behind for a four-week program. But it's worth it to not get injured, and this sets you up to be safe and ready for our third totally customizable template, the HB Strength Training Template, which we will introduce to you in Week 3

If you have been training regularly but doing mostly intense exercise and metabolic conditioning, if you are just getting back to training, or if you are brand-new to training, you will follow the HB Hormone Reset Template. If you've been overdoing it, this template will help to reset your hormones by bringing down the exercise intensity while still keeping you active, or if you've been more sedentary, this template will boost you up to a safe and effective level of exercise.

Quick Recap on Strength Training Options This Week

Option 1. If you're injured, postpartum, or have never healed your core and floor, even if it's been years that you have been postpartum, you'll do the HB Core+Floor Recovery Template 5 times per week for 3 weeks. The HB Core+Floor Recovery Template is an exception when it comes to our 3 times per week strength training recommendation as it's intended to be done 5 times per week for 3 weeks as a therapeutic approach to heal and strengthen your core and floor. Our other two templates, however, do follow our 3 times per week strength training recommendation. You'll find the layout of the HB Core+Floor Recovery Template on page 251, which includes detailed explanations of each movement along with pictures and instructions for what is prescribed.

Option 2. If you've been training hard, are brand-new to training, or are just getting back to training but are not injured or postpartum, you'll do the HB Hormone Reset Template 3 times per week for Week 1 and Week 2. Then you'll move on to the HB Strength Training Template, which you will be introduced to and taught to customize in Week 3. This workout targets common weakness in women such as lower lats, glutes, and hamstrings as well as being cortisol normalizing for all women. Do this workout three times per week for two weeks. Then you'll move on to the customizable HB Strength Training Template in Week 3. You'll find the layout of the HB Hormone Reset Template on page 265, which includes detailed explanations of each movement along with pictures and instructions for what is prescribed.

We have a couple more things we would like you to be mindful of before you dive into your first workout. First, be sure to do a dynamic warm up rather than static stretching to activate and prime the muscles that you will be using for your workouts and to signal proper movement patterns. Essentially, a dynamic warm up helps to increase blood flow and nervous system input to your muscles and to your core and will help to improve posture and overall alignment, which will optimize performance and help keep you safe during your workout. To break it down, you need your central nervous system to know that you are about to move, so a light jog and/or a few hamstring and quad stretches aren't sufficient. You'll notice right away how much easier it is to move and activate your core after you do our Dynamic Warm Up for the first time! You will also notice that, minus the Kegel exercises, the Dynamic Warm Up is very similar to the HB Core+Floor Recovery Template. This warm up can be used daily to continue to help heal the core and floor, and it should be used as your warm up prior to each workout. How to do our Dynamic Warm Up can be found on page 258.

Second, we understand you might be entering into this program with an existing injury and undergoing rehabilitation such as physical therapy. In this case always include any particular rehab or recovery work you've already been instructed to do by your physician, physical therapist, chiropractor, or other healthcare provider.

#hangrybitchfix

Be mindful of pelvic position. Aim to not be anterior, which is typically the default, but rather try to keep neutral throughout the day. Continually check in on your alignment: stacking of shoulders over lower ribs over hips. Be especially mindful of pelvic position, tight core, and joints stacked as you do the squats of daily living such as getting in and out of a chair, off the toilet, picking something up from the floor, or getting something out of a low drawer.

`5-4-3-2-1` 2 Liters (or More) of Water per Day

While hydration needs can vary from woman to woman depending on activity level and stress response (yes, stress changes hydration needs, as does blood sugar), all women can start with two to two and a half liters of plain water spread throughout the day. You might find water to be boring, but remember: you're more likely to be a Hangry B*tch if you avoid it or, worse, end up drinking something like diet soda instead.

Sparkling Water can be an awesome replacement for diet soda or soda. Add a squeeze of lemon or lime or choose the unsweetened flavored options. Sparkling water can help women get that sparkly, cold hit that they are used to getting from their favorite sugary or chemically soda.

Sparkling water *can* help keep you hydrated, but because of the carbonation, we tend to drink it more slowly and therefore don't drink as much as we would with regular water. Sparkling water should only account for about half of your water intake; keep a full bottle of regular water close by to drink throughout the day to make sure you are also drinking enough of the good stuff!

Finally, if you notice that sparkling water makes you a bit gassy or if you know you have digestive issues, we suggest you lay off the bubbles. Sparkling water can cause some irritation to the digestive tract as well as the bladder. If you're going through LaCroix by the case and find that you're peeing constantly or getting a bit bloaty, consider cutting it out entirely and see if these issues improve.

Caffein is a stimulant that can create further havoc on your adrenals and brain chemistry if you're stressed out and tired. Coffee can also create some additional stressors if you are sensitive to it (as many women unknowingly are).

We get it; this is a tough one, but during this phase of the plan, you can have no more than one caffeinated beverage per day, and we suggest that you skip it entirely if you can. Also, take an honest look at your need for caffeine. Are you nonfunctional without it? Do you go out of your way to get your fix in the morning? Do you need several cups to get through the afternoon? Do you actually feel tired AFTER drinking coffee? Do you have insomnia? Do you have more cravings for sugar or more coffee after drinking it? We'll tell you what adjustments to make in the coming weeks, but for now start by analyzing your caffeine habit.

If you're currently drinking several caffeinated beverages and are worried about withdrawal side effects, start by switching to half decaf for your coffee or tea and then wean yourself off it over a few days until you're having no more than one cup of caffeinated coffee or tea by the end of this week.

Soda is another health and hormone no-no, but many women are still reaching for these sugary—or, when it comes to diet soda, chemical-laden—pick-me-ups. The sugar and calorie content in regular soda is through the roof, and diet is hardly a better option due to the ingredient aspartame, a neurological stimulant. Both regular and diet sodas are chock-full of phosphoric acid, which wreaks havoc on women's bones, teeth, and metabolism. Chuck the soda this week, and ideally for good!

Finally, Alcohol. We get it—a glass of wine or two at night is sometimes the one thing you look forward to after a day of being a Hangry B*tch. You're tired or frustrated and just looking to "winedown." However, alcohol, although it feels like a stress relief, can actually be super stressful on your body and can majorly disrupt your sleep as well as your estrogen balance. But we recognize that avoiding that glass of wine, especially on a special occasion or date night, can also be stressful. Girl, we will meet you halfway. During the reset you'll be booze-free, but you don't have to avoid it forever. Let's focus on hormone healing and see where alcohol fits in for you for the long haul. If during this week you notice a marked difference in sleep quality, mood, energy levels, or cravings, you may be someone who just can't tolerate alcohol all that well. Cutting back or stopping for thirty days can be a huge eye-opener for how alcohol actually affects your body, as it may not be delivering the stress relief you thought it did!

5-4-3-2-1 1 Daily Commitment to Rest, Recovery, and Real Self-Care

Rest and Recovery

If you are still not getting those seven to eight hours of restful sleep, bump that bedtime up another fifteen minutes. Make that to-do list for tomorrow and whatever didn't get done today, simply let it go. All the stress in the world doesn't change what is still left undone or what is on the agenda for tomorrow. Also a quick reminder to do the sleep hygiene basics: make sure your room is cool and dark, keep the lights at home low during the evening or wear blue-light-blocking glasses, and/or use filters on your computer or phone.

We will talk about cortisol-related sleep trouble next week, but if you've tried both the sleep hygiene suggestions and the herbs and nutrients given on pages 39 and 41 and are still not able to fall asleep or stay asleep, it's time to talk about your brain chemistry and neurotransmitters. GABA (gamma-aminobutyric acid) and serotonin are both important brain chemicals that enable you to relax and unwind, and they counter some of the effects of cortisol abnormalities, which we'll get to next week. Below are the signs of trouble with both GABA and serotonin and a few supplement ideas to help.

Common Symptoms of GABA Deficiency:

- Feeling anxious or panicked or overwhelmed for no reason
- Feeling knots in your stomach, dread, or doom; inner tension or excitability that's difficult to turn off
- Having a restless mind or racing thoughts that you can't turn off when you want to relax
- Worrying or feeling guilty about things that didn't used to bother you

Herbs that boost GABA include valerian, chamomile, and passionflower. You can also take GABA itself, which is often most effective in the form trademarked as "PharmaGABA" (take 100–200 mg). Glycine (take 3 g one hour before bedtime) may also help boost GABA. If this increases anxiety and sleeplessness, you likely have some issues converting the amino acid glutamate to GABA; this can be worth exploring with your functional medicine doctor. See www.sarahanddrbrooke.com or the Supplement and Testing Resources (page 382) for more info on our favorite products.

Common Symptoms of Low Serotonin:

- Having "the blues" or feeling depressed (and perhaps feeling guilty that you aren't happier)
- Losing enjoyment and pleasure from things you used to enjoy
- Feeling more susceptible to pain
- Being more prone to anger than you used to be, even when unprovoked
- Feeling worse in gray, overcast weather

Herbs and nutrients that boost serotonin include 5HTP (take 50–100 mg at bedtime) and St. John's wort (take 300 mg at bedtime). Inositol is another great serotonin supporter as it can be relaxing and it is also great for female hormone issues of many sorts; try 1000 mg at bedtime. Serotonin-boosting supplements can give you very vivid dreams, which can make you wake less rested the next day. In this case, take earlier in the day or avoid. Do not take supplements that boost serotonin if you are also taking MAO inhibitors or SSRIs (selective serotonin reuptake inhibitors).

Real Self-Care

Remember, it's how you do self-care that matters even more than what you do. Having a best friend, cheerleader, biggest-fan voice in your head instead of a relentless critic is real self-care. We've given you a variety of tools to help cultivate self-care, including the Five Pillars, meditation, and mantras. This week we want you to add at least one more minute of meditation to your practice. Of course, if you're ready, you can add ten or even thirty, but add at least one more minute daily. Follow our guidelines for how to meditate on pages 36–38 or use a guided meditation of your choice.

Let's talk more about the ongoing meditation we want you to be practicing throughout your day: mantras. Mantras can be used during your meditation, but we also want you to use them to create changes in your mindset throughout the day. We love mantras because they are an easy way to wrangle the runaway (and often negative) thoughts in your head, and they are not time-consuming. We suggest saying your mantra five times in the morning, as you sit down to each meal, and at bedtime. You can also say them on your walks as part of a moving meditation—we call this a #mantrawalk. Try incorporating this mindfulness tool during your walks and don't be surprised if you find yourself craving more #mantrawalks—it's easy to want more of the blissed-out feeling you have when you're done! It's the best.

Wondering what your mantra should be? It can be anything that gets your head in a positive place and motivates you to create the life you want. Keep it positive and keep it simple. Here are a few of our absolute favorites:

Thank you.

I love you.

I matter.

Or try one from this list of Happy Babe gems, noting that some of the most powerful mantras start with "I am":

I am healthy.

I am letting it be easy.

I am worthy.

I am supported.

I am enough.

I am my best friend.

I am choosing to nourish myself.

I am choosing to shine.

I am choosing grace (or I am choosing to give myself grace).

We used some of our favorite concepts to create these mantras, such as choosing grace over guilt when you mess up or make a choice that doesn't work well for you, nourishing over punishing when it comes to our approach to the gym and nutrition, shining over shrinking when it comes to being who you are (our fifth pillar), and simply being your best friend (the fourth pillar). These mantras are ways to practice the Five Pillars and further incorporate all the goodness of this program into your daily life, but by all means make them your own, too!

If you're really struggling to find a mantra and none of these jive with you, think of what it feels like to be a Hangry B*tch. What's the opposite of that for you? That is how you WANT to feel, so make that your mantra. You can use the same mantra every day or change it up—whatever feels right to you.

#hangrybitchfix

The mantra we suggest for this week is "I got this," especially because this first week can feel a little overwhelming. Luckily, we have a pillar to cover that problem! And when you're in doubt, the mantras that are always applicable are "Thank you" and "Everything is OK."

You Can't Be in Real Self-Love When You're Utterly Overwhelmed

We presented the Five Pillars in chapter 3, and you should be already working away on the first pillar, Find and Commit to What Works for You, which we will help you tune in to more during Week 2. This week we're focusing on the second pillar, Opt Out of Overwhelm. The strategies to practicing this pillar are learning to really set your priorities as well as living in gratitude. You'll be taking on one additional pillar per week, but we don't expect you to manage each of these huge areas in just seven little days. However, by dedicating one week to each pillar, you'll start to hone in on how all Five Pillars will eventually become a perspective to live your life by for years to come.

Get Grateful, Girl

As we mentioned in the second pillar, a great way to Opt Out of Overwhelm is to have a gratitude practice. We'd love for you to take a little time each morning to write down or even say out loud what you're grateful for. This is a wonderful tool, and by all means please do it. However, what we're really talking about here with being more grateful is not just the morning ritual of making a list, but truly LIVING in gratitude. Not that temporary bliss you get while rattling things off or writing them down but rather experiencing that feeling all the time, or at least way more often than not. Truly living in gratitude helps to mitigate that gnawing feeling of lacking something that you might desire.

We want you to be literally moved to tears if you stop and think about what you have right now, even if you also want something more. Sheryl Crowe summed it up perfectly, "It's not having what you want; it's wanting what you've got." So that's the tool: sit and get yourself weepy about what you have that you're grateful for. As you do this daily or even a few times a week, you will start to be more keenly aware that what you have right now is more than enough, and you'll be feeling more gratitude more of the time. The more you do it, the more you begin to *live* in gratitude.

#hangrybitchfix

If you're having trouble feeling that big-time gratitude, try to think back to a time when you wanted exactly what you have right now. It's amazing, right? So often we take for granted the things that we may have spent years wishing and hoping for. A great example is kids. Perhaps you can remember wishing to become a mother and all the joy and anticipation that comes with that; and now you're here with those dreamed-of kiddos, and yet it's so easy to lose out on moments we wished for when we are so busy being stressed out or wishing things were different or "more than" what we finally have. There's truly always something to be grateful for when we snap ourselves into being right here, right now.

Your Top Five

The other tool for opting out of overwhelm is learning to set your priorities. This sounds straightforward but, believe us, it's not. Half the time we don't even know whose priorities we're setting. We may have inherited a value system from our parents or have had events in our lives that have made us feel less-than, all mixed up with societal as well as internal pressures to appear a certain way or to have certain things. We end up chasing our tails, trying to do the things that truly matter to us along with a whole bunch of crap that really doesn't.

To avoid getting pulled in a thousand different directions, each day you will keep no more than five priorities; we call it your Top Five. If your to-do list is longer, that's fine—if you get to more than your Top Five you'll feel like a rock star. If you don't, you are officially off the hook. Your Top Five priorities can be the same day to day or they can change (you can even just set one or three); the point is to have no more than five priorities for the day that truly matter to you.

Establishing a Top Five ensures that you complete what matters to you most each day while also acknowledging that you are not Superwoman, and that's fine. Plus, it ensures that you won't waste precious energy on priorities that aren't even yours.

Use These Questions to Help You Set Your Top Five:

- Does this value or importance belong to me and do I want to keep it?

- Does this activity favorably impact who I want to be in the world?

- Does this positively impact my family or most important relationship?

- Does this further my life purpose? (This can be your work/job or some other purpose or "work" you feel is yours to fulfill.)

- Does this positively impact my health?

We are painfully aware that with this first week alone we just gave you—a woman with too much to do already—several more things to do! But we also know that you wouldn't have picked up this plan if you weren't ready for some change. So before you take on everything in Week 1, first it's time to let something else go. You have to make room for these new habits that will create the change you're looking for without creating overwhelm.

There are so many things that we think we have to do, but when we get honest about it, a lot of these things simply aren't as important to us as we thought. Let these go. Other things may need to get done, but they make you miserable. In this case we can have someone else do them or we can get help with them. We will challenge you each week to choose to Opt Out of Overwhelm by taking one obligation off your plate.

We know . . . scary, right?

Scary or not, you will continue spinning your wheels if you don't address all sources of stress, and being overbooked, too busy, or spread too thin are most definitely stressful! Overwhelm is often overlooked in hormone books, diet plans, and even books on stress itself, but we firmly believe it is absolutely key not just to pile on more stuff to do but rather to make room for the new by getting rid of some of the old. Consider this spring-cleaning for your life. If you can afford it, hire it out. If you can get help with it, ask. If you can just stop doing it altogether, just stop. If your palms are sweaty just thinking about this idea, go back through the value questions above or get clear on your options:

What can you delegate? Honestly, are you the best person for this task or is your time better spent doing what you are most amazing at?

What can you hire out or share with someone? Think laundry, house cleaning, meal delivery, childcare, pickups or drop-offs, etc.

What is something you HATE doing? How can you stop it like yesterday or at least start working toward getting out of it? It's an energy suck to do things you hate—and of course this is stressful and wreaks havoc on your hormones!

What is something you FEEL is important but when you ask yourself WHY you do it, you don't have a great reason?

Finally, can you change how you feel about the stuff you are doing? Can you simply decide to not let your day-to-day tasks make you so stressed out? Can you just breathe and let it go, do what you can and simply move on? Usually we put way too much emphasis on all the little things that come up during the day when, instead, we can simply decide to not let these things get us so worked up.

Most women are scared to give up some responsibilities, whether you're a control freak or a people pleaser or just never took the time to really think about it; we are asking you to be brave enough to do it! Also, many women spend a lot of time thinking about how they do way too much, feel totally overwhelmed, and hate their current schedules and obligations, but they have never practiced voicing their need for support or change. We are often surrounded by more support than we realize with our families and friends, but unless we open up our mouths and speak our truth we will never be heard. Women are really good at holding up the world and appearing on the outside as if we are doing it with ease, but inside we are dying. We know this story well, because we've been those women. Beginning to use your voice to speak your truth and to put your self-care first is scary, but you can do it. Say out loud to those who need to hear it what you need to have situated differently in order for you to truly be OK. Say it with compassion, conviction, and honesty and then create your Top Five and stick to it like your health depends on it, because it does.

As Easy as 5-4-3-2-1! Here's a Quick Recap

5 Walks per Week Plus 5 Minutes of Breathing Work per Day. You should ideally walk at a leisurely pace for 45–60 minutes, out in nature if possible. You can use a mantra while you're walking and turn it into a moving meditation we call a #mantrawalk. Practice your restorative breathing after your strength training.

#hangrybitchfix

Walking is considered low-intensity cardio, but it's also an important part of your hormonal recovery and reset as you start your journey to being more of a Happy Babe. Walking, like sleep, is a hormone reset button so we know it takes some time, but it's key to your hormonal balance. Also, if you're doing it as a #mantrawalk and working on maintaining a healthy perspective, then it's also part of your mindfulness and mindset work. Nothing better than a two-for-one deal!

---

4 Meals per Day. They should be roughly the same size and include 25 g of protein per meal and at least 1–2 large handfuls of veggies at each meal, shooting for a pound a day total. Your meals should also include some healthy fat and two of your meals should include approximately 4–6 bites of starchy carbs; all food needs to be from the Hangry B*tch Reset food list (pages 106–09).

3 Strength Training Sessions per Week. You will be doing the HB Hormone Reset Template this week (and next week), always starting with the Dynamic Warm Up. Alternatively, if you are newly postpartum, injured (back, hips, neck), or otherwise have a weak core and pelvic floor, you will be doing the HB Core+Floor Recovery Template 5 times per week for 3 weeks, then you'll start the HB Hormone Reset Template 3 times per week for 1 week. This alternative doesn't perfectly follow the 5-4-3-2-1 template, but we want you to start here in order to get you healed up and ready to train for the rest of your life.

2 Liters (or More) of Water per Day. Some can be sparkling water if you tolerate it well. Watch excess caffeine, keeping coffee to one cup per day if you choose to keep it and avoid alcohol for the next four weeks.

1 Daily Commitment to Rest, Recovery, and Real Self-Care. This includes trying to get eight hours of restful sleep if you're not already there, adding one more minute of meditation, and choosing a daily mantra (use ours or write your own). You'll also be working on the second pillar, Opt Out of Overwhelm, using the tools of living in gratitude, setting your Top Five priorities by using the value questions, and choosing at least one thing to let go of (get one to-do off your list by delegating or just giving it up). Finally, if you find yourself in a really bad spot, use one of our Twelve Tangible Tools—we'll teach you three per week starting right now!

When It's Really Tough, Turn to the Tangible Tools

If this is all totally new to you, we know it can feel like a lot. We promise that once you get the hang of it, this new way of life will feel great. If you're a little type A (like us), embarking on a big change such as this one might have you worried about getting it perfect: "What if I mess this up? What if I fail? What if I am out somewhere, away from home and don't know what to eat? What if I miss a workout? What if I get overwhelmed and mess up the friggin' second pillar?"

Hold on! First, you probably will mess it up! It's totally new, it's a lot to implement, and let's face it: life happens. All you can do is give it your best each day. Let yourself off the hook if it doesn't go perfectly—grace over guilt. That said, planning ahead can really help; you can schedule your workouts on your calendar and treat them like a hair appointment you'd never ever cancel, you can prep food ahead of time to save loads of time and stress during the week, and you can get your act together to get into bed on time. Also, practice what we call "optimism light": assume you'll be successful and totally rock this (optimism), but expect some hiccups along the way (hence "light").

As we mentioned in chapter 3, we know we've given you a lot of support around the Five Habits and a complete perspective framework with the Five Pillars, but chances are you'll have a day when it seems, despite all of your resources, it's still all totally falling apart. No matter how solid this plan is, real life still happens and there will be those really stinkin' rotten, tough days. Since stress management is paramount to you healing your hormones and regaining your happiness, we have urgently stressed the importance of daily meditation and utilizing a mantra. This is like going to the gym every day; you get stronger and stronger as time goes on, and the practice of mindfulness builds upon itself. However, it takes time! As you practice and these tools take hold, when anxiety and stress get the best of you, we want you to turn to the Twelve Tangible Tools. These are our in-the-moment, losing-your-sh*t tools to help you see another perspective, calm down, and trigger your parasympathetic nervous system (get out of fight-or-flight), reset your mindset so you can get back to what matters to you . . . and not act like a total Hangry B*tch, because don't we all know how much we regret that later? These tools will help you see another option for how you're responding to the present stress and get yourself more easily through it, just like a Happy Babe would.

We'll be teaching you three tools per week. You don't have to use them all, but we wanted to give you a ton of options to try so that you can find the ones that are really helpful to you. We've found through our years of helping women that stress management is extremely important but highly individual. What works for one woman may just agitate another woman further, so try them all, take what works, leave what doesn't, and modify and improve upon them in ways that are unique to you. The tools for Week 1 are the Emotional Freedom Technique, or EFT (aka tapping), the Timed Tantrum, and 2X Out Breathing.

EFT (Emotional Freedom Technique). This technique commonly called Tapping, utilizes specific wording that you speak out loud as you tap on a series of acupuncture points. It essentially gives a voice to the craziness and fear in your head combined with gently stimulating acupuncture points. Not only does this harness the power of acupuncture (without the needles or driving to an appointment), but it pulls you out of your head and connects you with your body by having you focus on the negative emotion you want to work through. For a video demo, visit www.sarahanddrbrooke.com.

Timed Tantrum. Often the best way through a bad feeling is to just feel it by really indulging in all the yuck of it. With this tool you get sixty seconds of pouting/complaining/freaking out and then you're done. Give yourself permission to just feel crappy/cranky/ticked off/scared/etc. about whatever the yuck might be but promise yourself you can't stay there for more than a minute. (OK, ninety seconds if you have to, but no more.) Or if you're better with writing than stomping your feet, you can opt to journal it. This is a free-form, stream-of-consciousness open dumping of everything in your mind. Get it onto paper so it can stop running around in your mind; what you need to do here is feel, let yourself really feel it and trust you will survive it. Set a timer for sixty seconds and let it all flow; then let it go. Having a time-out room is a great idea, especially if you have kids. Simply say "I need a time-out," make your way to your time-out room (we like the bathroom for this), set your timer, and have at it. Sometimes it helps to really localize in your body where you feel the emotions you are feeling. As you are "in it," notice where you feel the painful stuff—in your chest, your stomach, your head, your throat—just notice, feel it, and let it come up and through you.

2X Out Breathing. This tool is amazing and works right with your physiology. When you're stressed, scared, or flipping out, you're locked into your fight-or-flight, sympathetic nervous system. By breathing out for two times as long as you breathe in, you will trigger that calmer side of your nervous system, the parasympathetic. You simply breathe in for 4 counts and then out for 8 counts. This is actually effective in just sixty seconds but feel free to do it for three minutes. The good news is, you can do this anywhere: in your car, in line at the grocery store, while cooking dinner, in a meeting at work, you get the point. At any time you can check back in with yourself and bring your emotions back to baseline simply by remembering to breathe.

Whew! Please rest assured each of the coming weeks WILL NOT be this dense with information. From here on out, for each week there will be a few more tools and lots of ways for you to tweak the Five Habits/5-4-3-2-1 framework for the hormone issues you're dealing with. You may have several hormone issues or just one. You'll find out for sure what you're dealing with in the next chapter after taking our quiz. Before the end of this week, be sure you take the quiz so you'll know what parts of Week 2 will be applicable for you.

Oh, and by the way: You got this. You totally got this.

Reminder: Check in Daily or at Least Weekly with the Hangry B*tch Scale

Score yourself from 0 to 3 on each item below, 0 meaning you are 100 percent rocking it in this area and 3 meaning it's a disaster. Aim each day to keep your Hangry B*tch score less than 5. If your score is less than 5, you know your hormones are happy, your mindset is right, and you are engaging in REAL self-care (i.e., living by the Five Pillars). If your score is over 5, assess each area and use the tools we've given you thus far (and know that every week we'll give you more tools) to feel better!

ACES Are Balanced. Your appetite is not too high or low, your cravings are minimal and well managed, your energy is even and adequate, it's easy for you to fall asleep and stay asleep.

Tolerating Exercise Well, Not Under- or Overtraining. You are not feeling that energy is depleted after exercise or showing any signs of RAMP (reluctance to train, aches and soreness, moodiness, and puffiness; see page 83).

Feeling Positive and Peaceful Overall. You are using meditation and mantras, choosing a positive perspective more often than not (listening to best friend voice), experiencing little to no stress, anxiety, and overwhelm.

Able to Stay Present in Your Life. You are using meditation, mantras, and third pillar tools for full-engagement living, and you are feeling little to no distraction from the present moment.

Being Who You Are. You are confidently speaking your truth and engaging in activities solely because they bring you joy and help you feel more like yourself.

The Hangry B*tch Hormone Quiz

Congratulations, you've gotten started with Week 1 of the Hangry B*tch Reset, which means you're going to want to be ready by Week 2 to understand how to take the Five Habits we have taught you (the 5-4-3-2-1 framework), and customize them to meet your own unique hormonal needs. In order to know exactly how to do that, you'll need to take our Hangry B*tch Hormone Quiz. Your quiz results will determine how to navigate Week 2 through Week 4 by helping you to hone in on your most important hormonal imbalances.

Before you dive into the quiz we want to prepare you for the likely possibility that you have multiple hormone issues. You might already know that you have more than one imbalance and have been confused about how to help yourself, as the advice you may have been given was for a single hormonal issue. Unfortunately this advice often counters that for another hormone issue. As an example, if you have insulin issues, you might have been told to exercise a lot and eat less, but if you have weak adrenals, you might have also been told to eat frequently and not exercise at all. Many women have both issues, and these opposing suggestions create more stress and frustration. Rest assured that most women are in this camp of having multiple hormonal imbalances, and clearing up all the confusion is one of the main reasons we wrote this book! We'll guide you through what to do in this case by teaching you the order in which you can address your hormones to ensure that you tend to them all without sacrificing one for another; we call this the Hormone Hierarchy and it looks like this:

Low cortisol and/or low thyroid

High cortisol

Insulin resistance

Estrogen: Progesterone Imbalance

Don't worry about how it works yet; we'll lay it out for you throughout the rest of the book so you'll easily be able to honor this hierarchy.

Now you're ready to take the quiz. Here's how:

- Simply answer YES or NO to each symptom question and record the number of YES answers in the total line for each section.

- Three or more YES answers in any section indicate an imbalance with that hormone to some degree.

The Hangry B*tch Hormone Quiz

Section 1

YES NO

☐ ☐ Do you require coffee to get going in the morning or keep going in the afternoon?

☐ ☐ Does your energy dip between meals, and do you then come alive again after eating?

☐ ☐ Are you irritable, cranky, or light-headed when you miss meals, or between meals?

☐ ☐ Do you have to eat every two hours or are you someone who forgets to eat entirely?

☐ ☐ Is your appetite low in the morning, particularly for protein, and/or do you feel nauseous in the morning?

☐ ☐ Do you crave sugar or starchy treats between meals?

☐ ☐ Do you crave salt?

☐ ☐ Do you have difficulty staying asleep, and when you wake do you find it hard to go back to sleep?

☐ ☐ Are you excessively fatigued and sensitive to stress (think burnout)?

☐ ☐ Do you have hot flashes or palpitations (when you feel your heart beating)?

☐ ☐ Do you have sensitive digestion, alternate between loose stools and constipation, or have a diagnosis of IBS?

☐ ☐ Are you sensitive to bright lights (for example, do you always need to wear sunglasses when outside)?

☐ ☐ Do you have low blood pressure (below 110/70) or do you get dizzy when standing up?

☐ ☐ Do you have low fasting blood sugar (below 85)?

TOTAL YES ANSWERS _____

Section 2

YES NO

☐ ☐ Do you awake tired even after seven or more hours of sleep?

☐ ☐ Do you suffer from depression?

☐ ☐ Is your hair falling out (increased hair shedding)?

☐ ☐ Is your skin dry?

☐ ☐ Is the outer third of your eyebrow thinning?

☐ ☐ Do you have elevated cholesterol even with a good diet?

☐ ☐ Do you tend toward constipation?

☐ ☐ Do you take thyroid medication but still have difficulty losing weight or still have low thyroid symptoms?

☐ ☐ Do you take thyroid medication and the dose is continually being increased over time?

☐ ☐ Do you feel you're becoming more sensitive to foods (increased food allergies or sensitivities)?

☐ ☐ Do you feel puffy in general or notice water retention more days than not?

☐ ☐ Do you awake stiff and achy or feel generally inflamed?

☐ ☐ Do you have difficulty recovering from exercise or injuries?

☐ ☐ Are you in a cloud of brain fog (can't concentrate or think clearly)?

TOTAL YES ANSWERS _____

Section 3

YES NO

☐ ☐ Do you hold most of your body fat around the middle?

☐ ☐ Do you awake tired even after seven hours or more of sleep?

☐ ☐ Do you sweat easily or without effort?

☐ ☐ Do you have GERD, ulcers, or "bad digestion"?

☐ ☐ Do you have difficulty recovering from intense exercise?

☐ ☐ Do you awake tired and achy?

☐ ☐ Do you have difficulty falling asleep (feel "tired but wired")?

☐ ☐ Do you retain water easily, feel and look puffy (especially in the morning)?

☐ ☐ Do you have high blood pressure (over 120/80)?

☐ ☐ Do you mostly crave sugary, fatty, salty treats?

☐ ☐ Do you have sugar cravings after eating?

☐ ☐ Do you have high fasting blood sugar (over 99)?

☐ ☐ Is your menstrual cycle irregular or getting longer? Or can you miss a period when you're stressed out?

☐ ☐ Have you had trouble conceiving?

TOTAL YES ANSWERS _____

Section 4

YES NO

☐ ☐ Do you get sleepy after eating?

☐ ☐ Do you crave sweets or starches after eating?

☐ ☐ Do you prefer protein breakfasts (e.g., an egg omelet) because you get hungry quickly after carb-heavy breakfasts (e.g., cereal)?

☐ ☐ Do you have belly fat?

☐ ☐ Is your waist measurement larger than your hip measurement?

☐ ☐ Are you losing your hair on your head, or even your arms or legs?

☐ ☐ Are you in a cloud of brain fog (can't concentrate or think clearly)?

☐ ☐ Do you have high cholesterol or is your total cholesterol more than double your triglycerides?

☐ ☐ Do you have high blood pressure (over 120/80)?

☐ ☐ Do you have high fasting blood sugar (over 99)? Or a hemoglobin A1c over 5.6?

☐ ☐ Are you in perimenopause or menopause, and finding it harder to lose weight?

☐ ☐ Do you have to urinate frequently (more than you should for how much water you drink)?

☐ ☐ Do you have a diagnosis of PCOS (polycystic ovarian syndrome), type 2 diabetes, metabolic syndrome, or prediabetes?

TOTAL YES ANSWERS _____

Section 5

YES NO

☐ ☐ Do you have water retention before menses (you can gain two to three pounds with your period)?

☐ ☐ Do you have heavy or painful periods?

☐ ☐ Are your breasts painful or tender with your period?

☐ ☐ Do you have breast or ovarian cysts?

☐ ☐ Do you have fibroids or endometriosis?

☐ ☐ Have you had difficulty getting pregnant?

☐ ☐ Are you in perimenopause or menopause?

☐ ☐ Do you feel agitated or irritable before your period?

☐ ☐ Do you get headaches of even migraines with menses or ovulation?

☐ ☐ Is your cycle shorter than twenty-one days?

☐ ☐ Is your cycle irregular or longer than thirty-five days?

☐ ☐ Do you have spotting before menses starts?

☐ ☐ Do you have a diagnosis of PCOS, endometriosis or fibroids?

TOTAL YES ANSWERS _____

Interpreting Your Results

For a detailed definition of each hormone's function, refer to pages 14–18.

Section 1: Low Cortisol

If you have three or more symptoms in this category, you are likely having trouble with low cortisol at least a few times a day and possibly throughout the day. This is often called "adrenal burnout" or "adrenal fatigue," but remember: cortisol problems are really a brain-based issue where signals from the brain to the adrenals are not coordinated properly, rather than you having a pooped-out adrenal gland that can't make cortisol. HPA axis dysfunction is a better term, and based on this quiz you're dealing with it! But semantics aside, cortisol is super important.

When cortisol is low it's the definition of "Hangry B*tch" as you have a very hard time keeping your blood sugar up between meals as well as overnight. You also have a very hard time tolerating exercise, especially more intense exercise, you may feel fatigued and achy; and your ACES are decidedly out of whack. You'll learn how to support this hormonal issue starting next week with regards to meal timing and frequency. We'll teach you how to exercise to heal your adrenals instead of hurting them and tell you which supplements can help as you implement all of these changes. Low cortisol along with the next hormone issue, low thyroid, are your most delicate hormonal imbalances, so you will always default to low cortisol or low thyroid advice first, even if you find you also have other hormone issues. You'll literally be building yourself back up by creating a very solid foundation for your health, hormones, and life as a Happy Babe!

Section 2: Low Thyroid

If you have three or more symptoms in this category, it means your thyroid hormone levels are likely not optimal and a thorough thyroid blood workup from your doctor is a good idea. If you have any symptoms from the latter half of the list (the last seven symptoms), then you should also be screened for Hashimoto's disease (ask for TPO and TAA antibodies from your doctor). For more info on testing visit www.sarahanddrbrooke.com/lab-guide or see our Supplement and Testing Resources on page 382.

It's shocking how many women deal with the fallout of low thyroid. Many women are untreated, as they don't fit the classic lab pattern of hypothyroidism, and others are missed entirely because only one marker of thyroid function, TSH (thyroid stimulating hormone), is ever checked. So don't be alarmed if you've had your thyroid assessed and were told "all good" and then you scored high on the thyroid section of the quiz. Not being assessed thoroughly is sadly very, very, very common, and because of this many women continue to struggle with hormone imbalance, lack of energy, and fat loss and are simply internally deteriorating because every single one of our cells needs thyroid hormone to do its job and to repair itself.

We've already covered in detail the function of the thyroid (on page 16 if you need a refresher), including autoimmune low thyroid, aka Hashimoto's disease, but it's important to remind you here that the thyroid can also impact your female sex hormones directly at the ovary and because hypothyroidism also slows the workings of phase II enzymes in your liver, meaning estrogen detoxification is often compromised. This of course means more estrogen dominance. Low thyroid may also be the cause of some of your issues in section 5 of the quiz, and among the toughest fat-loss challenges we see involve women with both PCOS or menopause and a thyroid problem. You will have a fight on your hands if fat loss is a goal, but we're here to help you win!

Section 3: High Cortisol

If you have three or more symptoms in this category, your cortisol is likely high, at least at certain times of the day. Keep in mind that you can also be dealing with low and high cortisol at the same time, as it can be low at certain times of the day and high at others, making your quiz results initially look confusing to you. But rest assured, if you acknowledge both issues and follow the hormone hierarchy, addressing each in due time, you'll do great.

High cortisol can happen intermittently as you go through a stressful time, but most women reeling with symptoms in this section are dealing with some type of chronic stress issue. When you're locked into constant high stress, frequent cortisol release leaves you puffy and having trouble with all of your ACES. In particular, if cortisol is elevated at bedtime, you can feel tired but wired when you want to go to sleep. Your craving for sugary, fatty, and salty foods is on full tilt, you may have a very exaggerated response to stress, and you probably gain weight easily (the latter is especially true when insulin is high as well).

Section 4: Insulin Resistance

If you have three or more symptoms in this section, you are likely dealing with insulin resistance. For a full description of insulin's functions and insulin resistance, refer to page 15.

Symptoms such as increased appetite or cravings for sweets or starches after you eat, or getting sleepy and needing a caffeine pick-me-up after meals, or overall trouble with energy and/or fat gain indicate that you either release too much insulin in response to eating (hyperinsulinemia) or your cells don't heed insulin's message well (to let the sugar in) so you secrete more and more of it to get that message across (insulin resistance). Either one of these two issues can lead to the other.

Insulin profoundly affects progesterone, estrogen, and testosterone, so trouble here can absolutely also lead to period problems, hair loss, facial hair growth, and acne. Insulin will also drive inflammation, making it a significant player in heart health and your longevity overall.

Like cortisol, insulin is absolutely vital for life, but when it's elevated or not working properly you have a much harder time controlling your ACES (especially the first three). You are also primed to store fat, especially when cortisol is elevated as well. You are, though, great at building muscle, so there is an upside here, as many women can struggle with this. Also to note, insulin resistance is often thought of as something only women with PCOS or diabetes have, but you could have mild to severe insulin issues even without a diagnosis of overt insulin resistance from your doctor. No matter where you are, diet and exercise can make a big impact. We'll dive into how to manage this in the weeks to come!

Why does insulin resistance happen? You can eat your way here, stress your way here, or you may have a genetic predisposition (like Dr. Brooke). When genetics are at play, this is your metabolic Achilles' heel, and while it can be managed, a poor diet or high stress will always make it worse. If stress and/or diet are the causes, your recovery will be easier.

Section 5: Estrogen Excess with Normal or Low Progesterone

Once again, if you answered yes to three or more of these questions, it's likely you are having issues with excess estrogen coupled with normal or low progesterone. See the "Ladies, Meet Your Hormones" section on pages 14–18 for more info on these two hormones.

In general, we suffer when progesterone or estrogen is either too high or too low. Also, the balance of estrogen and progesterone with each other will always have an effect on the balance of other hormones such as insulin, cortisol, and thyroid.

Without estrogen, you're likely to lose your strength and vitality and gain body fat as you lose your metabolic reserve; muscle mass decreases and you get more carb sensitive as well. This is in part why most women find that as they cross thirty-five, forty, and enter perimenopause, what used to work for them starts to fail miserably. For example, although lots of cardio and other intense exercise might once have helped you maintain or lose weight, as you enter middle age they can actually cause weight gain. Women may also find they need to lower their carb and alcohol intake and that dietary indiscretions in general are harder to bounce back from. Estrogen also helps keep the hunger-regulating hormone leptin in check and serotonin higher. Without it you'll tend to have more anxiety or depression, increased appetite, and cravings for sugar and carbs; thus, it impacts your ACES directly. Can you say PMS-related chocolate cravings? That's low estrogen talking.

But you can also have too much of a good thing, known as estrogen dominance. Estrogen can be overtly high due to conditions such as ovarian cysts, taking any estrogen-based medication (i.e., birth control pills), excessive alcohol, being overweight (body fat produces estrone, another form of estrogen), increased exposure to environmental estrogens (from various sources including dairy products, plastics, parabens), or when estrogen isn't metabolized and excreted properly by your liver and intestines and you get an excess of highly active estrogen metabolites. Estrogen dominance can also occur not only from absolute estrogen excess but also in relation to low progesterone, meaning it is at least relatively higher than progesterone during the second half of your menstrual cycle when progesterone should be higher. Both types of estrogen excess can happen during perimenopause as hormone production and metabolism become increasingly erratic. No matter the cause, estrogen dominance can cause a range of symptoms including breast tenderness, heavier or more frequent periods (perhaps even fibroids), bloating and weight gain, and difficulty losing fat.

Low progesterone can quickly leave you feeling puffy, can contribute to weight gain, and can put your ACES totally out of whack, including increasing your carb cravings and increasing your sensitivity to all of life's stressors. When it comes to body composition, progesterone supports estrogen's action on fat loss by working to keep cortisol's fat-storing effects under control, particularly around your middle. Progesterone can become low from a wonky cycle or anovulation (such as while breastfeeding, during perimenopause, or if you have PCOS), during times of stress, and after menopause.

Progesterone dominance is less common than estrogen dominance or progesterone deficiency but worth mentioning as it can give you a murky picture of estrogen-progesterone balance. It can occur from taking progesterone-boosting supplements (i.e., vitex), synthetic progestin medications, having a progestin-secreting IUD (Mirena, Skyla), or using topical progesterone cream. Also, relative progesterone dominance can occur when estrogen is very low. Excess progesterone can create insomnia or anxiety as well as increased appetite or hot flashes. If you continue to experience symptoms of excess progesterone after you've worked to balance estrogen and progesterone by following the suggestions in this plan or you're using synthetic or other forms of progesterone, this would be an issue warranting further investigation with a functional medical doctor.

While imbalances here will largely be resolved by honoring insulin and cortisol first, there are some unique metabolism challenges that arise when estrogen and progesterone are imbalanced—ones that most diet and exercise advice fails to acknowledge. We have specific adjustments for this imbalance in the coming weeks, and we'll really dig into estrogen and progesterone during Week 4.

Ladies, It's Complicated . . .

Based on your quiz results you have now determined the main hormone issues that are causing your emotional, health, and metabolic woes. As we mentioned before the quiz, many women have imbalances in more than one category, and because your hormones are so intricately connected, imbalances in one quickly lead to imbalances in another. Unfortunately, most women usually have been feeling badly for five or more years before getting the insight and help they need. Given all that, it's no surprise that you might be dealing with multiple hormones gone haywire, as these main hormone imbalances have a big ripple effect across your metabolism.

For example, thyroid issues often perpetuate issues with cortisol and vice versa. It is also common to have both insulin-resistance issues and high cortisol, or to see symptoms of both high and low cortisol. Low cortisol or high cortisol can also lead to insulin resistance over time. As well, you can have normal thyroid lab levels but test positive for Hashimoto's antibodies and still experience all the low thyroid symptoms such as brain fog, decreased exercise intolerance, hair loss, and fatigue. As you can see, these hormones are hugely interdependent. Finally, a lot of these hormonal issues can look alike! Let's take this array of symptoms, for example: fatigue, hair loss, inflammation, and difficulty losing weight. These all could result from low thyroid, insulin resistance, or high cortisol.

Also, please note that while this book is focused on insulin, cortisol, thyroid, estrogen, and progesterone, these are not the only hormones involved in hunger, cravings, and fat loss. Other key players include glucagon, growth hormone, adiponectin, ghrelin, neuropeptide Y, and leptin. However, getting the key players in balance will (for the most part) set the other hormones right. The tools you'll gain through this program will help you focus on the two hormones you have the most control over, cortisol and insulin, which will help you create a positive, balancing effect across your entire hormonal landscape.

Hangry B*tch Quiz Confusion

You may have noticed that some symptoms (fatigue's a biggie) can be the result of several different hormone issues, and you may also have issues with multiple hormone symptoms. Not surprisingly, you may be unclear about what you should focus on! Let us help you feel less anxious about that: focusing on the 5-4-3-2-1 main Five Habits will help you to normalize insulin and cortisol as well as thyroid, estrogen, and progesterone nuances, and this will take you a long way toward setting all of your hormones right and resolving your most troublesome symptoms like lack of energy.

One of the biggest reasons you may have issues with multiple hormones or feel that you can't get a clear picture of your hormonal imbalance is inflammation, which can cause your symptoms to paint you a rather murky picture. Fortunately, this entire plan focuses on decreasing inflammation as well.

If you find yourself experiencing a slew of symptoms related to various imbalances and you don't feel things are resolving by following the advice laid out in our four-week plan, consider getting tested with your medical provider or find a functional medicine physician to shed more light on your hormone issues. (Again, for more info on testing get the free guide at www.sarahand drbrooke.com/lab-guide or see Supplement and Testing Resources on page 382.)

But What If You Feel Crappy, Have Every Issue in This Quiz, and Yet Your Lab Results Are "Normal"?

There are typically two scenarios where we see this happen. The first and per-haps most frustrating are the discrepancies in how different doctors inter-pret lab results, as each practitioner may have a different idea of what an ideal value is. Remember, just because your labs might show that your hormones are within a normal range on a blood test on a Tuesday at 8 A.M. while at your doctor's appointment, this does not mean that they are at an optimal level over-all or functioning ideally. Not to mention there are many different ways to "test" your hormones. Unfortunately, what's done most often with testing is merely looking at a level of a hormone in your blood on a certain day while not looking at the bigger picture, including how effectively and safely that hormone is metabolized (i.e., estrogen), or if there is enough active free hormone pres-ent (i.e., thyroid, testosterone), or is it around at the right time (i.e., daily with cortisol, monthly with progesterone). Such testing misses the intricacies of how your hormones work best and how you could be feeling better.

The second scenario has to do with inflammation. As we mentioned earlier, inflammation could be affecting all of your hormones, creating low hormonal symptoms, while your lab tests remain within normal ranges.

Inflammation: The Great Hormone Mess-Maker

We touched on the problems of inflammation in chapter 2 and you may have heard that inflammation is at the root of nearly all chronic illnesses in the Western world; however, acute inflammation is a vital part of our immune sys-tem. When we've been injured or have an infection, inflammation is how we get the troops (white blood cells, oxygen, nutrients, etc.) to the places in our body we need them. Unfortunately, as inflammation becomes chronic it can damage healthy tissue and create several vicious cycles of hormone disruption, including triggering persistent cortisol release, worsening insulin resistance, creating estrogen deficiency or dominance, and hindering thyroid function. As with so many issues of modern womanhood, chronic inflammation is a case of too much of a good thing.

The immune system uses its own hormone-like messengers, called cytokines (protein structures that are basically the hormones of the immune system), and prostaglandins. Depending on the particular cytokine or prostaglandin, inflammation will be turned on or off. Prostaglandins are active lipid (fat) compounds that are the end product of our essential fatty acid metabolism. We make them from essential fatty acids that we eat or supplement with (such as omega-3 and omega-6) via enzymes called desaturase and elongase. Therefore, what we eat directly impacts inflammation, either because we have an immune reaction to it (think food sensitivities) or because it feeds an inflammatory prostaglandin pathway. There can also be genetic differences in our fatty acid–metabolizing enzymes that make us more prone to inflammation (for example, women with PCOS are more prone to inflammation due to differences in these enzymes).

Like cytokines, prostaglandins can be pro- or anti-inflammatory, and not only can they screw up the actions of hormones such as estrogen and thyroid but they also have hormone-like actions themselves. Prostaglandins have a significant impact on our HPA axis; are key regulators of reproductive processes including ovulation, implantation, and menstruation; and are necessary for proper hormone-receptor signaling. You can think of prostaglandins as the traffic cops of hormone orchestration as well as having hormone action themselves.

Next to stress (which ironically can cause inflammation), inflammation is the biggest hormone mess-maker out there. It is notorious for hindering the actions of all your hormones in one way or another and is often the culprit when your lab tests show normal levels of hormones but you have all the low hormone symptoms. This is in part because inflammation affects the intra-cellular transcription that happens after a hormone binds to a receptor. As we mentioned in chapter 2, you can think of a hormone as a key and a receptor as a lock. When there's inflammation present it's like someone put gum in the key-holes. The key eventually gets in and opens the lock but it's a slowed, sluggish, inefficient process, if the process even happens at all.

Inflammation can also cause hormone problems peripherally, in that it disrupts the microbiome of the gut, which will in turn affect estrogen, thyroid, and cortisol balance. And as we said above, inflammation is great at triggering vicious cycles of hormone problems, so once it's turned on, widespread disruption occurs rapidly. An unhealthy gut due to inflammation quickly creates food sensitivities, gut infections, and local immune activation, which all results in triggering more inflammation. What's potentially worse is that with all of this inflammation, the body is primed for leaky gut and a translocation of lipo-polysaccharides (which are a component of large gram-negative bacteria living in the gut) into the systemic circulation, triggering a low-grade infection and a ton of inflammation. This subsequential inflammatory soup happening in the gut goes on to then impact hormone balance in a variety of ways, including having a negative effect on thyroid hormone metabolism as well as ramping up production of an inactive form of thyroid hormone called reverse T3 (the latter also happens with high cortisol).

In short, inflammation is a metabolic deal-breaker and can become chronic for many different reasons:

- Under- or overexercising

- Food sensitivities

- An unhealthy gut due to infections, increased intestinal permeability, dysbiosis

- Stress

- Lack of sleep

- Injuries

- Too much alcohol

- Blood sugar problems

- Taking acid-blocking medications regularly. If this is you, it is pretty certain that you have some gut-based issues, as your gut microbiome (which thrives in an acid environment) is likely out of balance.

- Antibiotic use can create gut-based inflammation by disturbing your normal gut bacteria.

- Any type of chronic immune burden such as chronic viruses (EBV, Epstein Barr, for example), chronic gut infection (candida, for example).

- Any type of autoimmune or inflammatory condition such as Hashimoto's disease, Grave's disease, rheumatoid arthritis, celiac, Crohn's disease, ulcerative colitis, or lupus.

- Diabetes, PCOS, or any other issues with insulin resistance or elevated glucose, which create advanced glycation end products (AGEs) that are inflammatory. Having too much glucose or fatty acids around—think having just eaten a big slice of cheesecake or a doughnut—easily triggers inflammation for anyone, but it is worse if you have insulin resistance.

- Overconsumption of bad fats (trans fats) such as margarine, vegetable shortening (i.e., Crisco) and processed seed oils, including soybean, cottonseed, sesame, rice bran, rapeseed, corn, peanut, or the two worst offenders in the bad oils department: canola and sunflower oil. Keep in mind that you may get more of these than you think if you frequently eat in restaurants. These oils are higher in omega-6 fatty acids than omega-3s, which promotes inflammation. In addition, heating them, both during the manufacturing process and while cooking, damages the fatty acid bonds, which further increases the potential for inflammation.

- Use (current or past) of hormonal birth control. Taking the pill, for example, can quickly create deficiencies in vitamin B6, CoQ10, calcium, nicotinic acid, magnesium, and zinc, most of which are required for the proper production of prostaglandins via the enzymes elongase and desaturase. Research on the pill has shown that it increases inflammation, and this may be part of the reason why.

- Having a high exposure to endocrine-disrupting compounds found in plastics and pesticides on our food, or preservatives and fragrances in our body and hair care products. These endocrine disruptors can mimic hormones by binding their receptors directly or by competing with your own hormones for a receptor. They can also directly bind to human tissue, which creates a foreign body, an antigen that our immune system attacks. This can increase existing autoimmunity and also create further inflammation.

Do You Smell Smoke?

After reading all this, you may be wondering how inflammation is currently affecting your hormones. Here are two common tests, available through any doctor, that can assess inflammation:

High-Sensitivity C-Reactive Protein, or hs-CRP. Is a reflection of IL-6 (a proinflammatory cytokine). The normal range is 1.0 to 3.0 mg/L. While values above 3 are the most concerning, ideally your hs-CRP should not be greater than 1.0. This is not a perfect test—you can have normal CRP and still have elevated IL-6 or other inflammatory cytokines, which can be measured in your blood as well—and it is not routinely ordered by your primary care provider.

Erythrocyte Sedimentation Rate, or ESR. Indirectly measures the degree of inflammation in your body. Once you give a blood sample for the test, it's put in a tall, thin, vertical tube. Then the rate of fall (sedimentation) of your erythrocytes (red blood cells) is measured. You want your results to be below 15 mm/hr. However, normal values for women are 0–29 mm/hr.

However, even without testing, you will likely be able to tune in to many signs of inflammation because it has such far-reaching consequences. Inflammation can create symptoms such as the following:

- Digestive trouble, ranging from pain to gas and bloating

- Bowel movement issues ranging from constipation to diarrhea

- An increase in food sensitivities

- Skin trouble, including acne, eczema, psoriasis, rosacea, hives, or itching

- Fatigue directly due to inflammation or due to inflammation's impact on your other hormones such as cortisol and thyroid

- Allergies or sensitivities to both food and environmental antigens

- Puffiness, particularly in the face and around the eyes

- Gum disease or bleeding gums while brushing or flossing

- Brain fog, depression, poor memory or concentration (These are symptoms of brain-based inflammation. Any hormone problems can also be a manifestation of brain-based inflammation, as inflammatory prostaglandins will directly impact the hypothalamus, the command center that orchestrates the glands that make our hormones [ovaries, thyroid, adrenals, etc.]. Note that it can be hard to test for brain-based or central nervous system inflammation because of our blood-brain barrier.)

- Increasing body fat, particularly more body fat around the middle, is both a cause and result of inflammation This midsection visceral belly fat is considered a hotbed of inflammation.

- Pain of any type, including any injury, headaches, tendinitis, or achy or painful joints

- PMS, menstrual migraines, or painful menses.

- Increasing reactions to smells or jewelry or foods. These reactions can be a sign of sluggish detoxification in the liver, which may be caused by inflammation. This can create headaches, skin issues, worsening digestive problems, and hormonal issues such as hypothyroidism and estrogen dominance.

- Estrogen dominance may be related to inflammation impacting the liver as estrogen must be detoxed, or rather "biotransformed" into various metabolites, some with the ability to damage DNA. Sluggish detox pathways will also hinder our elimination of environmental endocrine disruptors, including estrogen mimickers, creating more estrogen dominance as well.

- Difficulty losing weight can be due to inflammation and environmental compounds known to hinder fat loss and metabolism called obesogens.

Now that you are more familiar with the culprits that can cause chronic inflammation as well as the symptoms, don't forget to assess inflammation yearly at the very least, but certainly do so more frequently if you are experiencing signs of inflammation and/or symptoms of low hormones.

This Quiz Is the Gift That Keeps on Giving

We encourage you to keep taking this quiz every four weeks or so, and you can keep taking it indefinitely. Returning to the test will show you in real time how your symptoms are improving! If you're working with a functional medicine provider, you can also get routine follow-up lab testing to ensure things are getting and staying in balance. When it comes to your daily or at least weekly self-check-ins you'll have your ACES to guide you as well as the Hangry B*tch Scale (page 96).

Week 2

What Carbs Are Making You Hangry?

Last week you embarked on Week 1 of the Hangry B*tch Reset, you tuned your antenna inward and learned how your appetite, cravings, energy, and sleep are among the many ways your hormones talk to you every day. This week you'll start to make adjustments that will address any issues you're having with your ACES by working to achieve well-balanced blood sugar, which leads to much better energy and the ability to regulate what you eat. In other words you'll have less ravenous hunger, fewer cravings for all the wrong things, and will be less of a Hangry B*tch and more of a Happy Babe.

The work you do this week will largely be focused on insulin and cortisol, as they are the main drivers of blood sugar, which profoundly impacts hunger and mood (read: when imbalanced makes you hangry). If after taking the Hangry B*tch Hormone Quiz you didn't find any obvious cortisol or insulin issues, this week will still be a game changer as these two hormones have a profound regulatory effect on literally all of your other hormones. Finally, and perhaps most empowering, this week you will also let go of any low carb/high carb, good carb/bad carb confusion and do something revolutionary: find your perfect carb intake, aka your very own unique carb tolerance.

Last week you started eating four meals per day, which might have been a meal less or maybe one more than what you were doing previously. Now that you've gone through Week 1 and your metabolism has been spurred out of complacency, it's time to start customizing the plan to what works best for YOU when it comes to when and what to eat. This week you will be given specific suggestions for manipulating your meals and meal timing based on your Hangry B*tch

Hormone Quiz results; following these suggestions, you will fine-tune your metabolism and mood via your blood sugar. You took the quiz, right? If not, go back to chapter 7 and do that right now. Don't worry, we'll wait. . . .

The quiz highlighted which of your hormones are showing signs of imbalance, and this knowledge will help you implement the strategies in this chapter

Hangry B*tch Hormone Hierarchy

Low cortisol and/or low thyroid

High cortisol

Insulin resistance

Estrogen-progesterone

As you go through the plan from here, follow the solutions and suggestions for the highest-priority hormone issue first (especially if there's a contradiction in recommendations), and as you heal the highest-priority hormones, you'll follow the recommendations for what's next. If you do have multiple issues, the good news is that when you follow the hormone hierarchy, you'll start to see improvements in the hormone issues further down the hierarchy, and that's exactly why it's laid out in this order. If you only have one hormonal issue, simply skip the advice for those that don't apply to you.

We totally understand that all of the hormone information we're teaching you can feel like you've unexpectedly enrolled in a fellowship in endocrinology, but here's the thing: most books on hormones help you balance one hormone but not others (think the cortisol diet or the thyroid solution–type books). When you have issues with more than one hormone yet the advice for how to exercise and eat for one totally contradicts the advice for another, what's a Hangry B*tch who desperately wants to feel better to do? We have the answer. You simply honor your more delicate hormonal imbalance first until its symptoms improve and then you move on down the list, always following our hormone hierarchy.

that are right for you. Remember that you may have multiple hormone imbalances or you may just have one or two. Given that, you won't necessarily make each adjustment suggested for each of your imbalances all at the same time. For example, if you have signs of low cortisol but not high cortisol, you'll skip the high-cortisol suggestions and just do the low-cortisol suggestions. How about if you have both low cortisol and insulin resistance? You'll honor the low-cortisol suggestions first, and once your cortisol is more normalized (i.e., your Hangry B*tch Quiz results or your lab tests indicates it is resolved) you can move on to the insulin resistance suggestions.

What's the Biggie About Blood Sugar?

Learning how to balance your blood sugar doesn't sound nearly as sexy as intermittent fasting, keto, or (insert the latest hormone or weight-loss diet here), but blood sugar is absolutely fundamental to your metabolism and how you feel every day. In fact, without good blood sugar control, it would be tough for you to ever feel better or get any results from those other diets. Like most women, when you feel like a Hangry B*tch, you not only want something to change, like fast, but you can also feel a little desperate—desperate to feel like yourself again and desperate to see some results. We 100 percent understand how enticing a super cool new diet with an advertised revolutionary promise can sound; however, what we see time and time again is that a lot of these diets, even the well-researched, solid, and generally effective ones can actually be really, really tough and ineffective for women with out-of-balance hormones.

For example, intermittent fasting can be great if you have insulin issues but a disaster if you have low cortisol or low thyroid. We are all way more complex than a one-size-fits-all diet can handle, and, chances are, if you are reading this book, your most delicate hormones are struggling. Following our plan will help you lay an amazing foundation for balanced hormones and optimal health, and down the road, once you've healed those delicate hormones, if you decide you want to try fasting or keto or want to make specific adjustments for fat loss, you'll be well set up to finally achieve sustainable results. We don't believe for one second that our approach is the only game in town, but we do know that when women take their wonky hormones on an aggressive diet that radically shifts their metabolism they will usually crash, end up feeling more wiped-out and frustrated than before, and be unable to sustain any results they might have momentarily achieved. What should be encouraging, however, is that after going through this program you will be ultra-tuned in to your hormonal cues so you'll know how to monitor what your hormones think of any diet, not just this one, which is the most empowering tool we could ever offer to you, and one you can use for the rest of your life. So for now it's back to the basics of blood sugar.

Your Main Blood Sugar Hormones: Insulin and Cortisol

As we explained in chapter 1, insulin is an anabolic (build-you-up), storage-type of hormone. It shuttles things like glucose and other nutrients out of your bloodstream into a cell so they can be utilized. One of insulin's key jobs is to lower your blood sugar, whereas your stress hormone cortisol (along with epinephrine and glucagon) will raise it. Insulin is triggered following a meal in order to deal with the rise in blood sugar from food or from your stress response. When your blood sugar gets too low—that is, when you skip meals or go too long (for you) without eating—cortisol causes a blood sugar rise by liberating stored sugar from your muscles and liver. Basically, both food and stress (via cortisol and epinephrine) raise your blood sugar, and insulin lowers it back down.

This mechanism works with varying degrees of efficacy in each of us. Some of us secrete an appropriate amount of insulin for the meal we eat while others secrete too much initially (hyperinsulinemia) or over time (insulin resistance). When you become insulin resistant, your cells can't heed the message to let sugar in; your body's response is to release more and more insulin because blood glucose still remains too high. Insulin resistance, or hyperinsulinemia, will trigger symptoms after you eat such as getting sleepy, craving carbs, or wanting to keep eating even though you're really not still hungry. When this happens, not only is it hard to control your appetite and cravings, but it also quickly spurs fat storage and hinders fat burning. Some of us are genetically prone to insulin resistance, while others have diet and lifestyle habits (overeating, overcarbing, overstressing, undersleeping) that have created it, and some of us may have both factors going on!

Clearly, you don't want to repeatedly secrete too much insulin by frequently overeating excess carbohydrates or overeating food in general. As we are going to show you in this chapter, the amount and types of carbohydrates you'll be able to eat will differ based on your unique metabolism and genetics. We also want you to be mindful of insulin surges. These surges happen in response to big meals, excess sugar or carbs, or simply repeated blood sugar highs and lows. When these highs and lows occur, your blood sugar gets too high so you secrete a bunch of insulin; it then plummets back down and cortisol is released in order to get it back up—all in an attempt to rebalance your blood sugar but making a metabolic mess along the way.

Why We Need to Get Off the Insulin Roller Coaster

Insulin surges from erratic blood sugar, overeating, over-carbing, and over-stressing trigger inflammation and make hormonal imbalances and autoimmunity (if you have it) even worse. Insulin surges can have exaggerated effects in women who already have female hormone imbalances, such as perimenopausal women or those with PCOS. For these women, a large release of insulin can increase ovarian production of testosterone, disrupting estrogen-progesterone balance and often hindering ovulation and causing a host of nasty symptoms, such as PMS, breakouts, unwanted hair growth (on the lower stomach, arms, face), head hair loss, and irregular menses.

Insulin surges also upregulate an enzyme called aromatase found in body fat that increases estrogen and could cause or worsen estrogen dominance, leading again to greater estrogen-progesterone imbalance and difficulty losing fat. So, as you can see, this is about a whole lot more than just a few sugar cravings!

These larger releases of insulin, for any of the already-mentioned reasons, will increase inflammation, throw your ACES out of whack, and turn on all of your fat-storing mechanisms, ultimately slowing efforts for fat loss.

You may be thinking, "Huh . . . I thought this insulin convo would really only apply to me if I'd been diagnosed with diabetes or maybe PCOS." This is a huge misconception; insulin issues are a spectrum with many shades of gray, rather than a black-and-white lab test diagnosis. Your lab tests may not show high fasting blood sugars or an elevated hemogloblin A1C or another verified marker of insulin resistance, but you do have some degree of insulin trouble if you have any of the following signs and symptoms listed below. In this case you're likely overshooting your insulin's capacity to manage your blood sugar:

- Getting sleepy or lethargic after eating
- Craving sugary or starchy foods after meals (a craving that is not relieved by eating something sweet or starchy)

- Wanting to keep noshing after a meal even though you know you've eaten plenty

- Feeling that your energy is low overall

- Having a difficult time losing weight

- Breaking out, having unwanted hair growth on face or body or losing hair on the crown or temples in cases where insulin is aggravating testosterone such as with PCOS

Finding Your Unique Carb Tolerance

Unfortunately, there isn't one set serving size or exact carb type we can suggest for you that will help you avoid this blood sugar nightmare. That's because you have your own unique hormonal imbalances, and therefore you have your own Unique Carb Tolerance, or UCT. Your job this week is to find your UCT accounting for your own imbalances with cortisol and insulin per the Hangry B*tch Hormone Quiz.

To find your UCT, begin tuning in to the following symptoms of low or high blood sugar after eating each meal:

Symptoms of Higher Blood Sugar/Insulin Resistance
Check for these symptoms within 30 minutes after you eat.

Feeling fatigued, sleepy, or lethargic

Experiencing brain fog or feeling cloudy headed

Craving sweets or starch after eating

Sweets craving not relieved by eating them

Increased hunger after eating

Increased thirst (in general)

Frequent urination (in general, not necessarily after meals)

Symptoms of Lower Blood Sugar/Low Cortisol
Check for these symptoms between meals.

Feeling ravenous

Irritability

Craving sweets

Fatigue, relieved by eating

Blurry vision

Need caffeine to keep going

Poor memory

Light-headed

Shaky

Now that you know what symptoms to look for, you'll have to be a bit of a detective to find your UCT, but the reward is knowing exactly what carbs work best for you and how much you need in order to keep your ACES normalized, maintain your ideal body composition, and/or lose fat, if that's your goal. So, with your best Sherlock Holmes attitude, let's do this.

Pick one allowed carbohydrate (starches/fruits) from the Hangry B*tch Reset Diet list on page 107 and eat approximately ½ cup of it with a combo of protein, fiber, and fat. Here's an example: choose sweet potato as your carb and eat ½ cup along with a mixed green salad dressed with olive oil and vinegar and 25–30 g of chicken breast. Watch for the symptoms listed above immediately after eating, two hours after eating, and as your next meal approaches. If within thirty minutes of eating you feel sleepy or cloudy headed, crave sugar or caffeine, or want to keep munching even though you don't feel hungry, your body is telling you that this was too much of this type of carb for you. To retest, eat the same meal at approximately the same time of day with less sweet potato—say ⅓ cup—and see how you do. For example, if you ate your first test meal for dinner at 6:00 P.M., eat your second test meal of the same foods the following day at approximately the same time but with the lesser amount of sweet potato.

On the other hand, if you find that immediately after the meal with the ½ cup sweet potato that you feel fine, but you become ravenously hungry, irritable, cranky, or light-headed within one or two hours, then that particular amount and type of carb also didn't work so well for you.

How to Adjust Based on Your Symptoms

Post-Meal Symptoms

Right after eating, if you get symptoms of sleepiness, cravings for coffee/stimulants, or cravings for more starches or sweets, try cutting the amount of sweet potato back by half or by at least two bites at the next test meal of mixed greens salad and chicken.

If this doesn't help, add more fiber (one more handful of veggies) and be sure you're getting 25–30 g of protein in that meal. Continue decreasing the carb amount or change carb sources until you find what works best.

Between-Meal Symptoms

One to two hours after eating, if you have symptoms such as cravings, ravenous hunger, irritability, lightheadedness, or crankiness, at the next meal increase your protein and fiber slightly (for example, eat a bit more chicken and a bit more greens) but do not adjust the amount or type of carbs yet.

If these adjustments do not relieve your symptoms, add a touch more healthy fat (olive oil or avocado or a few nuts, for example) to your next meal. If the added fat does not work, then up the amount of sweet potato by two bites at the next meal. Reactive symptoms between meals can indicate low-cortisol issues or reactive hypoglycemia, and we will show you soon how to specifically combat this scenario.

Continue this experiment, eating different types and amounts of starches or fruit from the Hangry B*tch Reset Diet food list. This may seem tedious, but most women find that they get in tune with their symptoms within a few days and can then infer how they will feel for multiple types of carbs based on one carb reaction. We suggest you do these challenges for breakfast and dinner only, and eat just protein and vegetables for your second and third meal of the day. You'll be able to figure out which other meals can include carbs, as well as meal frequency and timing by the end of this week depending on your Hangry B*tch Hormone Quiz answers for low cortisol and insulin resistance.

If you're trying to do this experiment with more processed foods like breads and foods that contain sugar, you'll notice that your symptoms will be more severe, which is why these foods made the "what you won't be eating" category on your Hangry B*tch Reset Diet food list in the first place. However, you'll also notice that you might have some troublesome symptoms after consuming "healthier" carbs as well. For example, while legumes or quinoa are often touted as the best carbs out there, you may not do so great with them. With this in mind, and with the exception of sugar, we want to instill the notion that no carb is really "bad" or "good" but rather that there are some that might not be the best for you and your goals, and since you will likely have some of those "not the best for you" carbs on occasion, we want you to get out of the good/bad model and into the "no one's just like me" mindset. When you're done with this four-week program, and if you're ready and you want to, feel free to add some of the no-go carbs on this plan. Experiment with grains and legumes and see if they actually do work well for you, or if they do not. Remember, this isn't about any one-size-fits-all diet template, it's about teaching you how to know what does and does not work for you and to help you avoid being too dogmatic when it comes to food.

Still Not Sure About Your UCT?

Most women glean a lot of insight with this protocol, with the exceptions of gut infections, inflammation, food sensitivities, and high stress. Even if you haven't 100 percent nailed it in a week, you should at least be close. However, if you feel that you just can't read your UCT symptoms clearly yet or they seem to be sending mixed signals, your hormones may be more out of balance than you realized. If this is the case, it can be hard to get a clear-cut answer based on symptoms alone. This is why telling a woman experiencing significant hormone haywire to "just listen to her body" or "eat intuitively" often doesn't work. Her body may be telling her to eat cupcakes for breakfast and chips, salsa, and a margarita for lunch. Intuitive or not, we know those habits won't help heal your hormones. In time, as you follow this program and your hormones heal, it will get easier and you'll be able to tune in more clearly; don't worry. The end goal

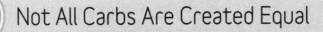

Not All Carbs Are Created Equal

Many women find that the most troublesome carbs for them include anything with a lot of sugar or gluten (bread, pasta, cookies, cakes, muffins, etc.) because of the inflammatory proteins found in gluten and the insulin-stimulating starch component of wheat amylopectin. While these foods are not on the menu in our plan, at some point after you wrap up this program, it's likely that you'll occasionally have some sugar again, including miscellaneous grains and/or legumes, and you may return to gluten-containing foods, at least on special occasions, so be sure to go back to this experiment of finding your UCT to see how your hormones react to these foods, which are often stressful for your body. You may decide that it's not worth going back to some of these foods, even on the rare occasion, based on the severity of your symptoms.

is to be able to use your ACES but if they seem murky and you can't hone in on how to find your UCT, we've got a great tool: the glucometer.

You can get a glucometer online or at your local pharmacy without a prescription (ask, because they are usually behind the counter) or, if you have any documented blood sugar problems or insulin resistance, your doc can write you a prescription and your insurance should cover it. Brands we recommend are OneTouch Ultra and ReliOn.

At first, you will feel like you're sticking yourself all day (because you kind of are), but it won't be like this for long—a week or so usually is sufficient to find your UCT. In fact, you may want to buy only one vial of strips. If you hate poking yourself, get the lancing device that looks like a pen to make it easier. If you don't mind pricking yourself, save yourself the money and just buy a box of disposable lancets. Prick any finger just off to either side of the center of your fingerprint, about a third of the way between fingerprint center and the edge of your fingernail. This tends to be the least painful area, and be sure to rotate fingers so you don't get a sore spot. All good? OK, here's how to utilize a glucometer:

First, check your fasting glucose by taking a reading ASAP after waking; before any food, drink, or exercise; and before you do much of anything at all, because cortisol will raise your blood sugar. It's great to get a fasting reading to better assess cortisol and insulin in the morning as well as to establish your baseline. Ideal readings are from 85–95 mg/dL. Readings above 99 are in the prediabetic range; readings above 120 are in the diabetic range. There is some debate about how low is too low. Conventionally, hypoglycemia is diagnosed at 65, but many people struggle with low blood sugar in the 65–80 mg/dL range, so most functional practitioners use 85–95 as the ideal range. Wherever your range might be right now, don't panic. By sorting out your UCT and getting on top of your blood sugar, you should start to see your readings fall more within the normal range.

Next, check again at the start of each meal. Keep some notes and write down how long it's been since the start of your last meal. By three hours after you should be back below 100 or to your baseline/fasting reading.

You will also check it one hour after the start of your meal; you want it to be no higher than 140 mg/dL. And then again at two hours after the start of your meal, you want it to be no higher than 120 mg/dL. Between meals, if you're dipping below 80, you may be feeling symptoms of low blood sugar, including irritability, ravenous hunger, lightheadedness, cravings, fatigue, or forgetfulness.

To adjust your UCT based on your glucometer readings, start with a test meal such as the example given previously (½ cup sweet potato, mixed green salad with olive oil and vinegar, and 25–30 g of protein). You'll want to either slightly increase or decrease the amount of carbs you eat at your next test meal depending on whether your readings are showing a spike or a drop in your blood sugar. For example, if one hour after a meal you're spiking to 140 or higher, or if after two hours after a meal you're not 120 or below, that amount or type of carb didn't work for you. If this is the case, decrease the amount of carbs by a few bites at your next meal. Furthermore, if your readings aren't back to your baseline (ideally below 100) by three hours after eating, this would be another scenario where you would decrease the amount of carbs at your next test meal. If between meals you're dipping down close to or below 80 be sure to make certain you are eating at least 25–30 g of protein and that you have an adequate amount of fibrous veggies (at least a few handfuls) at your next test meal and consider increasing your carbs by a few bites. Essentially, you will treat a blood sugar reading that was too low between meals the same as you would if you were experiencing the between-meal symptoms as described on pages 151–52, such as irritability, intense hunger, fatigue or cravings, and you will treat blood sugar readings that didn't lower to the recommended ranges the same as you would if you were experiencing the after-meal symptoms as described on pages 150–51, such as cravings, sleepiness or increased hunger. Also be sure to try testing your blood sugar during this experiment with different carb options as well, and remember there are some types of carbs that just don't work for you in any amount.

While you are working on finding your UCT it might be helpful to journal how you are feeling throughout the day so that you can start to see a pattern. Often we are so used to feeling awful that it's hard to correlate our symptoms with our food, so if you can start to take note of specific symptoms throughout the day it's easier to remember what foods or carbs might have triggered what symptoms and take note of any particular patterns. We know this sounds like yet one more thing to do, but after just a couple of days of taking notes, we promise it will be so much easier to get a handle on your UCT and what does and does not work for you.

Here's what we want you to track in regard to your ACES and blood sugar monitoring while you continue on your Sherlock Holmes duty of finding your UCT:

1. How did you feel upon waking? Were you nauseous, starving, anxious? Did you have a low appetite for protein, or a low appetite in general?

2. What did you eat at each meal? It's OK to approximate portions but try to keep a pretty close watch on things; sometimes the difference in being able to really tune in to your UCT will be just a few bites. For example, you might find that butternut squash is just fine if you have

½ a cup, but ¾ of a cup is just enough to tip you over the "blood sugar edge." Counting your bites (for example, three bites of sweet potato or ten bites of an apple) is a very easy, non-measuring sort of way to keep track and thus adjust at your next meal.

3. How did you feel at the start of the meal? Were you ravenous, nauseous, not hungry, a little hungry, or were you having cravings?

4. How did you feel at the end of the meal and for about thirty minutes after? Were you tired, hungry, craving caffeine or sugar, or having brain fog?

5. How do you feel one or two hours after the meal? Were you hungry, tired, or having cravings?

6. How did you feel at bedtime? Did you fall asleep easily, did you wake up several times in the night, and how easy was it for you to fall back asleep?

7. Finally, make a note of anything that feels "off" to you throughout the day; you think you'll remember, but it's so much easier to match it with the symptoms if you have it written down.

Now you are armed with the tools you need to help you tune in to your ACES and get closer to finding your UCT. It may take you more than a week to really nail down your UCT, but we find most women sort it out within two weeks. Finding your carb tolerance will help all your hormones get into better balance because insulin and cortisol have such a far-reaching effect on all the other hormones.

When You Can't Trust Your Cravings

For most women, this experiment is filled with light bulb moments that help them finally figure out how much and what type of carbs to eat. For some, however, their symptoms are not so clear-cut. If you're getting utterly confused because no matter how many of the allowed carbs you eat or don't eat or how diligent you are about using your glucometer to see what your blood sugar is doing and you're still getting some brain fog, low energy, cravings, or other symptoms after eating, here are some things to think about:

Food Sensitivities and Leaky Gut. We mentioned earlier that foods like gluten can lead to increased inflammation in many of us. While the most egregious offenders for inflammation and food sensitivities are not on our Hangry

B*tch Reset Diet at all, the truth is we can get sensitive to pretty much anything we eat frequently, thanks to a disrupted gut microbiome, an unhealthy overall environment, genetics, hormonal issues such as hypothyroidism or chronically elevated stress and cortisol, medications (such as antibiotics or antacids), or autoimmune disorders. When we eat a food we're sensitive to it causes a wave of inflammation that will make us feel like we're in a fog—both in our brains and bodies. We feel tired and sluggish, similar to how we feel when we overeat or overcarb. See page 385 for how to fix that gut.

Gut Infections. Critters such as candida are notorious causes of cravings for sugar and carbs as well as lower energy overall. A possible indication you have a candida infection is a low total white blood cell (WBC) count (less than 5.0 X10E3/uL) with a higher neutrophil and low lymphocyte count on the differential. This pattern can indicate other chronic immune challenges but is very commonly seen with candida. Your doctor can test you for IgG, IgA, and IgM candida antibodies; if these are elevated, it indicates candida overgrowth somewhere in your body. However, if your WBC count is low, testing for candida antibodies can show a false negative, and it may be that you've got a chronic immune issue of various types including both chronic infection and autoimmunity, so be sure to also have your doctor check total levels of IgG, IgA, and IgM as well as candida antibodies. You can also investigate candida with a urine test, looking for D-arabinitol (a waste product of candida), or by doing a comprehensive stool test available from Diagnostic Solutions and Genova, which are functional medicine labs not likely to be ordered with your regular physician. Again, see page 385 to deal with gut infections and leaky gut and see Supplement and Testing Resources on page 382 for more info on testing.

Inflammation and Stress. We already know that these two are hormone messmakers. We'll talk more about stress when we look at modifications you need to make if you came up low or high cortisol on the quiz, but know that your cravings and appetite can be off-kilter due to inflammation or stress and have less so to do with the amount of carbs you're eating. If things don't seem to be making sense as you try to find your UCT, look for signs of inflammation and get tested: ESR and hs-CRP are tests you can get with any doctor. Please note these are not perfect tests and sometimes we see normal hs-CRP and still have inflammation afoot, but it's worth testing. When it comes to stress, this program will do a ton to help you resolve stress, starting with the Five Pillars and throughout the next three weeks as we teach you to manage both low and high cortisol with diet and exercise changes.

Now that you've taken the Hangry B*tch Hormone Quiz and you have the tools you need to work on finding your UCT, it's time to customize your exercise, diet, and stress-management tools.

Start Your 5-4-3-2-1 Program

5-4-3-2-1 5 Walks per Week Plus 5 Minutes of Breathing Work per Day

Hopefully you already have one week of walking five times per week under your belt. If for any reason you didn't implement that habit fully during Week 1, let's do it now. If you found that after taking the quiz you uncovered low-cortisol or low-thyroid issues and after trying five walks last week you felt a little worn out, continue to work on finding a sweet spot that doesn't cause you to overdo it. We want you to move every day, so it's best to adjust by shortening the time that you walk rather than cutting out any days.

As for high cortisol, insulin resistance, and estrogen-progesterone issues, walking is an incredible tool for getting more activity (optimal for insulin resistance) and normalizing cortisol (great for low or high cortisol as well as estrogen and progesterone issues). We really can't encourage the walking enough, or have we? Hah!

The five minutes of breathing work daily stays the same. Remember: this not only helps you get into proper position so that you can do the strength training but also helps avoid a load of aches and pains in the neck, shoulders, hips, and low back. This is also an important part of triggering your parasympathetic nervous system and lowering stress overall. Proper breathing: so simple but so good!

#hangrybitchfix

While we are asking you to do only five minutes of restorative breathing per day, this is one area where more is actually better. For a reminder of how to do restorative breathing, you can find the description on pages 103–04. Remember, you can do restorative breathing in your car at a stoplight, while waiting in line, and by all means when you're sitting at your desk all day! As a bonus, say a mantra while you're doing it and you'll be well on your way to being a Happy Babe!

5-4-3-2-1 4 Meals per Day

In Week 1 we suggested that you eat four protein- and veggie-based meals per day, roughly the same size. This week you're already working on finding your UCT, but you're also going to adjust your meal frequency based on your quiz results. Meals still need to contain loads of veggies, aiming for that one pound per day spread throughout your meals, and 90–100 g of protein is still the minimum to hit each day. Your Hangry B*tch Hormone Quiz results with regards to insulin and cortisol will determine how frequently you eat and at which meals you have your carbs. We have a few suggestions for thyroid and estrogen tweaks as well. Remember the hormone hierarchy on page 145 and if you have multiple hormone issues, always follow suggestions for the most delicate hormones at the top of the hierarchy first. When you come to an adjustment below for a hormone issue you don't have, just skip it.

Low Cortisol

Finding your UCT will help you with low-cortisol issues, and eating four meals a day that are roughly the same size may work perfectly for you. However, since your cortisol response isn't perfect, among your biggest stress battles is keeping your blood sugar up without food between meals and throughout the night. If eating four meals a day isn't working, you can instead do five mini meals that are roughly the same size, still keeping within the guidelines of 90–100 g of protein for the entire day as well as a pound of vegetables. These frequent meals are a necessary part of healing. Fiber is also crucial. Therefore, including vegetables at every meal is an important habit to get into. Furthermore, using a fiber powder, such as cleanse + balance from Better by Dr. Brooke, can go a very long way toward ensuring your ACES are in check.

To manage low cortisol, you will most likely need to eat a smattering of carbs (ones you know work well for you based on your UCT experiment) spread throughout the day rather than eating larger servings at only a couple of meals or skipping them altogether. Start with ¼–⅓ cup, or four to eight bites, of a carb that works for you at each of the four meals (or at three of your five meals).

Another issue with low cortisol is that you may have very little to no appetite in the morning, especially for a protein-based breakfast. We typically do not recommend protein shakes as they are often made from whey (dairy), peas, or rice, which are all no-gos for now. However, a protein shake can actually be a good option here since with low cortisol it's so important that you stay ahead of a blood sugar crash that will ultimately further stress your delicate system even more. So finding a source of protein such as a shake that you can tolerate in the morning, even if not entirely optimal, is better than not eating protein at all. Options that you can try include collagen peptides (while not a complete protein source, they can work for the duration of this program as a shake) and/ or bone broth protein powder. (Relax; it tastes like a protein shake and not like a hamburger!) Alternatively, you can use actual bone broth, homemade or purchased, for an easy-to-stomach protein in the morning while your adrenals are healing and low morning cortisol is resolving. We have help for you in this department with several "breakfast soup" recipes in our Hangry B*tch Food Fix section on page 316. Also be sure to reference our Supplement and Testing Resources or www.sarahanddrbrooke.com for bone broth protein powder and collagen powder recommendations.

With regard to energy and cravings, low-cortisol ladies often are the ones who forget to eat altogether or go too long without eating. You're fine one minute and then all of a sudden find yourself feeling irritable, shaky, cranky, light-headed, nauseous, sleepy, low in energy, or forgetful—basically a Hangry B*tch. By the time you get these symptoms, you've already gotten into a bad spot, triggering stress hormones and subsequent insulin, and now you're on the blood sugar roller coaster.

A major key to your success will be using the strategies we've mentioned such as eating more frequently and having food prepped ahead of time to prevent yourself from getting to the point of getting hangry and turning to foods that you know don't work for you.

Nutrients and Herbs for Low Cortisol

Supplement suggestions for low cortisol include 500 mg pantothenic acid per day plus 50–100 mg licorice root (standardized to 20 percent glycyrrhizic acid) in the morning and possibly at lunch as well. Some people find benefit from doses of licorice root as high as 400 mg but you should not exceed 600 mg per day without supervision or take it if you have hypertension. The other game changer for low cortisol is electrolytes. See www.sarahanddrbrooke.com and our Supplement and Testing Resources on page 382 for our favorite brands.

Our other suggestion for both high and low cortisol is adrenal adaptogens, which help your body adapt to stress by restoring communication between your brain and adrenal glands. These are among our best tools to heal as we're looking to resolve as many sources of stress as we can. These amazing natural compounds can be used if your cortisol is high or low, which is helpful if your symptoms seem unclear or if you haven't had testing to confirm. *Panax ginseng* and *Withania somnifera* are ideal adaptogens for low cortisol.

Panax ginseng (aka Korean ginseng) is ideal for regular exercisers as it helps utilize fatty acids over glycogen (stored sugar), taking a huge load off the adrenals as far as keeping blood sugar normalized. It improves stamina, energy, and performance. You can use up to 3 g per day.

Withania somnifera (aka ashwagandha or Indian ginseng) works very similarly to cortisol itself, making it great for low cortisol and low blood sugar issues. However, because of this it can be too stimulating for some. This herb is also great for the thyroid. The dose is typically 200–500 mg of a standardized herb containing 1.5 percent with anolides, taken once or twice daily.

Low Thyroid

Finding your UCT and honoring any cortisol issues when it comes to meal timing is the first step in fine-tuning what works for you and your thyroid. This is super important because going too low-carb or too low-calorie can decrease your active thyroid hormone levels (T3), and that's the last thing a tired metabolism needs.

Your next step is to manage inflammation, as far and away the vast majority of low-thyroid issues in the Western world are due to an autoimmune issue known as Hashimoto's disease. With this condition your body makes antibodies to proteins or enzymes in the thyroid that attack these parts of you as it would a virus or bacteria. As this attack goes on and your thyroid tissue gets destroyed you will most likely become hypothyroid in time. If that's not enough, the immune system activation when you have these antibodies is enough to produce common low-thyroid symptoms such as fatigue, brain fog, and trouble losing weight—even if your thyroid lab testing is normal. For your thyroid, and this autoimmune issue, one of the best things you can do is heal your gut (see page 385 for our gut-healing regimen) and get clear on which foods are causing inflammation. Inflammation can be both a contributing factor as well as fallout of all autoimmune issues including Hashimoto's. We'll talk more about reintroduction of these culprit foods later; for now, just know this is a case where staying on the Hangry B*tch Reset Diet for longer than four weeks and/or investing in food sensitivity testing might be incredibly helpful.

Another important aspect of thyroid nutrition—one that is rarely talked about but that we've mentioned already—is fat quality and POPs (persistent organic pollutants). These metabolic disruptors accumulate in our own body fat and that of the animals we eat. They have been shown to hinder thyroid function via several mechanisms: decreasing thyroid hormone production in the gland itself, decreasing conversion of T4 into active T3, and increasing the breakdown of active T3 hormone, all in all contributing big-time to a sluggish thyroid. So with low thyroid it's very important for you to be extra mindful of our recommendations around animal fat intake, opting for mostly lean proteins such as chicken, turkey, fish, lean grass-fed beef, and lean bison and keeping fattier cuts of meat to one or two times per week only.

But what about all those "bad-for-your-thyroid" foods you've seen on Google, like broccoli and Brussels sprouts? The old-school adage that the natural compounds, called goitrogens, found in some plant foods will hinder your thyroid is not inaccurate, but it's an unlikely scenario. Goitrogens block iodine uptake into the thyroid, so the theory is solid, but in practicality there's little chance you'd ever eat enough of these foods to hinder good thyroid function. Furthermore, cooking deactivates goitrogens, so a light steam or sauté of your Brassica veggies will also negate any goitrogen issues. The exception here is possibly soy. Someone who drinks a soy milk latte, has soy protein shakes, and eats tofu all day, every day, could possibly eat enough soy to create a goitrogen effect, but if that isn't you, then there's no need to worry, and soy is on the "no" list of foods anyway for this program.

Nutrients and Herbs for Low Thyroid

While there's no supplement that can replace thyroid hormone medication when you need it, there are a few nutrients that can be helpful for a low thyroid. First, be sure your multi or other supplements contain at least 30 mg of zinc and 200 mcg of selenium to boost active thyroid hormone production. You can also utilize ashwagandha, as it has a favorable effect not only on cortisol but also on thyroid.

Another thyroid booster is *Commiphora wightii,* also known as guggul. This herb increases conversion of T4 to active T3. The dose is typically 750 mg daily. If you have Hashimoto's disease, using 1–3 mg of turmeric per day can help lower inflammation and antibodies. And don't forget that a healthy gut is vital for good thyroid function, so be sure you do our gut-healing protocol! See page 385.

With all of the above suggestions, if you're taking thyroid medications, be sure you speak with your doctor before starting any thyroid supportive supplements and get frequent labs drawn if you are using lab testing to monitor their effectiveness.

High Cortisol

Because of the intimate relationship between cortisol and insulin, finding your UCT is key to normalizing both high and low cortisol; however, there are a few tweaks you can make to the recommendation of four meals per day if you have high-cortisol issues.

You may do better on just three meals a day instead of four, but probably won't do well on less than three or on plans like intermittent fasting. This is because the time between meals is essentially a mini fast. Ordinarily that's no biggie—it actually can be a good thing to not be eating constantly. However, when you're in a chronic stress/elevated-cortisol situation, you have less control over appetite and cravings, so you can easily find yourself overeating if you skip meals entirely or go too long without eating. To complicate matters, when you're high cortisol you typically have an exaggerated insulin response to food in general so you should try not to eat too frequently or overcarb either. This high-cortisol and high-insulin combo wreaks havoc on all aspects of your ACES, raises inflammation, and is unfortunately a perfect scenario for fat storage (especially at the belly). Elevated cortisol can make it very tough to fall asleep, so saving your starchy carbs for dinner is usually your best bet as they help lower cortisol so you can more easily fall asleep. We recommend you eat 30 g of protein, some healthy fat, and loads of veggies (think several handfuls) at breakfast and lunch and skip the starchy carbs at these meals. Then have a ½ cup serving or about 8–10 bites worth of allowed carbs (adjust based on your UCT symptoms) with your dinner while opting for a leaner protein choice like chicken, bison, turkey, or fish. This combination will keep both insulin and cortisol happy as well as boost serotonin, thus increasing your chances of falling asleep easier.

Nutrients and Herbs for High Cortisol

Magnesium can help your elevated cortisol and normalize your stress response. Keep in mind that you may need much more than the RDA of 300 mg of magnesium daily to balance elevated cortisol. See pages 29–30 for assessing your magnesium need with testing but consider supplementing with 300 mg spread over divided doses per day, up to about 1200 mg total if you have elevated cortisol. Because chronic stress is inflammatory and can leave you achy and puffy in the morning, omega-3 fatty acids can be very helpful; take 2–6 g per day. Phosphatidylserine is excellent at lowering cortisol, high doses (usually 400 mg one or two times per day) are necessary to achieve this effect. This nutrient should not be taken with psychotropic medications. For high cortisol–related sleep issues (wired at bedtime), try passiflora (mentioned on page 387) and magnolia bark (*Magnolia officianalis*), which is typically taken at a dose of 225 mg at bedtime.

And of course with elevated cortisol, it's adaptogens to the rescue! One of our favorites is rhodiola, which prevents stress-induced catecholamine (adrenaline) activity, benefits the heart by reducing adrenaline-induced arrhythmias, enhances cognitive function and mental fatigue, and protects against the immune-lowering effects of long-term stress. If you get sick frequently when under stress, this baby is for you. The optimal amount is 100–300 mg daily of a product with 3 percent total rosavins.

Stressed-Out Cravings

Cravings go with stress like buttercream frosting goes with cupcakes or ketchup goes with fries. When you're dealing with elevated cortisol and craving those fatty, sugary, or starchy carbs, opt instead for the following hack that uses cocoa powder. Cocoa powder will have a dopamine-like effect in your brain, decreasing the food-seeking behavior by boosting PEA (phenethylamine), and it can really nip those sugar cravings.

Try this: add 1 heaping tablespoon of raw organic cocoa powder to a mug and pour in boiling water. Mix well and sweeten to taste with raw stevia or monk fruit extract. To make it a bit creamier use ⅔ cup boiling water and then top with unsweetened almond milk or just finish your cup with a splash of coconut milk. This works wonders for balancing your chemistry, and it's liquid chocolate—need we say more?

To kill those ice cream cravings, meet your new friend: coconut butter. This velvety goodness with the consistency and taste of frosting makes a great low-carb snack and appeases the creamy/fatty desire for something that can creep up with stress. Try coconut butter packs from Artisana: just knead, tear open, and squeeze out. They are super-convenient—great for travel, your gym bag, and the car. If you're up for something more adventurous, be sure to have this treat on hand: Mix together 2 cups coconut cream or coconut butter, ¼ cup almond butter, and 1 teaspoon cinnamon and, if desired, sweeten with your choice of raw stevia or monk fruit. Line a rimmed cookie sheet or a baking dish with foil, parchment, or wax paper and pour in the mixture; it should be about ¼ inch thick. Put it in the freezer for at least 30 minutes. Cut with a knife or break with your hands into bite-size pieces and keep on hand for those "moments." A little goes a long way with these, so a small bite is all you'll really need!

Holy basil (tulsi) is another great option as it improves a sense of well-being, helps normalize blood sugar, and, like Panax ginseng, can be great for those of us who train regularly, as it increases physical endurance. A good starting place for most people is 300 mg per day spread over a few doses. Finally, Eleutherococcus (Siberian ginseng) also optimizes the function of the HPA axis when under stress. You can take it in capsule form or try ⅛ teaspoon of solid extract one to three times daily. Doses are typically 100 to 200 mg of a product standardized to 0.8 percent eleutherosides. It's best to take eleutherococcus earlier in the day: think breakfast and lunch, and maybe early afternoon as well. Taking it too late can affect your ability to fall asleep. Avoid this if you have high blood pressure.

For adaptogens as well as most herbal medicines, a combination product that blends several together is typically best. For more info on products, see our Supplement and Testing Resources on page 382 and visit www.sarahand drbrooke.com.

Insulin Resistance (and/or Hyperinsulinemia)

Finding your UCT will be job number one, and doing this will eliminate most sugar, starch, and stimulant cravings. But before we go on, note that this is lower down on the hormone hierarchy, and if you have low cortisol or low thyroid, you may have to tweak the insulin resistance suggestions a bit to honor these more delicate imbalances first. If you are OK with cortisol and thyroid, the Hangry B*tch Reset recommendation of four equally sized protein- and veggie-based meals is likely perfect for you. Another option is just three meals instead of four, but your focus should be to not eat too frequently or too much at any one sitting in order to avoid stressing your insulin system. When it comes to carbs, you can get away with a lower-carb diet in general. Remember that you can utilize protein for fuel as it converts to glucose to be burned, so if you go low carb just make sure you're never getting less than that 100 g of protein per day. To avoid going zero carb when you do go low carb, you can opt for ½ cup or an eight- to ten-bite serving of a starchy carb at your dinner meal, skipping those starchy carbs at breakfast and lunch. And with insulin resistance, you simply can't go wrong eating more fibrous veggies. Fiber is an insulin-resistant girl's best friend. Start by adding another handful of vegetables to each meal and see how you fare, and for the times when you can't get in more veggies (travel, low appetite, or an empty fridge), try using a plant-based fiber powder (see Supplement & Testing Resources, page 382, for our fave fiber powder).

Nutrients and Herbs for Insulin Resistance

There are some excellent nutrients that lower blood sugar and improve insulin sensitivity; some of them are as effective as prescription medications. One example is berberine, which can be taken with meals. A typical dose is 200–500 mg per meal. Minerals such as vanadium (100–200 mg per day) and chromium (500–1000 mcg one to two times per day) are helpful, as is the antioxidant alpha-lipoic acid—look for the R form and take

200–600 mg per day. With elevated cortisol, a higher dose of omega-3 fatty acids (2–6 g per day) is helpful for a few months. You can also utilize inositol (d-chiral and myo forms) if you have PCOS. Visit www.sarah anddrbrooke.com and our Supplement and Testing Resources on page 382 for more info and brands we love.

Do You Have Blood Sugar Double Trouble?

If you noticed on the quiz that you have both low cortisol and insulin resistance, we'll tell you this right now: this is perhaps the toughest combination when it comes to managing blood sugar. You will have trouble if you overcarb, undercarb, eat too frequently, or don't eat often enough.

If you find that you have trouble with both lowering your blood sugar (insulin) and keeping it up (low cortisol), meaning you get symptoms after eating but also can't easily go three hours without eating, then you have to manage both of these issues but make sure you follow the hormone hierarchy by honoring low cortisol first. With that being said, four meals a day will most likely be best, and they should all be about the same size. Lucky you; that's what you did during week 1 so you're already halfway there. You may also want to include both the 25g of protein and about three or four bites of starch at every meal—and, again, fiber is your BFF here. It's super important here to be diligent about making sure you are eating veggies (optimally) or fiber powder in conjunction with your protein and fat every single time you eat.

Even with your best efforts with food timing, carbs, and amounts, you will likely need to take some extra steps to control your blood sugar this week:

- Support your adrenals with adaptogens and likely licorice and electrolytes as well, in addition to some basic insulin nutrients such as the balanced+beautiful multi available at www.sarahanddrbrooke.com.

- Get to work stat on addressing all sources of stress, be that lifestyle stress, inappropriate exercise, lack of sleep, being too busy, a bad relationship, finances, or something stealthy like an undertreated thyroid condition, autoimmunity, anemia (borderline or overt), or even chronic infections.

Estrogen-Progesterone Imbalances

You guessed it—finding your UCT will also do wonders for your estrogen-progesterone balance. This is especially true if you have issues like PCOS or if you are going through perimenopause, as cortisol and insulin have specific importance to your estrogen and progesterone issues, which we will target more during Week 4.

For now, we have a few estrogen and progesterone tips for you with regard to food. When it comes to progesterone, you can make the biggest impact by dealing with cortisol problems because progesterone is often the second domino to fall (after insulin) when stress is high. Unfortunately, low progesterone also makes you more stress-sensitive, so it's yet again another hormonal vicious cycle, but the solution is to deal with cortisol issues first. Progesterone is also unfavorably impacted by insulin resistance, as we see in the case of PCOS. Again we'll dig into that more in Week 4, but for now know that progesterone will respond well to you restoring better balance and function to insulin and cortisol.

With estrogen, your biggest nutritional dial movers are fat quality and fiber. Thank goodness we've survived and come out the other side of the fat-phobic 80s, but many of us have swung too far in the other direction and are overdoing fat—especially if we're eating lower-carb. With the resurgence of a higher-fat diet we've upped our bacon and red meat consumption by a whole lot! Of course you need fat for many reasons; it increases satisfaction and provides fat-soluble nutrients (A, D, E, and K). However, not only does fat quickly rack up the calories for many women, but animal fat contains a lot of hormones and endocrine disruptors, so it's worth being mindful.

As we've already mentioned, substances called POPs (persistent organic pollutants) and normal metabolites of the animal's own hormones make their way into our bodies when we eat a diet high in animal fat. This isn't necessarily an issue for everyone or even every woman, but it can be a big deal for some, especially if you are already dealing with estrogen-progesterone imbalance.

So if you have estrogen-progesterone issues, you'll be better able to normalize your estrogen balance; reduce estrogen dominance–related symptoms like PMS, sore breasts, and painful periods; and spur fat loss if you lean toward lower animal fat consumption. Consider eating fattier red meat or bacon just one or two times per week and otherwise sticking with leaner proteins like poultry, fish, bison, and lean pork and keeping your plant fat intake up.

It's also vital to have a healthy gut when it comes to estrogen issues. Problematic bacteria in your gut make an enzyme called beta-glucuronidase, which can disrupt your body's ability to detox and get rid of estrogen and other environmental gunk via the gut. This is one more reason to consider the gut-healing regimen on page 385 as well as sticking to foods that help you balance your hormones and gut bacteria. Taking probiotics with *Lactobacillus* and *Bifidobacterium* and/or eating fermented foods like sauerkraut as well as limiting fattier meats will also help. Finally, we're giving one more big push for fiber. Once estrogen has been metabolized by your liver, it's on its way out via the large intestine, and daily bowel movements are vital to getting rid of those problematic estrogen metabolites completely lest they get back into circulation and act again.

OK, you're well on your way to dialing in and getting closer to being a Happy Babe! Now on to the rest of the Five Habits. This week is heavy on the adjustments to the second variable (the four meals per day, content and frequency) in the 5-4-3-2-1 structure, but now we'll touch on what to do about the other habits.

5-4-3-2-1 3 Strength Training Sessions per Week

This week, continue with your current workout, be that the HB Core+Floor Recovery Template (five times per week) or the HB Hormone Reset Template (three times per week). Next week we'll introduce the HB Strength Training Template and show you exactly how to manipulate it based on your hormone issues.

If this is your second week doing the HB Hormone Reset Template, you'll transition to the HB Strength Training Template next week. If you are doing the HB Core+Floor Recovery Template, you'll stick with this for a full three weeks and then transition to the HB Hormone Reset Template for two weeks before moving on to the HB Strength Training Template. For next week, go ahead and read that chapter and get acquainted with what's coming for you in a couple of weeks with your fitness plan, but don't make adjustments just yet to your workouts. You won't be "behind" on our four-week program: this is a lifelong program, and by taking the appropriate steps to heal, you'll be well prepared when the time comes to lift more and lift heavier. There will be some minor tweaks to the other parts of our 5-4-3-2-1 template during Week 3 that will apply to those of you who are doing the HB Core+Floor Recovery Template, so keep progressing with the rest of the program. Just understand that you won't start the HB Strength Training Template until you complete three full weeks of the HB Core+Floor Recovery Template followed by at least two weeks of the HB Hormone Reset Template.

Is Histamine Hindering Your Hormones?

Histamine is typically associated with stuffy noses and watery eyes, but it's actually a big player in our hormone balance as well. Histamine is an important part of our immune reaction to something like a bee sting, plant pollen, or a peanut. It is stored in immune cells (mast cells and basophils), and when we have an injury or insult, the cell dumps those contents and cause blood vessels in the area to leak, getting important immune cells to the area. This creates the typical swelling and puffiness we see with something like hives or swollen red eyes with allergies. Histamine also causes itching.

It also is an important neurotransmitter in the brain as part of our sleep-wake cycle (this is why some antihistamines make you sleepy), plays a role in how we perceive pain, regulate our body temperature, and keep our hormones balanced. Histamine acts as a neurotransmitter in the uterus as well and appears to play a role in sexual arousal. It is active in the gut, causing parietal cells in the stomach to secrete stomach acid, and it plays a role in intestinal motility.

Histamine intolerance can develop when you are unable to clear histamine or if you're having an exaggerated histamine release in your body. An excessive buildup of histamine can be caused by many things, ranging from infections (chronic viruses or gut issues such as SIBO), overzealous or unstable mast cells dumping histamine too often and inappropriately, or when enzymes that normally clear out histamine from your system are running sluggish. Enzyme sluggishness can be due to genetic variances or any number of epigenetic (lifestyle) factors that have slowed your ability to clear histamine, causing excess histamine symptoms.

For any of the following issues, histamine may be the culprit, and you do not need to have every symptom on this list to have a histamine issue:

Itching

Irritability

Insomnia

Menstrual irregularities (abnormal cycle timing, excessive cramping)

Headaches (more extreme cases: migraines, seizures)

Flushing

Rapid heartbeat

Profuse sweating

Seasonal or food allergies

Urticaria or prickly heat

Exaggerated response to mosquito bites (large, very swollen, very itchy)

Runny nose or bloody nose

Car sickness, motion sickness, or seasickness

Nausea, vomiting, stomach pain, or loose stools

Known gut infections, such as candida or SIBO

Chronic viral issues, such as EBV

GERD or heartburn

Asthma

Chest tightness or shortness of breath

Increased sex drive and libido

Skin issues, including acne, hives, eczema, and psoriasis

Don't worry; you can usually get out of histamine trouble largely by using diet strategies. Visit www.sarahanddrbrooke.com for foods to avoid, recipes, and more info about this increasingly common issue. We've also covered this multiple times on the *Sarah & Dr. Brooke Show*!

5-4-3-2-1 2 Liters (or More) of Water per Day

Whether you are easily drinking enough water or struggling to get it down, you may have noticed that it seems like you pee out everything you put in. If so, electrolytes are a simple game changer; it's a shame they are associated mainly with athletic performance or a hot day at the beach. It's important to start using electrolytes daily, especially if you have high or low cortisol, insulin resistance, PCOS, have histamine issues or nighttime urination, or you notice you are peeing out all the water you consume. You may have heard that Himalayan sea salt in water is useful for adrenal support and low cortisol. While this works for some, most women need a full spectrum of electrolytes beyond sodium, such as potassium. Refer to Supplement and Testing Resources on page 382 for recommended electrolyte brands.

5-4-3-2-1 1 Daily Commitment to Rest, Recovery, and Real Self-Care

Rest and Recovery

If you're rocking bedtime and waking rested and refreshed, don't change a thing. If not, you can probably guess what we're going to say, right? Bump that bedtime up by another fifteen minutes if you're still shy on sleep.

If the Hangry B*tch Hormone Quiz showed that you have high cortisol and you have a hard time falling asleep, be sure you have some carbs at dinner. This will cause an insulin release, which will shuttle amino acids, including tryptophan, into the brain so you can make serotonin and melatonin for better sleep. Also, remember when insulin is high it means fuel is plentiful and cortisol will naturally be lower, so this insulin boost will help to lower high bedtime cortisol. We suggest ½ cup of allowed carbs (but find what works for you within your UCT) at dinner for both high cortisol and insulin resistance. If you haven't employed some of our supplement strategies for sleep (pages 41 and 43) and high cortisol (pages 162–64) do that now.

If you uncovered low cortisol on the Hangry B*tch Hormone Quiz then you will want to be sure that you don't go too long between dinner and bedtime. If you have dinner more than three hours before bed, you may need a protein-based snack close to bedtime. Try making this part of your four- or five-meal-a-day plan. Also, be sure you're having a small serving of carbs with at least three of your meals, including both lunch and dinner.

If you have an estrogen-progesterone imbalance, when it comes to sleep you may be suffering thanks to low estrogen or low progesterone. By all means, address the cortisol issues as well, but see also page 116, where we talked about serotonin and GABA support, because when your female hormones wane, your brain chemicals can suffer. Low estrogen can cause you to have low serotonin, and low progesterone can create a low GABA situation, which can make getting a full night's sleep very challenging.

Real Self-Care

You've been encouraged to add an additional minute to your current mediation practice. So no matter where you started, by the end of this week you will be meditating for at least two whole minutes a day. Two little minutes may seem like a dinky meditation plan, but one of the biggest reasons women don't meditate is time. When it comes to meditation, something truly is better than nothing, and even a few minutes of actually doing it instead of stressing that you can't find a half an hour to meditate is a big win.

We obviously are not going to hold you to adding just one minute; if you're ready, expand your practice of meditation as your schedule allows. Many women find that committing to a solid fifteen to thirty minutes of meditation in the morning can be life changing.

Finally, continue opting out of overwhelm by taking one more thing off of your plate. See pages 120–21 for support.

It's Getting Hot in Here

This week you will be focusing on our third pillar: Full-Engagement Living. We all struggle to be fully present because this kind of presence opens us up to a lot of intense feelings, both good and bad. We can feel discomfort when we are totally "in the moment," and we often want to avoid that sensation even when the moments are good. This week we are going to encourage you, as we say on the *Sarah & Dr. Brooke Show,* to "put your toe into the hot water." What this means is that if you want things to be different, you have to experience all of the feelings that are part of a fully lived life; you have to really feel them. So don't be afraid to put your toe, then your foot, and then your whole self into the hot water and soak for a bit. It's OK to go slow, but know that the sooner you immerse yourself, the sooner you'll realize that dipping that first toe in won't actually kill you and you're safe to climb all the way in, and safe to face whatever it is you might need to face. As you marinate in the uncomfortable, you'll see more clearly how to take the next steps.

As we aim to be fully present and engaged in our lives and with the people we love, the sh*t will come up. The things we can no longer hide from the people we want to be closer to will pop to the surface, so we have to be bravely who we are and straightforward and honest about our perfections and imperfections. In order to be more present and fully engaged, we also have to be totally straight with ourselves. This is harder than it sounds! The amount we tiptoe around, ignore, and flat-out lie to ourselves about what we really want vs. how we actually are in the world is astonishing. It can be painful to look at the truth about what's not working in our lives and our role in it. We aren't saying that other people can't be big jerks (or worse), but our only control in any terrible situation (or any situation at all) is how we choose to react to it.

Start by making a list of where you feel uncomfortable, ill at ease, agitated, annoyed, frustrated, and disappointed in your life. Without placing blame (even if there is plenty to go around), look at who you are being in the situation. Ouch—we know that water is hot! It's OK. We're all human, and the behavior we complain about in other people often looks a lot like (or exactly like) our own behavior. This can sting a bit, but this type of radical responsibility gets you out of complaining mode and right back into a position of power. Guess what? You can always change how you see a situation and how you behave in it—even when other people are still being jerks. Does it make it more fun when they are jerks? Not really, but your head is held up higher, your cortisol goes down, and you feel better about who you are—and that's powerful healing for your mind and your hormones! Also, most of the time those around us are inspired by us being better and step up themselves. Either way, you know you're doing your best, and that helps you relax and spend your mental energy somewhere else.

Having a hard time seeing where you can show up better? Look at the situations that make you want to eat cookies; binge-watch TV; pick a fight with your partner, parents, kids, or friends; drink wine; shop; spend hours staring at Facebook; or punish yourself at the gym so you don't have to think about your life. What are you trying to escape or avoid? There's your answer. We know this is hard, and it isn't talked about much by fitness and hormone experts, but we are going to talk about it a lot. In chapter 2 we illustrated that there are many stressors we are clear on and many we don't even know about. You might not be 100 percent conscious of how stressful it is on your hormones to be in a state of constant agitation, frustration, and unhappiness, but truth be told it is downright exhausting and negatively impacts our physical and emotional health when we are not speaking our truth or not being the kind of person we want to be in the world and when we complain about the same stuff day after day. So take time this week to see where you can put yourself back in the driver's seat in situations and relationships that have gotten into a bad, frustrating spot. Yes, it's getting hot in here, and we know it can be scary, but we promise you that as you get comfortable, just like in a bubbly hot tub, it will start to feel pretty good. Your hormones will thank you for your vulnerability and bravery as you enjoy your new life as a Happy Babe. This is a big one, but we know you can do it.

Marinate in It

We live most of our life on autopilot, with uncontrolled thoughts driven by insecurity and fear bouncing around in our brains. Both meditation and mantras are great tools to get you more conscious, more present, and give you some control over what thoughts occupy your mind. Changing how you think, how you see the world, and how you talk to yourself takes a lot of conscious effort because it's likely that those tapes full of negativity and self-doubt have been playing on repeat since you were a kid. Mantras are an incredible tool to change these tapes into something more loving and helpful. In short, mantras give you the freedom to choose your thoughts rather than be ruled by them. Last week you chose one of the mantras we suggested or created your own, and you may just love it. If so, stick with it! If you haven't found one yet, here are our suggestions for this week:

> I am enough.
>
> I am worth it. (This one may take the edge off the overwhelm you may be feeling as you try to work this plan and find what works best for you and your hormones.)

If you're feeling a little like mantras are too fluffy or that you don't believe yourself when you say them, try this tool, called bridging. Simply be open to the possibility of things being different even though they may not be yet:

> I am open to being joyful.
>
> I am open to the possibility of feeling totally at peace.
>
> I am grateful for all the great things coming my way.

All a mantra needs to do is give you an anchor to what you'd rather be thinking and feeling. This is how you grease a new groove in your brain. Think of it as recording a new tape—one of your choosing. This new tape needs to get a lot of play if it's going to take hold, and that's why we want you to practice full engagement with it. Marinate in it—really immerse yourself in the feeling of what you'd rather feel. We want you to say or write the mantra five times first thing in the morning, five times as you sit down to eat a meal, and five times as you lie down to sleep. But if you really want to get in there and swim in it here's how:

- Set an alarm on your phone to go off on the hour with the mantra.

- Post the mantra on sticky notes around your home or car.

- Change the screensaver on your computer or phone. Or put a sticky note in these places, too!

- Change your passwords online or on your phone to reflect your new mantra.

- Buy yourself a coffee mug or small piece of art that represents your mantra.

- Simply repeat your mantra out loud or in your head as you wait in line, at a red light, or for water to boil. These moments can be a huge gift of time to record the new tape and focus on what you want to create.

More Tools for Being Fully Engaged

Now that you've gotten present to some of the uglier stuff and you're willing to put at least a pinky toe in that hot water, let's move on to some less-painful but still very happy-making ways to practice more full-engagement living. When we introduced this pillar in chapter 3, we mentioned that one of the best ways to be more present and engaged is to look people in the eye when you speak to them. If you're talking with a child, get down on their level. If it's a grown-up, look them in the eye as well, even if they dart their eyes away. This can feel uncomfortable for many reasons, including the fear of really being seen or the fear of what others think of us, or we may be disconnected, thinking about what we'll say next or judging what the other person is saying. Don't worry; we are all judgmental, scared, and unsure of ourselves. It's human nature, but the more we are fully connected with others and ourselves, the more we will be able to let go of all of these things that get in the way of our ability to be fully engaged and present in our own amazing lives!

The next tool is to step away from the cell phone. We've got the world in the palm of our hands these days and it's pretty cool, but it's also made us terribly disconnected from the real people sitting right there in front of us. We know you need your phone for a lot of things, but chances are you spend way too much mindless time on it and miss out on connection and productivity because of it. It will still be there for you to text your kids or sweetie or to pick up that important call or look up a restaurant for dinner, but let's minimize the temptation to get lost in social media or randomly surf the web. Here are some tips for cutting the cord with your cell phone:

- When you need to be focused on work or focused on your family or friends, put the phone out of reach—not in your purse or pocket but in a closet, deep in a drawer, or up on a high shelf. This way, you'll have to go out of your way to get to it.

- Place social media apps on your phone in a folder that's at the back of your phone (where you scroll right several screens to get to it). Label that folder something that reminds you why you're there. For example, on our phones that folder is labeled "What Are You Here to Do?" We are reminded that we are there to share news about our families with those we love or to share tips to live bigger, better lives with you. We are not there to mindlessly scroll to compare ourselves to others, or to engage in any other unhelpful habits that social media can trigger.

- Limit your time on social media in general and be very aware that it is designed to suck you in. Many women find that fifteen or thirty minutes per day is enough to keep them connected to their friends and interests, but not so much that they lose precious time in the real world. If you can't trust yourself, have your partner change your password so that only they can sign you in for your set time. As with any other habit, in time it will loosen its grip on you and you'll actually find it a bit unsettling when you do scroll. It's like when you stop eating a food that's been hurting you even though you enjoyed it—when you eat it again, it might taste good but it just doesn't feel like it's worth it anymore.

Finally, our favorite tool for being more present is to do something each day that can't be undone. We do so much daily that is immediately undone, like laundry or dishes, and we want you to be fully present when you are doing these things. In fact, we encourage you to make these things into a meditation just as we taught you to do the kitchen meditation on page 78. However, when we carve out time to do things that, unlike laundry and dishes, can't be undone we get the peace that comes with being fully immersed in something that we know will linger on. So create, write, draw, learn something new, paint, hug someone, make a memory with your kids or friends, or have a meaningful conversation. Every day, take a minute to create something that lasts—physically or even just in your mind—something that you know can't be undone.

This Week's Tangible Tools

Hopefully your mindset is shifting overall from Hangry B*tch to Happy Babe, but this is real life, and some days, despite your best efforts, you'll find yourself flipping out. To recap from last week, we'll be giving you three of our Twelve Tangible Tools each week. Try them all, keep what works, and disregard what doesn't. Here are the tools for this week:

Mindful Observation. Choose a natural object in your immediate environment and focus on watching it for a minute or two. This could be a flower, a house-plant, an insect, the clouds, a blade of grass, a leaf, a pebble or rock, a tree, the rings of your fingerprint, the veins on the back of your hand, your child's face, or even the stars or the moon. It simply needs to be created by the wonder of nature and not man-made. Just notice it; take it in. Simply relax into synchrony with whatever the object is for as long as your concentration allows. Look at the object with childlike fascination, as if you are seeing it for the first time. Visually explore every aspect of what it is. Allow yourself to be consumed by its presence. Allow yourself to connect with the energy of the object and its role in the natural world and notice how you feel after this exercise. Our guess is that you'll feel a whole lot more peaceful, connected, and alive.

The Flip-Out Mantra. When you feel totally out of control and like a bunch of crazy crap is happening to you all at once, you must remember that you can choose to observe the situation at hand, rather than getting caught up in the crazy and reacting without conscious thought. We are not what is happening to us; we are simply watching what is happening to us, and we can choose to react, how to react, or to not react at all. When you're in one of those moments and you feel scared or anxious and ready to lose it, here's the simplest mantra that will get you through:

Everything is OK.

Or try:

Everything is actually OK.

Or:

I am OK.

And if that feels too intangible, like you can't yet believe that things are OK now, you can use:

Everything will be OK.

Or:

I will be OK.

As you say this, choose to just be with the discomfort, knowing that you don't have to do anything right now, you don't have to react, you don't have to respond. Just let it be. Most important, keep your heart open during these times, even when it's incredibly painful. You can also use the mantra, "stay open" in order to allow the experience or feeling to come through you instead of distracting from it or reacting to it. This will allow you the space to feel what you need to and decide with an open heart and a clear mind how you should proceed.

Act of Kindness. Performing small, kind gestures throughout the day not only diffuses our stress but also contributes to overall better mental health. When you're feeling like life is kicking your butt on the regular, the best thing you can do is get out of yourself and do something kind for someone else. Open the door for someone. Buy the person in line behind you their coffee. Stop at a long-term care facility and drop off some flowers or, even better, stay for a visit. Give someone a compliment. Send a nice text message to your partner or best friend. Whatever else feels good to you in that moment—simple, on-the-spot, random, easy, small—these little gentle nudges of good will help you feel better and more alive. We promise.

Reminder: Check Your Hangry B*tch Scale

ACES are Balanced. Your appetite is not too high or low, your cravings are minimal and well managed, your energy is even and adequate, it's easy for you to fall asleep and stay asleep.

Tolerating Exercise Well, Not Under- or Overtraining. You are not feeling that energy is depleted after exercise or showing any signs of RAMP (reluctance to train, achiness or extreme soreness, moodiness, and puffiness; see page 83).

Feeling Positive and Peaceful Overall. You are using meditation and mantras, choosing a positive perspective more often than not (listening to best friend voice), experiencing little to no stress, anxiety, and overwhelm.

Able to Stay Present in Your Life. You are using meditation, mantras, and third-pillar tools for full-engagement living and you are feeling little to no distraction from the present moment.

Being Who You Are. You are confidently speaking your truth, engaging in activities solely because they bring you joy and help you feel more like yourself.

Aim for a score 5 or less. If you don't achieve it, pull out your tools and take care of yourself. Your health and happiness depend on it.

Week 3

YOUR Perfect Workout, Finally

Welcome to Week 3! This week we'll be customizing the third habit, strength training three times per week, by introducing the HB Strength Training Template. By now you've done at least the walking and either two weeks of the HB Core+Floor Recovery Template or the HB Hormone Reset Template. Where you'll go with your workouts this week will depend on your readiness: unlike most books that include an exercise plan, ours doesn't hold you to a twenty-eight-day or four-week standard.

The truth is that injury, pregnancies, and hormonal imbalances (especially problems with cortisol and low thyroid) place you in a unique spot when it comes to exercise. It is impossible for each woman who picked up this book to need the exact same exercise plan. We believe that exercise is powerful medicine that has to be used wisely—it's very easy to create hormonal issues or turn your current hormone haywire up several notches with the wrong exercise. Unlike most fat-loss plans, which can totally burn you out with low calories, low carbs, and loads of intense metabolic exercise, ours helps you find your perfect balance to heal your hormones first and then, if you want, move the needle toward fat loss. Furthermore, unlike other experts who say that if you're low cortisol or low thyroid you can't strength train or even exercise at all, we are going to *encourage* strength training and teach you how to use exercise to actually heal your hormones.

In chapter 5 we covered the importance of lifting weights, and not the little pink dumbbells (as adorable as they are) but real weights, in a way that moves multiple joints at once (called compound movements). This week we'll guide you to lift safely, and you'll learn how to squat under load, deadlift, bench press, press overhead, and more, with an emphasis on "heavy" and in a rep range designed to get you stronger.

What about the classic bicep curls or tricep extensions? These exercises aren't bad—in fact, you'll see them in our program, as many of these more isolated movements are included as auxiliary work in our HB Strength Training Template—but they sure as heck do not produce the same results if that's all you were to do. When you regularly strength train with the use of compound movements under heavy resistance, you spur more output of testosterone, growth hormone, and myokines that mitigate inflammation, support a leaner body comp, and promote longevity. Win, win, win.

With the HB Strength Training Template, your focus will be on completing the bigger compound exercises. If your hormones allow, you can move on to the part of our template that includes a metabolic circuit using lighter weights and some isolation exercises. Our practical experience confirms what research shows: when done right, these bigger compound lifts benefit even the most hormonally wiped-out and inflamed women because they don't overtax your metabolism or hormones. Instead, our prescribed lifts will spur some very favorable effects to get you on the road to better health and hormone balance. If you are afraid of overdoing it, rest assured that even if you're dealing with the most delicate hormone deficiencies (cortisol and thyroid), you'll know exactly how to exercise the right way for your unique hormonal issues by the end of this chapter.

So Where Are You?

If you've been doing the HB Core+Floor Recovery Template for the past two weeks, stay with it for one more week, then move on to the HB Hormone Reset Template for two weeks. You'll then be ready to begin the HB Strength Training Template, but go at your own pace. You can still follow the rest of the 5-4-3-2-1 habit suggestions for Week 3; simply come back to the HB Strength Training Template when you are ready.

If you have already done the HB Hormone Reset Template for two weeks, you'll start the HB Strength Training Template this week, alternating between two workouts that we will teach you how to create, for a total of three strength training sessions per week. You'll also be given the option of doing cardio exercises tailored specifically for each hormonal issue as well. Just be sure that you're prioritizing your walking and weight lifting before you add additional cardio, as these are the foundations of the health of your hormones.

If you've been doing the HB Hormone Reset Template for the suggested two weeks but feel like you need to continue here for another week before moving on to the HB Strength Training Template, that's fine; there's not a Hangry B*tch Fitness Plan finish line, and we'd rather you feel confident instead of rushing into anything you might not be ready for. In this scenario you will also follow the 5-4-3-2-1 habit suggestions for Week 3 and come back to the HB Strength Training Template at a future date.

Before we move on to the customization of your 5-4-3-2-1 for Week 3, we want to introduce you to our Hangry B*tch Strength Training Template.

The Hangry B*tch Customizable Strength Training Template

We've explained it a bit and hyped it a ton—now we'll finally show you what it is and, most important, how to customize this template for you and only you! You will be able to use this template to create endless workouts; however, we understand that this might feel like a lot of work and seem a bit confusing, especially if you are new to the strength training world. As far as fitness plans go, this one is actually pretty easy to follow compared to some of the more complex plans that are out there, but we know your time is precious, so we have some help for you. You can both create and customize your own workouts from this template based on your Hangry B*tch Hormone Quiz results (instructions to follow), or we have pre-programmed-for-you workouts that are customized for various hormonal issues, which you can find at www.sarahanddr brooke.com.

Again, we encourage you to do three strength training sessions per week, or two at a bare minimum. How long you train and whether you add in metabolic conditioning or other additional cardio will all depend on your Hangry B*tch Hormone Quiz results. You can find the specifics about our HB Strength Training Template on page 279 in our Exercise Templates resource along with pictures and thorough explanations of each movement we prescribe, so be sure to refer there prior to attempting your first workout. For now, we'll show you the template and how to use it and then teach you exactly how to tweak the template for your unique hormonal needs—always honoring the hormone hierarchy of low cortisol and/or low thyroid followed by high cortisol, then insulin resistance, and finally estrogen-progesterone imbalance.

We will also introduce you to our HB Movement Progression Guide (which you will find in its expanded form in the Exercise Templates resource on page 281), so even if you've never stepped foot into a gym, you'll know if you should start with just bodyweight movements or if you are safe enough to move on to dumbbells and kettlebells or the barbell. Finally, we will also teach you how to breathe and brace in order to protect your spine and be in proper alignment to lift, also found in our Exercise Templates section on page 279.

How to Use the HB Strength Training Template and Create Your Workouts

- You will create two different workouts and then alternate between those two, ideally doing three strength training sessions per week.

- You will change your programming every 4 to 6 weeks.

- Be sure to review all the exercise descriptions in the Exercise Templates section on pages 279–308 to ensure proper technique prior to attempting your first workout.

- Always begin your workout with our Dynamic Warm Up (page 258) followed by five or six breaths of Forced Exhalation (page 251), and then appropriately warm up your lifts as described on page 189.

Strength Training Glossary of Terms

Circuit. A system of training where you perform one set of an exercise and then move quickly on to the next exercise.

Rep (repetition). One complete motion of an exercise. If you lift a weight 5 times, you have done 5 reps.

Set. A group of consecutive reps. For example, if you are instructed to do 10 reps for 5 sets; that means you will lift that weight 10 times and that will be one set, then you will rest before you move on to the next set of 10 reps and repeat until you complete all 5 sets.

Workout. A generic term for an exercise session, but for the purpose of this plan a workout is one full series of prescribed exercises. For each phase of your training, which is four to six weeks long, you will be taught how to create two different workouts and rotate between them to get your three workouts in per week.

Your HB Strength Training Template consists of three different sections:

- Section A 5×5 is the heavy-lifting portion of the template.

- Section B is the metabolic circuit.

- Section C is auxiliary strength work.

Each time you work out you will do the Section A 5×5, and then be given the option to do either section B or C depending on your Hangry B*tch Hormone Quiz results.

Section A 5×5

How to Create Your Workouts

A1	A2	A3
Squat (goblet, dumbbell, or barbell)	Overhead press (dumbbell or barbell)	Step-up (bodyweight or weighted)
Deadlift (kettlebell, dumbbell, or barbell)	Bench press (dumbbell or barbell)	Bent row (single arm or barbell)
Weighted glute bridge or weighted hip thrust	Pull-up (assisted or not) or body rows	Static or reverse lunge (bodyweight or weighted)

How to Design Workout #1

- Pick one exercise from each group: A1, A2, and A3.

- A1 stays constant for your four-to-six-week program.

- Alternate between A2 and A3 each time you perform Workout #1.

Example of Workout #1

- A1 squat (stays constant)

- A2 overhead press and A3 step-up (alternate the movements each time you do Workout #1)

How to Design Workout #2

- Pick one different exercise from each group: A1, A2, and A3.

- A1 exercise stays constant for your 4-to-6-week program.

- And again, alternate A2 and A3 each time you perform Workout #2.

Example of Workout #2

- A1 deadlift (stays constant)

- A2 bench press and A3 bent row (alternate the movements each workout)

Here's a chart showing an example of two weeks of programming at the suggested 3 days per week using the two workouts from the selected exercises:

	Monday Workout #1	Wednesday Workout #2	Friday Workout #1
Week 1	Squat 5×5 (A1) Overhead press 5×5 (A2)	Deadlift 5×5 (A1) Bench press 5×5 (A2)	Squat 5×5 (A1) Step-up 5×5 (A3)
Week 2	Deadlift 5×5 (A1) Bent Row 5×5 (A3)	Squat 5×5 (A1) Overhead press 5×5 (A2)	Deadlift 5×5 (A1) Bench press 5×5 (A2)

How to Do Your Section A 5×5 Workout

1. Start with your Dynamic Warm Up and Forced Exhalation.

2. Appropriately warm up your lifts for your selected workout. How to do this is explained on page 189.

3. Begin your 5×5 by performing your chosen exercise from A1 for 5 reps, followed by the chosen exercise from either A2 or A3 for 5 reps. Repeat this rotation for 5 sets, resting as needed between sets. Once you complete all 5 sets of each movement, then you can move on to either section B or C.

Your Section B or C Workout

Now that you have created your two section A workouts, you'll move on to either the section B metabolic circuit or section C auxiliary strength work, choosing which one is appropriate based on your Hangry B*tch Hormone Quiz results.

Section B

Pick one exercise from each column to create a four-exercise metabolic circuit.

B1	B2	B3	B4
Lunges	Dumbbell flat bench press	Lat pull-down	Plank (20-second hold)
Glute bridge	Push-up	Single arm dumbbell row	Side plank (20-second hold each side)
Hamstring curls	Parallel dips (assisted or not)	Seated row	
Skull crushers	Bicep curl	Standing cable row	
Superwoman			

You'll do 8–10 reps of each of the four exercises unless otherwise specified (one from each column) for 3 sets, with little to no rest between. You will choose different movements from each column every time you work out.

For example for Workout #1 you might choose lunges, push-up, seated rows, and plank, and for your next workout you would choose four entirely different exercises from each column, and so on.

Section C

Perform the following exercises for 3–5 sets.

Remember to do these exercises at a normal pace that will not significantly raise your heart rate, with emphasis on technique.

Suitcase carry: 40 feet each way, alternating arms

Bilateral or unilateral glute bridge: 10 reps or 10 on each leg for unilateral

Lat pull-down: 10 reps

Plank hold: up to 20 seconds

From this template you'll end up with three different choices based on how you customize: you'll either do the Section A 5×5 alone, Section A followed by Section B, or Section A followed by Section C.

Here's a two-week sample template of the example workouts. You'll continue to follow this template for 4 to 6 weeks and then repeat the same design but with different lifts from A1, A2, and A3, being sure to continue to change your programming every 4 to 6 weeks.

Week 1

Monday: Day 1 Workout #1: squat 5×5, overhead press 5×5, followed by Section B or C

Wednesday: Day 2 Workout #2: deadlift 5×5, bench press 5×5, followed by Section B or C

Friday: Day 3 Workout #1: squat 5×5, step-up 5×5, followed by Section B or C

Week 2

Monday: Day 4 Workout #2: deadlift 5×5, bent row 5×5, followed by Section B or C

Wednesday: Day 5 Workout #1: squat 5×5, overhead press 5×5, followed by Section B or C

Friday: Day 6 Workout #2: deadlift 5×5, bench press 5×5, followed by Section B or C

Example of Two Weeks of Programming Including Sections B or C

	Monday Workout #1	Wednesday Workout #2	Friday Workout #1
Week 1	Squat 5×5 Overhead press 5×5 *Followed by Section B or C*	Deadlift 5×5 Bench press 5×5 *Followed by Section B or C*	Squat 5×5 Step-up 5×5 *Followed by Section B or C*
Week 2	Deadlift 5×5 Bent Row 5×5 *Followed by Section B or C*	Squat 5×5 Overhead press 5×5 *Followed by Section B or C*	Deadlift 5×5 Bench press 5×5 *Followed by Section B or C*

How to Use an HRV Monitor

If you tend to push hard in life, it can be super challenging to know intuitively when to rest and recover, especially if you have used exercise as your only form of stress management or if you have ever been competitive within the fitness arena. Some of you also might not yet be clued in enough to your body's cues to really be able to listen to whether or not you should train, and then you end up feeling wrecked as heck after a lifting session because what your body really needed was some time walking in the woods or soaking in a hot bath rather than pumping iron in the gym. This is where monitoring your heart rate variability, or HRV, can be a great tool. An HRV monitor basically measures the health of your nervous system and puts the data right in front of your eyes: YES I should train, NO this is a day for rest and recovery, or this is a day for something in between. This can be extremely useful as you work toward balancing your ACES.

An HRV monitor works by measuring the changes in time intervals between consecutive heartbeats. These varying time intervals are indicators of how your body is handling the current demands being placed on it. When you have greater variability between heartbeats, this is an indicator that your body is tolerating or recovering well from stress. When there is lower variability, this is an indication that you are not handling the inherent demands from inputs such as exercise, lifestyle, and/or all other internal or external events that cause stress. In a nutshell, using HRV provides you with some hard data regarding your autonomic nervous system and will ultimately help you understand whether exercise should be on or off the table for that particular day. Most HRV monitoring devices will instruct you to use the HRV device in the morning during a state of rest and will give you a color as an indicator of your current state of health; for example, you will see a green light to train, a yellow light to take it easy if you do decide to go to the gym, or a red light to make it a rest day.

An HRV monitor is kind of like your best friend voice. This cool little device will give you a clear picture of how you are dealing with stress and can help put to rest that Nasty B*tch voice telling you to just push harder.

There you have it! Your own strength training template that you can use for life! We will show you next how to make specific tweaks to the Hangry B*tch Strength Training Template based on your quiz results. Furthermore, we also want you to govern how you approach this template based on how you feel day to day. For example, if there's a day when you feel you can only do the Section A 5×5 exercises—whether because of your low cortisol, low thyroid, inflammatory issues or because you didn't sleep well the night before, you may be coming down with a virus, or are super stressed out for any reason—you can decide to skip Section B or C or decide to not work out at all. On days like this, you could always do only the Dynamic Warm Up or opt for just a walk instead.

Finally, we suggest you heed the advice to take it easy based on your ACES, the RAMP signs, or use a tool such as a heart rate variability (HRV) monitor. By now you may have gotten so tuned in to your hormone signals that you'll be able to easily use your ACES and RAMP to know when to back off and when you need to rethink your diet and exercise. However, sometimes we aren't able to honestly tell ourselves that we need to take it easy, and this is when HRV can be super helpful.

Heavy Is All Relative

We've been repeatedly referring to strength training—especially the 5×5 Section A—as heavy, but please remember, "heavy" is whatever is heavy for you right now. You want to challenge yourself and your muscles, trigger those lean hormones, but still always be able to move with proper form and avoid injury. What we consider heavy in our own personal squat or overhead press may be way too heavy or way too light for you. The point is that you should find what is challenging for you and push yourself to where you're working hard to complete the set but with good form and not in any way that is unsafe. If this style of training is new for you and you're unsure which weights to use and how to even begin to find what's heavy for you, you'll want to do the following:

First, for these Section A exercises—deadlift, squat, overhead press, bench press, and weighted glute bridge or hip thrust—you will need to find your 5-rep maximum weight, with one caveat: if you have never lifted weights before, we want you to first get comfortable with proper technique and form before you start pushing yourself with the amount of weight you are lifting or before you try to find your 5-rep max. See the HB Movement Progression Guide sidebar (next page) for more info.

Once you have achieved enough strength and proper technique to work your way through the HB Movement Progression Guide and you feel confident enough to start challenging yourself with more weight, or if you're already a

HB Movement Progression Guide

If you're new to strength training or unsure if you're ready to move from a bodyweight exercise to a dumbbell- or barbell-based exercise, follow this guide, mastering the first movement listed before moving on to the next. You can find a complete description of the progression with pictures in our Exercise Templates on page 281.

Squat. Air squat (body weight), goblet squat, dumbbell squat, barbell squat

Deadlift. Kettlebell or dumbbell deadlift, barbell deadlift (sumo and/or traditional stance)

Bench Press. Dumbbell bench press, barbell bench press

Overhead Press. Dumbbell press or landmine press (if lacking shoulder mobility), barbell press

Weighted Glute Bridge/Weighted Hip Thrust. Bodyweight bilateral glute bridge, bodyweight unilateral glute bridge, bodyweight bilateral hip thrust, barbell bilateral glute bridge, barbell bilateral hip thrust

seasoned weight lifter, it's time to find your 5-rep max. For those of you who are veterans and already have a good idea of what your 5-rep max is, instead of jumping right into the template, first carefully review the exercise descriptions starting on page 285 to be sure you are using proper technique and that you are breathing and bracing (how to do this properly is found on page 279) during your lifts. You might be surprised at how much faster you'll progress or how much better your lifts might feel by making a few of our suggested tweaks. Remember, we also have video instruction at www.sarahanddrbrooke.com.

Now, here's a general guideline to follow in order to find your 5-rep max. During your first few workouts, you'll determine what your working weight for your 5×5 should be for the following lifts: deadlift, squat, overhead press, bench press, and weighted glute bridge or hip thrust. With whichever lift you have chosen, begin your first lift with a weight that feels comfortable but doable, such as just the barbell or a light dumbbell, and perform a set of 5 with good form. Continue to add weight, whether using a heavier dumbbell or adding plates to the bar, until you feel like you are potentially at the maximum weight for your capability. Your 5-rep max is a weight that you can lift five times with good form but that would be challenging to continue doing while maintaining good form. For example, if you can easily complete 8–10 reps with the weight you are using to do your 5-reps, the weight is considerably too light for your actual working sets. This will give you a strong idea of your starting weight for next time and help you structure your sets for your future workouts. Be sure to keep a notebook and write down your numbers so you can continually keep track of where you're at! Free downloadable templates can be found at www .sarahanddrbrooke.com.

Now that you have a solid idea of your 5-rep max, the next time you work out you'll want to make sure you warm up well for your lifts. Your warm up sets should take place after you do your Dynamic Warm Up and are NOT part of your 5×5 workout, but what you'll do to get ready to perform your actual working sets.

Here are the guidelines we want you to follow for your warm up sets for the following lifts: deadlift, squat, overhead press, bench press, and weighted glute bridge or hip thrust.

How to Warm Up Your Lifts

Start with an empty bar or very light weight as compared to your 5-rep max and perform 1 or 2 sets of 8–10 reps. Add enough weight to be at 50 percent of your 5-rep max and perform 1 set of 6 reps. Next, add enough weight to be at 70 percent of your 5-rep max and perform 1 set of 2 or 3 reps.

Working Weight Percent	Reps	Sets
0 (light weight or empty bar)	8–10	1–2
50	6	1
70	2–3	1

Now you are ready to move on to your actual workout: 5 sets of 5 reps (5×5).

Your first set of 5 reps will be done at 75 percent of your 5-rep max. For your second set, perform your 5 reps at 85 percent of your 5-rep max. For your last 3 sets, perform your 5 reps at 100 percent of your 5-rep max. Rest as needed between sets, but no less than one to two minutes when you are performing your last 3 sets. If you're feeling unsafe either from fatigue or pain, do that last set of 5 back at 75–85 percent of your 5-rep max, and if you feel like you have done enough before you get to your last set of 5 reps, then listen to your body and STOP! This is not set up to be a punishing workout, and as you continue to listen to your hormones talk, it's important to be mindful of those messages. We want you to push yourself but not past capacity or ability, and every day might be different, so pay attention and listen to the feedback from your body on the days you are lifting.

For the exercises in both Sections B and C, keep in mind that the rep range is higher than the 5 × 5 Section A and that you will want to choose a weight that is not so heavy that you are unable to lift it for the prescribed reps but not so light that you can easily do several more than what is programmed.

Progressing with Weight

The whole point of this program is to get stronger, and in order to do so you'll need to continually increase the amount of weight that you lift. A good rule of thumb is to increase the weight of your lifts in the 5 × 5 Section A portion of your workout by 0–10 lbs. every time you lift. This is a safe and effective way to increase the load and thus your strength as well. You'll notice that your numbers in certain movements, like your deadlift, squat, and hip thrust, will go up faster than movements like your bench press and overhead press, which is why we give you the range of 0–10 lbs. to add at each session. You may be wondering why the range option includes 0 if this is supposed to be about progression. Ideally, you'll be adding weight each time you work out, however, we have given the 0–10 lb range because you will find that there will be days you are unable to add any additional weight due to periods of increased stress, lack of sleep, or other inevitable factors. Furthermore, at some point you will plateau with the amount you can add to each lift, and this is when you will want to drop the numbers in your weight down by around 10–15 percent of your current 5 rep max and then work your way back up and likely beyond where you plateaued by using the rule to add 0–10 lbs. each time you work out.

5-4-3-2-1 3 Strength Training Sessions per Week

The next step is to customize the Hangry B*tch Strength Training Template for your unique hormone issues and to make your workout work for you!

Low Cortisol and Low Thyroid

You will create your two workouts and aim to do your 5 × 5 Section A exercises three times per week and choose Section C in addition to Section A on any

How Long Should You Rest Between Sets?

The point of resting between your 5×5 Section A sets is to allow for adequate recovery for maximum output and performance during each set. You may be in a hurry to get that workout done and move on to the next thing, but you'll feel better in the long run, avoid injury, and make more progress in the gym if you honor this system. If you are starting to fail on your sets, it's a sure sign you are not resting enough in between. Here's an example of what we mean by adequate rest:

Perform 5 reps of your back squat. Rest two minutes, and then go back to your next set of back squats. Continue in this fashion until you are finished with your 5 sets of 5 reps of that particular movement. As a general rule for this template, use this rest pattern; however, on days when you are lifting heavier or you feel like you need more rest between sets, listen to your body and make adjustments to increase your rest period as needed. We recommend between two to five minutes of rest depending on how heavy you are lifting and how you are feeling overall.

given workout day if you feel up to it. If three times per week wipes you out, aim for just two times per week. As you heal, you can do the Section B metabolic circuit in place of Section C. Likely the first month or two using this template you'll be doing the 5×5 Section A only, or Section A and C only. However, if your ACES are improving, you have no issues with RAMP, and, ideally, your HRV monitor shows that you're having an optimal stress response, you can switch from Section C to the Section B metabolic circuit. Again, this likely won't happen during your first month or two on the template, and even after you are on your way to healing these two hormones, we still encourage you to take it day by day. Maybe one day per week you're able to do the full workout, Section A plus Section B, but your next session you're only able to do Section A plus Section C or only Section A. It's all good; the most important thing is that you are tuning in to your ACES and finally listening to your body.

You can also continue the five walks per week as you've been doing, but we don't recommend any additional cardio. You don't have the stamina for longer-distance cardio or have the oomph to do high-intensity interval training—and even if you muster up the energy to give it a go, you aren't getting that magic fat loss and longevity brew of cortisol, testosterone, and growth hormone to get the benefits of that intense training anyway! So focus on walking for thirty to sixty minutes (whatever is about five to ten minutes shy of wiping you out) and getting in the heavier lifts the 5 × 5 Section A, with plenty of rest between sets, 2–3 times per week.

Sometimes we need to hear things again so here goes: until your thyroid gets addressed and your stress response recovers, there will be no intense exercise for you, which means no metabolic conditioning. You'll start out with the template, keeping the focus on the 5 × 5 Section A followed by Section C. Continue to check in on what more you can tolerate as you progress—for example, try switching to the Section B metabolic circuit in place of Section C on one or two of your workout days and see how your body responds by monitoring your ACES and RAMP. As you consider adding more exercise, add it in small increments, meaning if you're going to choose the Section B metabolic circuit, just add one set or maybe two, but not four. See how you do and then consider adding more sets the next time or, if it was too much, take some away.

High Cortisol

You will also create two workouts to be done 3 times a week for 4 to 6 weeks. You can do both the 5 × 5 Section A and Section B metabolic conditioning of the Hangry B*tch Strength Training Template. You absolutely can keep the five walks per week, and we highly encourage you to do so! Remember, walking and sleep are your hormone normalizers. When it comes to other cardio, we suggest you avoid longer-duration cardio because it elevates cortisol in isolation of other hormones and you're already high cortisol so there's no need to dump in more. The combo of high cortisol and long-duration cardio can make you extremely catabolic, which means you'll be eating away muscle more than body fat, which is a lose-lose situation. While it's not done in the gym, sleep may be your most important "exercise" when you have high cortisol.

If fat loss is a goal, and if your ACES and HRV are giving you the green light, you can add some short sprint sessions or other metabolic work, but keep those sessions to ten minutes or less (see page 196 for how to sprint). If these sessions really wipe you out, trigger trouble with your ACES, or get your HRV in the red, then you'll need to back off for now as this type of exercise will just perpetuate the stress and inflammation you're already reeling from. Remember: stress and inflammation are the great hormone mess-makers.

Remember that you can be high cortisol and low thyroid, which is a tricky combo. In fact, high cortisol can make you hypothyroid by decreasing con-

Training with Low Thyroid

Low thyroid hormones are a metabolic deal-breaker: without sufficient thyroid hormone, you will continue to spin your wheels at the gym, suffer tendinitis and repeated or non-healing injuries, and further drive yourself into the ground. Because of this, having healthy thyroid levels is crucial for you, not only so that you get the benefit from exercise but also so you can recover from exercise as well as not have exercise become an additional stressor on your system.

Furthermore, if the cause of your low thyroid is Hashimoto's disease (or you have Hashimoto's with normal thyroid levels, meaning you don't need medication), or if you have any other autoimmune issues, there are some very specific considerations you need to make when it comes to exercise. If you don't heed these considerations, you will not tolerate the oxidative stress that comes as a normal consequence of exercise and will end up creating more inflammation and immune activation, thus destroying your tissues by attempting to do something "healthy" like exercise.

Consider supplementing with glutathione or n-acetyl cysteine, anti-inflammatory and antioxidant supplements such as resveratrol and turmeric, as well as mitochondrial nutrients. See the protocol for low exercise tolerance on page 199 and visit www.sarahanddrbrooke.com as well as our Supplement and Testing Resources on page 382 for more info and product recommendations. And be sure you're getting your thyroid adequately tested using the lab guide, free at www.sarahanddrbrooke.com/lab-guide.

version of T4 into active T3 thyroid hormone; by disrupting your gut balance, which conjugates certain forms of T3 hormone; and by spurring creation of reverse T3, which is inactive. In this case, we want you to honor your low thyroid first by sticking with 5 × 5 Section A and possibly Section C exercises two or three times per week and only switching from C to the Section B metabolic circuit as your thyroid symptoms allow. You should absolutely not do any other metabolic or high-intensity training in this case, but of course, walking is your BFF, as is sleep. Remember always to follow the hormone hierarchy (see page 145).

#hangrybitchfix

Don't skimp on your rest, recovery, and meditation time, especially if you are high cortisol. Walking and restorative yoga are excellent for high cortisol. Try to include restorative yoga a couple of times per week—even as little as fifteen minutes will do wonders. Also, with high cortisol, don't miss those five minutes of restorative breathing we recommend daily! Finally, the tangible tool called 2X Out Breathing (page 125) is a great one for high cortisol. This technique will trigger your parasympathetic nervous system and stop the fight-or-flight response—and you can do it anywhere!

Insulin Resistance

As with high cortisol, you can create your two workouts and do both the 5×5 Section A and Section B metabolic circuit exercises as long as you do not also have low cortisol and/or low thyroid. Never forget that hormone hierarchy! Those delicate hormones trump any advice for hormonal issues further down on the list. You can always take it day by day, but in general women with insulin resistance need more exercise and movement than the average girl because it helps normalize their blood sugar and hormones so significantly. But even if you have insulin resistance, you need to listen to your ACES, RAMP, and possibly monitor with HRV. If you're having a tough day, you can keep it to just the 5×5 Section A, possibly coupled with Section C versus opting for the Section B metabolic circuit. When it comes to cardio, as long as you don't have low cortisol or low thyroid, you can benefit from both traditional cardio (kept to no more than forty-five minutes) and higher-intensity intervals and metabolic conditioning or sprint work if you have additional goals such as fat loss. Always stay tuned in, however: Is this working? How are you feeling? How are your ACES? Either way, avoid opting for cardio over the Hangry B*tch Strength Training Template and walking, as these two do indeed give you the most bang for your buck.

Cardio Options If Your Hormones Dig It

As we've already mentioned, cardio (especially on its own) is not the most effective fat-loss tool, and too much of it is indeed hard on you. Cardio can burn some calories, boost serotonin, and exercise your heart and lungs, but hormonally it triggers cortisol without triggering testosterone and growth hormone, which are those lean fat-burning hormones you want exercise to give you. However, done right, cardio can be useful if you are not overdoing it for your adrenals and thyroid AND if you are also weight training.

Depending on your thyroid and adrenals, you'll tolerate various types of cardio, ranging from intense to steady state, better than others. If your hormones allow, here are the two main types of cardio you can consider: short metabolic sessions (high-intensity interval training, or HIIT) and more traditional steady state cardio.

#hangrybitchfix

Among the toughest hormonal conditions to manage when it comes to energy, meal frequency, and carb tolerance is the combination of low cortisol and insulin resistance. We see this very frequently in women with PCOS and women going through perimenopause. In this case, your best way to honor both hormonal issues is by eating every three hours with a few bites of starch, walking five times per week, and doing the 5×5 Section A exercises three times per week coupled with the Section C rather than Section B. Consider Section B only as your ACES and HRV monitoring allow. This is also a strong case for taking both insulin-supportive nutrients and adrenal support such as those we suggested on pages 164–65 and pages 159–60 respectively.

Metabolic/HIIT Cardio

If you are high cortisol or insulin resistant but do not have low thyroid or low cortisol, consider doing one or two short metabolic sessions such as high-intensity interval training that lasts no more than ten to twenty minutes and sprints that are no more than twenty to thirty seconds. Examples include stair, track, or treadmill sprints or sprints on a rower or stationary bike.

To monitor intensity, think WWW: warm, winded, and want to stop. The biggest mistake we see with women thinking they are doing HIIT is that their sprints are longer or not intense enough, meaning they can "sprint" for more than thirty seconds. The sprints we're talking about here are all-out bursts, where you are most definitely warm or hot (both your body and your muscles, meaning you feel a warmth or burning in the muscle), out of breath (winded), and can't keep going for more than thirty seconds (want to stop). You should

How to Sprint

We have three different sprint workout options for you laid out in the following chart. These are designed to get the most out of your sprinting sessions but to also keep you within a capacity that is safe yet effective.

Before you sprint, be sure you are warm! If you do your sprints directly after the Hangry B*tch Strength Training Template, you should be warm and ready to go. If you do your sprints on a day that you are not lifting, be sure to warm up well. Do the Dynamic Warm Up at least twice through as well as a light jog of 200 to 400 meters to prime your body for this type of exertion.

For each of the following sprint workout options, the walk back will be your rest period. When you begin, your first "sprint" should be at about 50 percent maximum effort. Assess how you feel on your walk back, and if you feel recovered after your initial sprint, perform your second sprint at 60–70 percent of max effort, then walk back and perform your third sprint at 70–80 percent max effort. If you are performing a fourth sprint, based on which option you choose, at this point you can sprint at 80–90 percent max effort. Make sure you are recovering well on your walk back and pay attention to how your body is responding. Always stop if something doesn't feel right. You can follow this exact same sprint template using either a stationary bicycle or a rowing machine if running isn't an option for you due to an orthopedic issue or injury.

Sprint Workout #1	Sprint Workout #2	Sprint Workout #3
Sprint 100 m	Sprint 200 m	Sprint 100 m
Walk back	Walk back	Walk back
(Repeat 4–6 times)	(Repeat 3–4 times)	(Repeat 3 times)
		followed by:
		Sprint 200 m
		Walk back
		(Repeat 2 times)

rest between sprints until you feel you can go again and give your all-out effort rather than doing a timed rest.

More Traditional Cardio

If you have insulin resistance but no low cortisol or thyroid issues, you can also do some steady state cardio (thirty to forty-five minutes at 65–70 percent of your maximum heart rate) or paced intervals (longer intervals that are not as fast or intense as HIIT), using rate of perceived exertion as a gauge.

Rate of perceived exertion, or RPE, is a measurement of the intensity of your activity, based on a scale of 1 to 10. RPE 1 is sitting on a couch at rest, RPE 5 is steady cardio where you can easily talk while you move, and RPE 10 is an all-out sprint.

Here's an example: Perform a five-minute warm up followed by twenty to thirty minutes of paced intervals—one minute at RPE 6 followed by one minute at RPE 8, then back down to 6 for one minute, repeated for twenty to thirty minutes. Cool down for five minutes or walk for twenty to thirty minutes afterward.

During this type of training, you're hitting two of the three W's: you're warm and winded, but you don't feel like you must stop. Your RPE will change over time as your health and fitness improve so it's a great tool to fall back on to gauge your ability. It will also change throughout your cycle and even day to day depending on factors like sleep, recovery, inflammation, and stress.

Consider after two weeks adding an additional thirty to sixty seconds to the RPE 8 intervals. So you would do one minute at RPE 6 and then one and a half to two minutes at RPE 8, go back to RPE 5 and repeat for twenty minutes, and then follow it with a cool down and/or walk.

Estrogen/Progesterone Imbalance

For this week you'll simply honor the cortisol, thyroid, and insulin considerations. If you don't have any issues in those other hormonal systems, simply follow the Hangry B*tch Strength Training Template doing the 5×5 Section A followed by the B metabolic circuit as well as the five walks per week. We'll offer some unique estrogen and progesterone caveats next week.

Easy Does It: How to Know When You're Overtraining

You know now that intense exercise is the secret sauce for fat burning, and most of us stress addicts love it! We're talking metabolic conditioning, high-intensity interval training, sprints, etc. When your cortisol is already elevated, however, you can have a tough time coming down from these high-stress bouts of exercise, but we know that some of you are wondering how and when you can get back to that type of training, and we get it.

Until you are no longer dealing with low or high cortisol or low thyroid then you simply have to keep intense training sessions to a minimum, if you do them at all. Most hormonal imbalances in women make us more prone to overtraining because we crave the high, and yet we are further driving ourselves into hormonal disarray with intense exercise. Most at risk are those with low cortisol, low thyroid, and high cortisol. HRV is likely your most accurate tool, but your ACES will tell you a lot as well. When your ACES are out of whack, remember: that's your hormones telling you, "Hey, I kinda hate your diet and exercise plan right now. Can you please knock it off?" So if you're in the low-cortisol, low-thyroid, and high-cortisol camp, this is our final plea to back off on the intense stuff for now until you have healed, really pay attention to your ACES and RAMP, and commit to what works for you right now, which is easy does it.

How to Adjust if Your **ACES** Get Unbalanced from Your Exercise Changes

In addition to HRV, always check in with that hormone talk:

A If your **appetite** increases or decreases, you're likely utilizing more cortisol and you should back down on cardio of any type or decrease the sets in the Section B metabolic circuit (or avoid them altogether). Stick with only the 5×5 Section A, and you can always opt to follow up your 5×5 with Section C if you feel up to it.

C If your **cravings** increase, you're also likely to be secreting more cortisol and need to follow the same recommendations above.

E If your **energy** is getting lower or becoming erratic, you're likely having a problem with cortisol or inflammation, so, again, back down on any cardio and metabolic work. This can also be caused by lowered thyroid or lowered cortisol. In this case, not only should you dial back the metabolic work, but you should also consider adding more carbs or spreading them out throughout your day.

S If you're developing more difficulty falling **asleep**, you may be getting more cortisol output from your training. Consider training earlier in the day and be sure you're having some starch at your dinner meal. Next up, as above, dial back the metabolic work. If you're starting to wake more frequently in the night you may be dealing with tanking cortisol; go back to all recommendations for low cortisol (see pages 190–92).

And don't forget the RAMP signs: reluctance to train, achiness or extreme soreness, moodiness, and puffiness. Both cortisol and inflammation are likely at play. In the meantime, consider this supplement regimen for improved exercise tolerance:

CoQ10: 100–200 mg 1 or 2 times per day

L-carnitine tartrate: 1–2 g per day

Creatine: 1000 mg 1–3 times per day (We recommend creatine magnesium chelate rather than creatine monohydrate for less digestive upset and ease of use.)

Resveratrol: 100–400 mg per day (antioxidant, anti-inflammatory)

Turmeric: 1–3 g per day (antioxidant, anti-inflammatory)

Electrolytes: 1 serving per day

Branched chain amino acids (BCAAs): 5–8 g per day (This amount is adequate for most women. Another guide is 100mg/kg body weight per day spread throughout the day. Taken before or during a workout helps with endurance, while taking them post-workout helps with recovery.)

Glutathione or NAC: Liposomal glutathione: 100–500 mg per day or 300 mg NAC 1–3 times per day (typical doses range from 600–2400 mg per day)

And to adequately support glutathione recycling after it's used as an antioxidant, be sure you're getting 200–600 mg of alpha lipoic acid per day or 200 mg milk thistle per day. Cordyceps is also helpful to support glutathione balance, and we love the cordyceps elixirs from Four Sigmatic. (Save 15 percent at www.us.foursigmatic.com and use code BETTEREVERYDAY at checkout.)

5-4-3-2-1 5 Walks per Week Plus 5 Minutes of Breathing Work per Day

For the five walks per week, no adjustments here unless you feel your ACES or HRV are indicating you need to back down. If that's the case and you are low cortisol or low thyroid and have added heavier strength training, then cut down on walking by five or ten minutes. As for the five minutes of restorative breathing daily: no change there; just keep doing it, especially post-workout!

5-4-3-2-1 4 Meals per Day

No major adjustments to this habit this week. If you're not already there, be sure you're getting closer to finding your UCT and ideal meal spacing. As always, be sure you're hitting that one pound of vegetables daily and 90–100 g of protein daily. If you've got all that nailed down, now is the time to start to branch out with your recipes! Nothing kills a good nutrition plan faster than boredom. Sometimes just a few quick additions to your kitchen tools helps up your "wow" factor in the cooking department and helps you start to enjoy cooking. We love to have a few special items in the kitchen, like a big, beautiful cutting board and, oh-so important, a sharp knife! Nothing is more frustrating than trying to chop vegetables with a dull blade, and using a knife that feels good in your hand while you chop on a gorgeous board really does make a difference! Also, little things like using fresh herbs turns a kind of blah meal into a "heck, yes!" meal.

5-4-3-2-1 2 Liters (or More) of Water per Day

No major adjustments in this habit this week; just keep pushing to get to an adequate amount of water and add electrolytes if needed per our suggestions last week. For a fun way to get your water in—especially if you're still struggling to ditch the sodas or sweetened flavored drinks—try one of our refreshing "spa water" recipes. To make a Strawberry Mint Mojito, combine 1 cup halved strawberries, ½ cup fresh mint leaves, one lime cut into thin slices, the juice of one lime, and 1 cup water in a bowl. Stir gently, lightly crushing the strawberries and mint. Transfer to a 1-quart Mason jar and fill the jar the rest of the way with water. Refrigerate for a day or two—then enjoy! You can use the same method with different ingredients to make a Cucumber Citrus Delight—combine ½ cup fresh basil leaves, ½ cup fresh raspberries, a large orange sliced into wedges, and a small cucumber cut in thin slices in a bowl. Stir gently to lightly crush the ingredients, transfer to a 1-quart Mason jar, fill with water, refrigerate, and enjoy!

5-4-3-2-1 1 Daily Commitment to Rest, Recovery, and Real Self-Care

Rest and Recovery

You guessed it: if you're still struggling to sleep because of hormonal or lifestyle issues, be sure you review the suggestions we gave on pages 38–44, and 116 and address any low or high cortisol issues that are affecting sleep. Also, if you're still having trouble getting your beautiful self into bed so that you're getting seven to eight hours of restful sleep per night, bump that bedtime up again by another fifteen minutes.

New this week, however, we would like you to start to pay attention to your rest days, or days off from the gym, now that your training volume and intensity have gone up. We all need days off, and if you are low cortisol, low thyroid, or high cortisol, these days become even more vital. If you're in the low cortisol and/or low thyroid camp, you need at least one day off between strength training days and maybe even two. Hopefully you can still walk five times per week, but, as always, watch your ACES, HRV, and thyroid lab testing to be sure you're not overtaxing yourself and that you are getting adequate recovery.

To bolster recovery, you may also want to include these habits:

Walking. Yes, we are broken records, and you should already be doing this at least five times a week, but we simply can't stress this enough. In addition to all the other amazing benefits of walking, it also happens to be one of the best tools to bolster recovery. Walking helps with lymphatic drainage; that is, it gets the muscles moving just enough to help remove any toxins or systemic waste from your system. So, in other words, are you feeling a bit inflamed from your workout? Then, you guessed it—WALK!

Epsom Salt Baths. Hot baths are indulgent, they feel good, and a long soak in the tub is a great time to do some meditation, say a few mantras, or read a good book just for fun. And, of course, Epsom salt baths are fantastic for recovery. Why? When you sweat, you're losing some electrolytes, and one in particular that most of us are deficient in happens to be magnesium. So soaking in a hot tub of water with a cup or two of Epsom salts (magnesium sulfate) will help replenish your system with this much-needed mineral. Epsom salt baths will aid in ratcheting down inflammation, relieving stress, and improving circulation, and, as an added bonus, they will soften your skin!

Foam Rolling. Foam rolling is a tool used for self-myofascial release, which helps improve movement by reducing muscular tension and soft tissue adherence that might be limiting mobility and functionality. Foam rolling also helps remove lactic acid buildup in your muscles, which will speed up recovery time and help decrease any muscle soreness—so we encourage you to pair a good foam-rolling session with a nice hot Epsom salt bath, and you will be in recovery-mode Happy Babe heaven! For a video demonstration, visit www.sarahanddrbrooke.com.

Finally, when it comes to recovery and training, we should talk briefly about post-workout nutrition and refueling from your workouts. For most women, a good meal after a workout that has plenty of veggies, 25–30 g of protein and some starch that works for you with your UCT is sufficient. While you will be more insulin-sensitive and tolerate more carbohydrates after a workout, you don't want to eat past your UCT and get symptoms of increased appetite, sugar or carb cravings, or start to feel sleepy. So your post-workout meal may include a bit more carbs than you normally eat, but we encourage you to bump it up slowly and monitor your blood sugar symptoms. This is a time when a protein shake can come in handy, as it doesn't require a lot of digestion and is therefore rapidly absorbed. Just watch that your protein shake isn't made to resemble a fruit sugar bomb, and, as always, honor that UCT. Another tool that can work well for you post-workout is branched-chain amino acids (BCAAs). These unique amino acids will stimulate insulin (and thus lower post-workout cortisol and zip right into those muscles for recovery). We recommend 3–5 g of BCAAs post-workout. Note that if your insulin resistance is significant, BCAAs can up your cravings and appetite, so, as always, listen to your ACES and do what works for you. See our Supplement and Testing Resources on page 382 for our favorite brands or visit www.sarahanddrbrooke.com.

Real Self-Care

This week you can give yourself at least one more minute of meditation time, and by all means keep using your mantras. Hopefully you've been doing your #mantrawalks regularly and have a few gems that make your heart feel at peace when you say them. If you're wanting a few suggestions for this week, let's focus on strength. Try "I am strong," "I am capable," or maybe just "I got this"!

If you're feeling a bit frustrated that you can't do certain exercises you love or that your hormones feel so out of balance, try "I am healing."

At the very least use "I am open to healing" or "I trust my body can heal."

Oh, and to continue to opt out of overwhelm, aim to take one more thing off your to-do list.

Love the One You're with (Um . . . That's You!)

The pillar we'll hone this week is a biggie: Be Your Best Friend. It's time to stop being your own worst enemy, slave driver, and critic and start being your own biggest fan, rah-rah cheerleader, and best friend. This is the perfect time for this pillar with everything we've told you in this chapter about overtraining, overdoing it, and eating or exercising in a way that could get you into trouble with your hormones. Oh, the bad behavior so many of us may have engaged in—especially when it comes to weight loss—when not our own best friend! These behaviors might have led you to treat your body in ways that have had some not so fun consequences such as injury, HPA axis dysfunction, triggered autoimmunity, and a tanked thyroid. You may also have lost your period, and of course there's the emotional fallout. We wish we could wave our magic wand over you and help you find your best friend voice right this very second. We have been right where you might be right now, and we understand how tough it can be to tune in to your best friend voice and well, it simply takes time and consistency to change how you treat and talk to yourself.

Getting in touch with your inner voices, the one that is kind and the other that is more critical, can be tough at first. You know there's a voice telling you some old tired and mean stories about who you are, and there's also one that's more supportive, assuring you that you've got it, but you likely struggle to know which voice you're listening to. Both voices give you advice all day. In fact, they both may have a lot to say about whether or not you should go to the gym today or if you should eat that or not—but their motivation and their tone are very different.

Tune In to the Tone

Your inner critic has a whiny tone and is typically full of excuses and justification, whereas your best friend voice may offer some tough love on occasion but she's calmer, more certain, and doesn't need to defend her advice. It's often easiest to see the differences in the tone of your internal dialogue when sh*t goes down. When you mess up, feel less than, feel frustrated, or flat out fail—what's the convo in your cranium then? We're guessing it's something like this: "I'm such a loser! How did I mess that up? I never learn! I'm lazy/crazy/[insert mean descriptor here]." Or the ever-popular "What the heck is wrong with me?" The real trouble happens next: you believe that voice! This voice you hear is a collection of disappointments, judgments, and fears that become who you think you are, but it isn't necessarily true. It's merely one version of a story you tell yourself about who you are, and unfortunately it's the voice you filter your sense of self-worth through every day. It's simply one perspective you see yourself from, and each moment is a chance to tune in to a different perspective.

So think back to a recent slip up or failure. What did you say to yourself? Now that you're tuned in to that voice, the next time she chimes in, try tuning in to it right in the moment. Rather than getting caught up in your same old story, just observe. Don't try to quiet, change, or avoid that voice. Instead, simply listen. The only way to change it is to get better at identifying it in the moment. Nasty B*tch in there is on repeat. She's been yapping at you with her unhelpful, hurtful jabber since childhood (or at least middle school!), she's smart, and she ain't going quietly. Get good at knowing what her shtick is so, in time, you can opt for a different perspective instead. Let's go back to the example of whether or not you should go to the gym today and see what each voice sounds like. Inner critic, Nasty B*tch voice sounds something like this:

"Yeah, you should go to the gym—you look like crap." (criticizing)

"You don't have to go to the gym today—you worked so hard yesterday!" (justifying)

"You should go to the gym, but not when it's crowded, cuz you'll be the fattest/most uncoordinated/out-of-place/skinny/weak/bulkiest/[insert your Nasty B*tch's fave insult here] person there." (comparison)

"Don't go to the gym. It's too hard, and why should you have to work out so much when so-and-so looks amazing and doesn't even have a gym membership?" (complaining, frustrated with the unfairness)

There are a lot of excuses, justifications, and defensiveness in her tone. There's a lot of engagement in the worst of the misery makers: complaining, justification, frustration with unfairness, and comparison. Do you see it? Sounds familiar, right? Now the best friend voice sounds a little more like this:

"Yeah, let's rock the gym today; your happiness and hormones get such a benefit from it! You're amazing and it's so great to see how strong you're getting. You totally got this."

Or on the flipside:

"You didn't get much sleep last night, and training on empty will not help but rather hurt your hormones. You're not lazy; you're respecting where you're at. It's all good; you're in this for the long haul, not just one workout."

The tone AND the motivation are totally different. The best friend voice has your best interest at heart. She has a reason, but not an excuse or justification. She sees the bigger picture (your overall health and hormone balance) and that you have worth, no matter whether you clock one more workout or not. If you're still struggling to tune in to this new, loving voice or if the critical one is just so darn loud that you can't find the best friend voice, think about how you speak to your child or how a loving mother would speak to you. Or how your real-life best friend treats you; she doesn't show up with a bottle of wine and a box of cupcakes when she knows you're two weeks into the Hangry B*tch Reset, does she? She's cool with joining you for a walk or learning how to do restorative breathing because she's just happy you're taking care of yourself. Or think about how we—Sarah and Dr. Brooke—would speak to you if we were right there with you! You know we'd be all about REAL self-care and a big dose of love. This week, get clear on the voice you tune in to most often and begin the lifelong process of being your own best friend more often than not.

This Week's Tangible Tools

Here are three more tools for those really tough moments. As always, give these a test run and keep the ones that work and leave the rest.

Get Grounded. This tool is so simple and it works. Go outside and put your bare feet on the earth or on the grass whenever you are feeling disconnected, flustered, and overwhelmed by the big stuff. This one act is what our heart and soul crave, and it's something we neglect far too often. Connect to the idea that what is troubling you feels so HUGE in your head but that in the grand scheme of the earth or, better yet, our incredibly expansive universe, whatever the "huge thing" is, it's actually quite small. Michael Singer, author of *The Untethered Soul* and *The Surrender Experiment* says:

> You're sitting on a planet spinning around in the middle of absolutely nowhere. Go ahead, take a look at reality. You're floating in empty space in a universe that goes on forever. If you have to be here, at least be happy and enjoy the experience.

It's not that what's going on in your world doesn't matter or that it's small in its importance to you, but when it doesn't feel like it's the biggest thing in the whole universe, it's more manageable and something you are confident you can handle.

Move It, Don't Lose It. Yes, we've been telling you to not overdo it and that crazy exercise can add to stress when you're already stressed out, but sometimes the right dose of exercise at the right time is exactly what you need to re-focus, regroup, and utilize that adrenaline pump that's inherent in a super stressful situation. This does not replace a workout—it's simply a quick burst of one to five minutes to put that stress hormone to work.

Do 5 quick sets of 5–10 bodyweight squats or push-ups or go outside for a super charged walk around the block. This not only puts your adrenaline to work but keeps you from yelling, eating something that doesn't work for you, or being unkind to yourself, and this quick burst of movement won't tax you or hurt your hormones. It will get you out of fight-or-flight mode and help you regroup your thoughts. You can follow this up with a couple of minutes of restorative breathing and say your favorite mantra to change your perspective.

Question the Truth. So often when we are playing out a stressful scenario in our heads, ruminating and filling in the blanks about what may happen, what so-and-so thinks, what this means about us, etc., we have to remember that all we're doing is writing a story. It's just one possible version of the truth—yet we react like it's the gospel truth handed down from on high.

In those moments when you're future tripping, worried what others think, or otherwise aboard a runaway thought train, use this exercise to get back to reality. This tool is derived from Byron Katie's four questions as part of what she calls The Work. In your mind, speaking out loud or writing it down, ask yourself her four questions:

Is This Thought True?

It may feel true, but is it? After you really look at your thoughts, often you can see holes in your thinking. Be careful not to fill in the gaps with more of the same story; just assess the truth of this thought or feeling.

How Can You Know It's True?

Look for any actual proof that your mental reality is the real world reality for you or anyone else. This is our favorite part of the exercise, because often it feels so absolute and real in our heads but there's little to no actual proof or evidence that you'd bet your life on. Here's an example: "My partner never supports my efforts to eat healthier." That's the thought, but when you look can you find at least one time when they did support your efforts? Or another example: "I'm lazy and I never go to the gym." Have you ever even once gone to the gym? Well, then the thought "I never go to the gym" is actually not a fact, and therefore not the truth.

How Do You Feel/React When You Think This Is the Truth?

This is the moment of yuck, the moment you have to really step into the hot water. You'll get present real quick to how bad it feels, how dysfunctional our behavior can get, how disconnected our actions can be from our true selves, when we believe what's going on in our monkey brain and live as if it's fact.

Who Would You Be, What Would You Do, and How Would You Act or Feel if You Didn't Believe This Thought?

In other words, what would life be like if you let that particular story about this situation, that person, or yourself go? Often it feels a whole lot better and you're reminded that this new version of the story, which is your authentic self shining through, is one you can adopt instead.

To learn more about Byron Katie visit www.thework.com. She offers some powerful stuff that goes very deep, but using just a quick rundown of these four questions can quickly get you out of a mental mess!

Reminder: Check Your Hangry B*tch Scale

ACES are Balanced. Your appetite is not too high or low, your cravings are minimal and well managed, your energy is even and adequate, it's easy for you to fall asleep and stay asleep.

Tolerating Exercise Well, Not Under- or Overtraining. You are not feeling that energy is depleted after exercise or showing any signs of RAMP (reluctance to train, aches and soreness, moodiness, and puffiness; see page 83).

Feeling Positive and Peaceful Overall. You are using meditation and mantras, choosing a positive perspective more often than not (listening to best friend voice), experiencing little to no stress, anxiety, and overwhelm.

Able to Stay Present in Your Life. You are using meditation, mantras, and third-pillar tools for full-engagement living, and you are feeling little to no distraction from the present moment.

Being Who You Are. You are confidently speaking your truth, engaging in activities solely because they bring you joy and help you feel more like yourself.

Aim for a score of 5 or less. If you don't achieve it, pull out your tools and take care of yourself. Your health and happiness depend on it.

Week 4

Female Hormones, Flames, and Fat Loss

This week you'll keep going with the Hangry B*tch Hormone Reset Diet as we help you determine your next steps. For your workouts, you'll also continue on with the HB Strength Training Template, or you'll consider starting it. Or perhaps you'll get on to the HB Hormone Reset Template if you've been doing the HB Core+Floor Recovery Template. As far as mindset goes, of course we'll have more tools for you as we shift focus to the last and perhaps most important pillar: Be Who You Are.

For the past three weeks, the focus has primarily been on insulin and cortisol control with the implementation of our Five Habits. This was intentional because, as you now know, these hormones significantly impact your other hormones. Insulin and cortisol must be on the mend before you can gain much ground with estrogen, progesterone, and, to some degree, thyroid. While you may not have these key hormones totally whipped into shape in just three weeks, if you've been humming along with this plan, you are definitely well on your way to feeling more and more like a Happy Babe. You have also made great strides with one other key player that doesn't get its fair recognition in the hormone conversation, and that's inflammation. Finally, if fat loss is your goal, you've laid an amazing foundation, but we'll give you a few more tips in that department this week as well.

Sexy Steroids

Nothing trumps balanced cortisol, thyroid, and insulin for creating better overall balance with your female hormones, estrogen and progesterone. There's also not much use digging a whole lot deeper into estrogen and progesterone if you are experiencing a lot of inflammation. Fortunately, you are likely dealing with less inflammation since you've been following this plan for the last three weeks. Furthermore, now that you've begun to address insulin, cortisol, and inflammation, you can now apply some unique nuances with exercise that will really help you capitalize on your amazing feminine hormones, estrogen and progesterone.

How to Train with Your Cycle

Let's recap how your female hormones affect your metabolism, starting with your girly anabolic hormone, estrogen. Estrogen is key for healthy bones and lean muscle mass. It also makes you more insulin-sensitive, so you can get away with consuming more carbs with fewer fat-gaining consequences, in addition to increased fat burning and increased muscle gain. Estrogen also keeps serotonin high, helping to keep your appetite level, cravings at bay, and sleep sound. Progesterone, on the other hand, tempers estrogen's proliferative nature with regard to your menstrual cycle and breasts. Without it you become estrogen dominant and your cycles get heavier and more irregular, and you may have more breast swelling and pain with your period as well as increased water retention that last week of your cycle. Progesterone also mitigates some of cortisol's stress effects, including that stress-induced increase in body fat, especially around the waist, and when it wanes you'll likely have more trouble balancing your ACES, particularly just before your period. When it comes to mood and sleep, progesterone is a gem, in part because it supports production of allopregnanolone, a very calming neuro-hormone, but also because it boosts GABA (your chill-pill neurotransmitter).

When estrogen is at its highest, typically days 7 to 14 or the second week of your cycle (sometimes called the Venus week), you can reap the benefits by training harder, doing more metabolic or aerobic exercise, and eating more carbs. This is a great week to push yourself in the gym with bigger lifts and more metabolic conditioning, and if you do push it in the gym, be sure you're fueling adequately for it. This is also the time when you'll fare better with dietary indulgences, as insulin sensitivity is increased and inflammation is lower. While we aren't giving you a hall pass to go crazy with food that doesn't work for you, we are mentioning this here because if indulgences do happen during this week, you'll simply tolerate them better. Estrogen lowers an inflammatory cytokine called interleukin-6, making it an important part of taming inflammation for women. You'll likely notice that this week of your cycle your skin is clear, your mind is bright, and your strength is high. On the other hand, if you notice that headaches, allergies, skin issues, runny or stuffy noses, dark under-eye circles, anxiety, or sleep trouble are worse during this time you may be dealing with histamine intolerance. Estrogen down-regulates DAO (diamine oxidase) enzyme production in your gut (this enzyme digests histamine) thus when it's higher you may see a worsening of symptoms. See pages 168–69 for more info on histamine.

#hangrybitchfix

Venus week is also when you will likely feel the most feminine, the most inspired, and, well, like a total Happy Babe. It's a great time to set up and start really grooving your mindset practices so that they are easier to stick to when estrogen wanes. It's also a great time to work on big projects that require all of your beautiful brainpower, as you'll be at your peak creative ability as well.

As for progesterone, it will be highest during the third week of your cycle, peaking around day 21. During the second half of your cycle, you will be less tolerant of carbs and sugars with a tendency for sugar (glycogen) and fat storage, due mostly to the lack of estrogen rather than the peak in progesterone. This is sort of a cruel joke because we all know that the week preceding our period is when we want all the ice cream. Be careful during this second half of your cycle to keep your wits about you and your ACES balanced, as this will help ease any female hormone–based cravings. During this time after ovulation, known as the luteal phase, which is generally two weeks long, you'll also be more catabolic in general, so intense exercise can be tougher on you, leading to more fatigue, loss of muscle mass, and a hard time with recovery. This is a good time to keep to less-intense training; still walking and lifting, of course, but being careful to not overdo it. In other words, this is generally not the time for HIIT or metabolic conditioning.

Now, all of this advice holds true IF you have a regular, normal cycle with normal timing and rhythm of estrogen and progesterone output. It also only holds true if you are not insulin-resistant, don't have low- or high-cortisol issues, are not hypothyroid or overly inflamed, and are not taking hormonal birth control. Common scenarios where this advice can't really be applied include being under high stress or having HPA Axis Dysfunction, Hashimoto's disease, or PCOS; or if you are going through perimenopause or are postmenopausal.

If you don't have the issues we just mentioned, and provided your other hormones are in balance (always remembering that hormone hierarchy), here's how to vary your training and diet according to your cycle:

Follicular Phase (first day of your period until ovulation, typically days 1–14). This is when you could include some metabolic conditioning (twenty to sixty minutes) or more intense exercise like a spin class or a CrossFit class. You can include some steady state cardio up to three times per week, or if you miss your longer runs or bike rides as well. However, don't neglect or trade these sessions out for your strength training sessions; these should still be done three times per week. If you are using the HB Strength Training Template, you can do both Section A and the Section B metabolic circuit. Nutritionally, consider adding more carbohydrates to fuel the increase in training, using a carb-protein-fat ratio of 40:30:30.

Luteal Phase (ovulation until next period, typically days 15–28). You will want to switch back to a bit lower carbs but bump up your fat and protein. Most women will find during this second half of the cycle that a carb-protein-fat ratio of 30:40:30 or 20:40:40 works best to manage their cravings and avoid weight gain. For your training, you will want to do your cardio-based exercises on the same day that you weight train in order to avoid your cardio being overly catabolic or skip cardio entirely. One option is to do the HB Strength Training Template just as it's laid out with the Section A followed by the Section B metabolic circuit. Another is to finish your strength training with some sprints. You will for sure want to do a walk daily, and avoid longer-distance activity or metabolic conditioning that lasts more than ten to fifteen minutes.

Again, this advice should really only be utilized when you have a normal cycle; that is, you bleed for four to five days, your period regularly comes for you in the twenty-eight- to thirty-day range, and you're testing normal for insulin, cortisol, and thyroid hormones per the quizzes in this book or lab tests. If not, keep sticking with the plan to resolve those hormonal issues.

The Other Sex Hormone

Next we want to talk about the other sex hormone we have yet to mention: testosterone.

Although estrogen is your main metabolic hormone, testosterone is important for you, too. Women absolutely need some testosterone for good energy levels, a happy and motivated mood, a healthy sex drive, healing and recovery, and, of course, for building lean muscle mass and burning fat. Without adequate testosterone, you can also have a hard time gaining or maintaining muscle mass, or healing and recovering from any injuries, as it's an important anabolic hormone.

The cause of low testosterone in women is almost always stress-related. So, once again, addressing cortisol issues will likely be your best bet for boosting your testosterone level to "just right." Another common cause of low testosterone is estrogen dominance, because excess estrogen will increase sex hormone–binding globulin (SHBG) and bind up free sex hormones, rendering them unusable, including testosterone. This means that the pill is pretty darn bad for testosterone because it automatically creates estrogen dominance and sends SHBG through the roof—sometimes indefinitely, even after a woman stops taking the pill. On the flip side, women can get a rebound elevation of testosterone when they come off the pill, creating a lot of breakouts, hair loss, and irregular cycles. Finally, if you are not getting your period due to menopause, hypothalamic amenorrhea, or premature ovarian failure, you are also likely to develop low testosterone and have low estrogen and progesterone, as your ovaries are not producing these hormones anymore and thus everything falls on the adrenals. If you're under any stress, this problem will of course be more pronounced as again resources for steroid hormone production will be steered toward cortisol as a priority. Your body, for better or worse, always wants to keep you alive rather than have a lean body composition, a baby, or a libido.

Not consuming enough calories overall can lead to low testosterone, and so can not eating enough of any one kind of calorie—protein, carbs, or fat. Lack of heavy strength training in your workout plan can also lead to low testosterone. You can bump testosterone with the hormone helper zinc (30 mg per day), adequate vitamin D levels (50–80 ng/dL 25-OH vitamin D on lab testing), and the herb maca (which boosts estrogen, testosterone, and DHEA). You will also want to address any estrogen dominance issues.

Now the opposite—excess testosterone and other androgens—is an even bigger problem. Excess testosterone can increase a woman's risk of heart disease and create a host of not-so-fun side effects, including acne, hair loss, facial hair growth, and trouble ovulating. This can occur as part of worsening insulin resistance or as part of the condition we're about to dive into: PCOS.

Our Prescription for PCOS

PCOS is one of the most misunderstood and yet most common female hormone issues, and it is the number one cause of infertility in the Western world. Like Dr. Brooke, you may know that you have PCOS, or you may have a suspicion but have not received a formal diagnosis because you don't 100 percent fit the criteria, or you've heard our least-favorite comment from your doc: "I'm not going to test for that because you don't look the part." (Sorry about that one, we hope this stops happening—soon.) However, the conventional treatments for this condition are very limited either way: the pill, Metformin if you have significant insulin resistance, and often the unhelpful advice to "just lose weight."

PCOS is a complicated hormonal issue because women with this condition have some degree of insulin resistance, often have excess androgens or are hypersensitive to them, and can have low progesterone and/or anovulatory cycles or HPA axis dysfunction. Women with PCOS also always have higher inflammation in general than women without this condition, and some experts are beginning to think inflammation is the root cause rather than a result of this condition. The vast majority of the time, women with PCOS also have other hormone issues, such as low thyroid, autoimmunity, and HPA axis dysfunction. There are also a couple of conditions that mimic PCOS, such as hypothalamic amenorrhea (typically due to stress, creating nonovulatory cycles, or due to other problems with the hypothalamus or pituitary), adrenal androgen excess, and congenital adrenal hyperplasia (rare). Furthermore, hypothyroidism can also look like PCOS on an ultrasound, with multiple small cysts on the ovaries—which is not to say a woman with PCOS can't also have a low thyroid problem, as many do.

While research is pointing toward inflammation being the root cause of PCOS, experts do not completely agree on what causes this condition, but we do know that genetics plays a role. We've heard this inaccurately described as a lifestyle disease, which is frankly an insult to a woman with PCOS. However, lifestyle factors, including diet, exercise, stress, and the resulting inflammation from not managing these factors, will profoundly impact this condition. As far as diagnosis goes, the guidelines from the Endocrine Society using the Rotterdam criteria for diagnosis mandate the presence of two of the following three findings:

Hyperandrogenism (testosterone, DHT, androstenedione, DHEA-S)

Ovulatory dysfunction

Polycystic ovaries (on ultrasound)

Plus the exclusion of other diagnoses that could result in hyperandrogenism or ovulatory dysfunction.

There is no one definitive diagnostic test for PCOS, but here are some of the findings or symptoms you can have as part of this condition:

Ultrasound to visualize the ovaries (twelve or more follicles on one ovary)

Elevated blood glucose testing or high hemoglobin A1C

Abnormal glucose tolerance testing or insulin level

Elevated lipids (cholesterol, triglycerides)

Elevated androgen testing (testosterone, DHEA, etc.) (Note: Androgen levels are not always reflective of symptoms, as many women with excess androgen symptoms, such as acne, hair loss, or facial hair growth, have normal androgen levels. The issue is that women with PCOS can be hypersensitive to androgens so they can simply get symptoms at lower levels.)

Elevated prolactin

Elevated AMH (anti-Müllerian hormone)

Low day 19 progesterone

High day 3 LH:FSH ratio (often very high in PCOS)

Hypothyroidism (low thyroid can look like PCOS on ultrasound but it's not) or Hashimoto's antibodies (a woman with PCOS has a three times greater risk of Hashimoto's)

Hirsutism (male-pattern hair growth on face, arms, etc.), skin tags, or acanthosis nigricans (patches of darker, thickened, velvety skin)

It's important to remember that not all women with PCOS present with the same symptoms. Furthermore, it's impossible to tell by looking at someone if they have any hormonal imbalances whatsoever, and this is certainly true with PCOS as well. There have been at least a couple of versions of PCOS established, such as the lean type and the heavy type, but we still need better characterization so that more women get the help they need with this complex and common hormonal issue. You may have some of the above symptoms but not all of them, so we encourage you to find a functional medicine practitioner who understands this condition very well or visit www.sarahanddrbrooke.com for more support.

There is also a complex set of hormonal implications stemming from the presence of insulin resistance and subsequent blood sugar problems, cortisol impact, inflammation, low progesterone, and estrogen dominance, as well as excess androgens. Most women with PCOS have multiple hormone issues, ranging from low thyroid to autoimmunity to the myriad female hormone troubles that can come with this condition. Women with PCOS also have multiple manifestations of inflammation that contribute to and worsen both digestion and liver biotransformation or detox abilities, and, you guessed it, this makes all of their other hormonal issues worse.

If you've been diagnosed with PCOS or your hormone quiz results indicated an issue with insulin resistance and estrogen-progesterone imbalance, there are a few special considerations for the Hangry B*tch Reset that will help you get better results:

You Are Stress-Sensitive. Due to both insulin issues, which create blood sugar ups and downs, and low progesterone, you are overall less resilient when it comes to stress. Because of this, you have to really make a commitment to do the things we've laid out in this book, like meditation, sleep, walking, and getting your training just right.

You Are Anabolic. Because of insulin resistance and excess androgens, you are good at putting on muscle and body fat. Even lean-type PCOS women will say that losing even a couple of pounds can feel almost impossible. This gets frustrating if fat loss or avoiding weight gain is a concern. Remember to always honor your UCT and if you also have low cortisol, see page 165 for how to navigate that tough hormonal combo. Finally, if you feel like you are bulking up as you start lifting heavier, rather than put down the weights, you need to dial in your diet, sleep, and stress.

You Need a Lot of Movement. If you have dialed in your stress and sleep, you can tolerate more exercise than most—again, however, honor low cortisol and low thyroid first if you have them. Daily walks are a must. This movement will help you to burn off excess fuel in your bloodstream and improve insulin sensitivity. You do, however, also have to be careful about overdoing it, so be sure you track your ACES and keep going back to the cortisol questions on the Hangry B*tch Hormone Quiz to see how you are doing. If cortisol and thyroid are doing fine, when it comes to fat loss or weight maintenance you will likely do well to include some metabolic training or short sprint–type work as well as some longer-distance cardio one or two times per week.

Your Diet Matters a Lot, Maybe Even More Than for Others. Because you've got two things working against you already—insulin resistance and inflammation—a diet that does not worsen either of these except on the rare indulgence occasion is oh-so important for you. When you do overshoot your UCT, eat something that causes inflammation, or otherwise end up eating something that doesn't work for you in general, you can use exercise to combat it. If you've had a big meal, overdone your carbs, or ordered that second margarita, be sure you get out for a thirty- to forty-five-minute walk. Your muscles will help soak up that extra fuel before it's stored as fat or has a chance to further perturb your blood sugar. This extra exercise after some indulgence is not a punishment for eating but a tool that works for your unique hormonal issues, so this should always be done with the attitude of self-support and love, not regret and shame.

Nutrients that support your PCOS metabolism will include all insulin sensitizers (see pages 164–65), things that address elevated inflammation such as turmeric and omega-3 fatty acids from fish oil, and herbs that support low progesterone and estrogen balance. See the suggestions at the end of this chapter for more info as well as our Supplemental and Testing Resources on page 382 for a recap.

#hangrybitchfix

In a similar vein to walking after a big meal, if you know you're going to indulge in a bigger meal or a celebration, you can get your muscles hungry by doing a workout before you eat. A quick weight or sprint session will also make you slightly more insulin-sensitive after exercise, which means you'll tolerate the extra carbs and calories better. Exercise, when done right, is really your best ally when you have insulin resistance. This is not about "earning a cheat meal" or anything like that, so be sure to keep your head in the game here and don't make this a cycle of exercise punishment for food reward. This is about honoring your unique metabolism and learning to work with it.

When Female Hormones Sputter and Stop: Perimenopause and Menopause

Perimenopause can be a frustrating time for women as their female hormones wane, but diet, lifestyle, exercise, and a few key supplements can really help smooth the transition and can allow you to rock the next phase of life. One of the biggest upsets women face during this hormonal transition is utter confusion about what they should be eating and how they should be exercising, especially when what has worked for them no longer does or suddenly makes their issues worse.

Initially, during perimenopause you are in a situation where estrogen is erratic, progesterone declines, and there's an initial rise in testosterone to pick up the slack. This is when hormonal symptoms like insomnia, hot flashes, night sweats, memory decline, and weight gain are at their worst. As your ovaries produce uneven levels of hormones, it's absolutely crucial that you manage your stress response (the adrenals will drive backup sex hormone production as ovarian production wanes), and you will undoubtedly need to reevaluate your UCT.

As we mentioned earlier in this chapter, estrogen helps you maintain lean muscle mass, burn fat, and tolerate carbs better by aiding in insulin sensitivity, while progesterone helps temper both estrogen and cortisol. What women often notice during perimenopause, because of the loss of estrogen and progesterone, is that they are more susceptible to weight gain and have a difficult time maintaining muscle mass. Many women notice more weight gain around the middle when that was not typical for them before and also notice that intense metabolic training or longer-duration cardio (spin classes, running, etc.) actually make them gain fat when before it helped them lose it—again, particularly around the midsection. In part this is due to worsening insulin resistance thanks to the loss of estrogen. Furthermore, intense exercise is now likely making you feel totally wiped out because of the decline of your two major sex hormones, leaving you more sensitive to all forms of stress, such as lack of sleep, inflammation, blood sugar problems, and of course the wrong kinds of exercise for you.

During perimenopause there is some initial increase in testosterone as well, which can be helpful for mood, energy, and body composition, but it can also cause unwanted issues like sprouting a few rogue chin hairs and problems with acne, and it can worsen insulin resistance, which, combined with waning estrogen, can increase weight gain. In time, of course, when estrogen and progesterone fall after menopause, testosterone will fall as well. But all hope is not lost, and your symptoms can be eased doing exactly what you're doing with this program: honoring your UCT, training with heavy weights, walking, avoiding excess cortisol-triggering types of training, addressing any unique metabolic stressors (such as anemia, inflammation, low electrolytes, and managing stress of all types via rest, recovery, sleep, meditation, and mindset).

Rest assured that you're well on your way to a better perimenopausal experience if you're reading this book in your twenties, thirties, or early forties. If you're already in perimenopause or on the other side, remember these key concepts about your menopausal metabolism:

Super Stress-Sensitive. Daily meditation, keeping up with the Five Pillars, and using our Twelve Tangible Tools and mantras to maintain a positive outlook, as well as ensuring good rest are paramount. You also need to honor your adrenals during this transition so they can nurture your female hormone balance as best they can to support waning ovary production. Adrenal adaptogens are a must during this time, and so is following our suggestions for low cortisol. Be careful with intense metabolic training, and it's likely best to skip the spin classes and long-distance runs altogether. Daily walks are vital, as they add that magic movement without perturbing your increasingly sensitive hormonal balance.

More Carb-Sensitive and More Insulin-Resistant. Even if you are not diagnosed with insulin issues on lab testing, you can utilize the insulin resistance suggestion on pages 164–65. In fact, following the low cortisol plus insulin resistance recommendations on page 165 is the best place to start for menopause. Of course, you should tweak your carbs or exercise as needed, using your ACES to guide you.

Less Anabolic. You are losing both estrogen and testosterone during this transition, so you're going to want to trigger growth hormone and as much testosterone as you can with heavy weight training for both bone density and muscle mass. Using the HB Strength Training Template will serve you well here, as will making sure you get enough protein.

Higher Inflammation, Tanking Thyroid. With the loss of estrogen, it's typical for women going through perimenopause to have increasing inflammation. This is also a common time for the thyroid to go kaput and for digestion to become totally off, in part due to an increased cortisol response or waning thyroid. Be sure you're addressing any sources of inflammation and that you have a healthy gut (consider the protocol on page 385), and get a thorough thyroid panel to catch any issues there as early as possible.

#hangrybitchfix

Aging can be a really emotional process for women; we lose so much of what we may have identified with in our younger selves and can feel an intense pressure to cling to youthful ideals. Maybe we miss having beautiful lush hair, smooth skin, a sharper memory, perky breasts, or a more hourglass figure. Or maybe we feel the sting of our children growing up and becoming more independent, or we feel a pang of jealousy around the new crop of younger women in our careers. If you're experiencing the changes that come with both time and declining female hormones, it's fine to mourn the loss of that. Honor and love the body that's changing now and pay respect to the woman you've been. Next, remember we're all headed to the same place—forty and beyond—right? (If we're lucky!) Don't sweat the gray hairs and changes in body shape but rather relish them as the next phase in your journey as a woman. Women experience such rich, wonderful, varied chapters throughout our lifespan, and while change can feel scary and stressful, much of this is remedied with a change in mindset. Honor the woman you've been and embrace the woman you are now thanks to who you were in your younger years. There will be new and wonderful things during this next phase in your life, different but equally as amazing. One of them is finding it easier to be who you are, this week's pillar!

Estrogen-progesterone imbalance is an area where natural medicine really shines. Here are a few suggestions to help you get into better balance:

Taking zinc 30 mg per day will help all of your sex hormones—estrogen, progesterone, and testosterone—be more balanced.

Utilize 300–1200 mg of magnesium per day. (We prefer magnesium glycinate, for its added calming effect.)

For estrogen dominance, nutrients such as DIM (di-indole-methane; 200 mg per day) can be helpful, as can overall support hormone detoxification, including glutathione or n-acetyl cysteine, methylation support (folate, B12, etc.), vitamin B6 (50–100 mg per day), and, again, our fave: turmeric (1–3 g per day). Green tea can also be used for estrogen-detox support; you can drink 4–8 cups per day or take green tea catechin supplements (200 mg per day). If you tend toward constipation, you can utilize calcium d-glucarate to aid in scooting estrogen metabolites out (1000–1500 mg per day). And be sure you're eating sulfur-containing vegetables such as onion, garlic, and all the brassicas (broccoli, cauliflower, Brussels sprouts, kale, etc.).

Low or fluctuating estrogen can be tempered with phytoestrogen herbs such as black cohosh (80–100 mg once or twice daily).

Low progesterone can be bolstered with chaste tree (aka vitex), typically given from ovulation (around day 14) until the start of the next period, in doses ranging from 200 mg or more per day.

For hot flashes, you can use a *Rheum rhaponticum* extract called ERr 731. We like Estrovera from Metagenics (4 mg per day) or Herb Pharm Rhubarb extract.

And, of course, take adrenal adaptogens and blood sugar support as needed. See our Supplement and Testing Resources on page 382 and www.sarah anddrbrooke.com for more info and products.

Fan the Flames If Necessary

Remember that inflammation is the biggest hormone mess-maker, and its effect may be more pronounced if you're perimenopausal, have estrogen dominance issues already such as fibroids or endometriosis, or have PCOS. So if your hormonal symptoms do not seem to be resolving after working this program for the last three weeks and implementing all of our suggestions, it may be wise to look at inflammation as the issue. Quick reminder about the hormone mess-making effects of inflammation: it disrupts the hypothalamus and directly impacts the HPA axis, which is the command center that orchestrates the brain and the glands that make hormones, including thyroid, ovaries, and adrenals. Because of this central control impact, inflammation can create problems with ovulation signals and menstrual irregularities or worsen existing hormone irregularities such as having PCOS and during perimenopause.

All hormones are affected by inflammation; thus, it can show up as a host of different symptoms related to all of the hormones we've taught you about:

High cortisol, as well as inflammation itself, is a significant stress, which causes more stored sugar release and thus insulin surges, and yes, more inflammation, creating a vicious cycle of cravings, sleep issues, weight gain, and further hormone imbalances

Blood sugar dysregulation via insulin and cortisol troubles make it difficult for you to manage your unbalanced ACES, and unfortunately excess glucose and fatty acids in the blood will also trigger more inflammation (another vicious cycle)

Low thyroid symptoms such as fatigue, weight gain, brain fog, hair loss, and menses issues

Low testosterone symptoms, such as low libido, depression, poor wound healing, and lower metabolism

Low estrogen symptoms, including low libido, loss of muscle mass, a host of cycle problems, and infertility

Low progesterone symptoms, including PMS, spotting, extended cycles, anxiety, sleep problems, water retention, miscarriages, and fertility problems

All of the above may occur even when your hormone test results are normal because even though you might have enough of a certain hormone, inflammation is hindering that hormone's activity. But rest assured that by following our plan, you're well on your way to managing inflammation through these important steps:

Get enough sleep, rest, and recovery.

Manage all sources of stress.

Balance your blood sugar.

Eat a diet that works for you in terms of blood sugar and low inflammation.

Exercise—not too much and not too little.

Avoid trans fats and processed seed oils.

If by this point on your journey to becoming a Happy Babe you feel like you have the program dialed in but you're still feeling inflamed, it may be time to employ these tips to topple inflammation:

Supplement with omega-3 fatty acids from fish oil, not flax oil. Many women, certainly those with insulin resistance, can have trouble converting the essential fatty acids in flax into the necessary omega-3s,

EPA, and DHA because of a sluggish delta-6-desaturase enzyme, so skip the flax oil and opt for fish oil. During high inflammation, higher doses are needed, so try 3–6 g per day for a few months.

Assess and treat any chronic infections (such as Epstein-Barr virus or CMV, cytomegalovirus) or gut infections (such as candida or SIBO) and be sure you've adequately healed your gut, which we've found doesn't always happen simply by avoiding common inflammatory foods. Again, see page 385 for our gut-healing regimen and our Supplement and Testing Resources on page 382 for testing info.

Consider food sensitivity testing with Cyrex Labs. Food sensitivities can be a source of stress caused by taking antibiotics, antacids, or NSAIDS; or due to a leaky gut; or genetics.

Look into histamine intolerance if you have not already. See pages 168–69 for more info.

Consider taking a broad-spectrum digestive enzyme (see Supplement and Testing Resources for options). Improve digestion in general by taking five slow deep breaths before you begin your meal and making sure that you are not wolfing down your food (taking twenty minutes to eat each meal is a good gauge). Even with these habits, you may have less-than-optimal functioning of your vagus nerve, an extremely important nerve that triggers digestive enzyme output and gut motility. (This can happen as a result of low thyroid, a head injury such as a concussion, or for other reasons.) You can stimulate the vagus nerve by singing, laughing, gargling, and gagging yourself—unpleasant but effective!

Turmeric is an amazing spice that you can include liberally in your food; however, if you have significant inflammation, a supplemental dose is warranted (1–3 g per day). Other potent herbal anti-inflammatories include boswellia, ginger, and resveratrol.

Antioxidants and bioflavonoids, such as pycnogenol and EGCG (found in green tea), are also beneficial.

Systemic enzymes can help "munch up" inflammation in your system and reduce your symptoms. These are taken between meals; see Supplement and Testing Resources on page 382 for brands we love.

Glutathione and glutathione recycling nutrients. See Supplements and Testing Resources for specifics, page 382.

Note to Our Hypothyroid Ladies

If you are dealing with low thyroid, you likely are also dealing with Hashimoto's disease and inflammation is a big issue for you. If this is you, you will be doing worlds better following this program, as we've tackled inflammation and stress from pretty much every angle. However, it's worthwhile keeping these considerations in mind:

You may need to stick with a longer-term low-inflammatory diet. It will probably be better for you to continue to avoid certain foods, such as grains and dairy, beyond the duration of this four-week program.

Healing your gut may be something you need to do occasionally versus just once, as you are prone to leaky gut as well as food sensitivities, and this creates a vicious cycle of inflammation.

You might benefit from the help of a qualified functional medicine practitioner. This is a case where you'll be well on your way with our program but may need some professional guidance to get you the rest of the way there.

What If You're Still Tired and Hangry?

You likely picked up this book initially because you felt tired and wiped out and were in an all-out fight with your hormones. As we've shown, inflammation can be a major culprit in your lack of energy, mental fogginess, and all manner of hormone troubles. We have helped you address inflammation and hormone imbalances with this plan, but if you are still experiencing symptoms, you may need to take things a step further and get some testing done. See our Supplement and Testing Resources on page 382 for more info and grab the free lab guide at www.sarahanddrbrooke.com/lab-guide.

Finally, Fat Loss

This was never intended to be another diet book or fat loss plan but rather a program to help you lower stress, regain your energy, and get you—and your hormones—happy again. However, something that can be very stressful for women is to not feel at home in their body, so we wanted to offer some help here as well. But first, a quick reminder: fat loss is not worth it if done in a way that makes your hormones hate you. The fallout is a more sluggish metabolism and hormone haywire that gets harder and harder to resolve the more you punish your system. It's seriously just not worth it to trigger an autoimmune condition, tank your thyroid and adrenals, wreck your gut, ramp up inflammation, lose your period—or your sense of well-being for that matter.

Anything done in the name of fat loss needs to be done with love. Read that just one more time, please. What we do to shed body fat needs to be done with the spirit of nourishment, not punishment. There is no ideal body type, just the one that represents the healthiest, happiest version of you. What we want for you from here on out is to view fat loss as something that you will do not to be "less" but rather to be more of the you that's already more than enough.

Fat Loss Versus Weight Loss

Before we get into the "how" of fat loss let's cover the "what." Losing body fat is not the same as losing weight, which can be water, muscle, or fat. What we want to do, of course, is make sure any weight that's coming off is primarily fat or excess water. The scale alone simply can't track this. There are several daily factors that will change the number on the scale, such as the amount of carbs you consume and your water consumption, as well as hormonal changes throughout the month. Furthermore, the impact of stress, sleep, and inflammation will also change that number, leaving you uncertain as to what variables of your plan you need to adjust. Because of these reasons, using the scale as your only fat-loss tracking tool is not only inefficient, but it can also be super frustrating and misleading.

Daily weigh-ins are a sure way to keep that Nasty B*itch in your head telling you what a slacker you are instead of allowing your best friend voice to encourage you and support you along your journey. If you absolutely feel that you need to keep using the scale as a way to monitor progress, we urge you to weigh yourself every four to six weeks instead of every single day, and never forget that the number on the scale is simply a measure of your relationship to gravity and not your worth.

In an effort to lose weight, you've probably done a lot of wacky things to your body already, which has wreaked havoc on you hormonally and metabolically, and although you've probably lost weight before, you've also most likely gained it all back, and then some. When you do a super restrictive and calorie-deprived diet coupled with crazy amounts of very intense exercise, your weight loss will almost always include some loss of muscle mass. When you eventually fail on said diet because your body is begging for you to feed it and stop running yourself ragged, you gain back all the weight, which means less muscle than before and even more body fat.

With that being said, losing body fat in a healthy manner does not result from a quick fix or a "lose thirty pounds in thirty days" diet. Your body, hormones, and thought process *must* get healthy first before your system will feel safe enough to lose any unwanted fat. This is yet another reason that measuring your progress on a scale on a day-to-day basis is seriously a bad idea, especially because we are asking you to lift weights, which will most definitely increase muscle. As we mentioned in chapter 5, when you start strength training there is a period of time when you might lay down some muscle before you start losing fat, which can translate to perceived fat gain. The number on the scale will reflect this and that Nasty B*tch in your head will tell you you're failing because of a number on a little flat box, when actually you are finally on your way to sustainable fat loss.

So instead of the scale, or in addition to it, we want you to use some different ways to track your progress. Taking measurements, for example, can be a very useful tool. We suggest you measure around your belly, making sure the measuring tape is placed right at the level of your belly button, take hip measurements, bringing the tape around the widest part of your hips. You can also measure your upper right thigh and the bicep area of your upper right arm in a relaxed state. When you initially take your measurements, take them first thing in the morning before you have eaten and not after a night of drinking alcohol or eating more sugar or carbs than usual, after a weekend of travel, or after a night of poor sleep. When you retake your measurements, make sure you do so under the same conditions you took them the first time and on the same day of your cycle if you're having one, and give yourself at least four to six weeks in between your measurements.

If tracking with measurements seems too daunting, then skip it and simply pay attention to how your clothes fit and how you see yourself in pictures but NOT the mirror. We tend to look in the mirror and see the same old thing we've always seen (which is why doing those mantras while you are getting ready in the morning is such a fantastic idea), but often we can see ourselves differently when we see ourselves in a picture.

Finally, if you heed our advice of ditching the scale for daily weigh-ins but you do end up weighing yourself after your first four to six weeks on our plan and feel like a failure because of the number you see, we invite you to not flip out but first assess how you feel on the plan and what else has changed for you. Are you feeling better? Have your ACES all improved? Are you less of a Hangry B*tch and more of a Happy Babe? Do your clothes fit a bit better? Are you happier? If you can answer yes to these questions, then you are progressing just fine! Remember how long it took you to get to the place where you needed the advice in this book and honor the fact that it might take your unique, wonderful, and special body awhile to decide it's in a safe enough space to lose fat, and that's OK! You are getting healthier and happier by the day, and that's what life is truly all about.

OK, now that you've stepped away from the scale and your mindset is ready for a sustainable and healthy approach to fat loss, we want to chat with you about how to use your ACES as a guide to make adjustments to the Hangry B*tch reset specific to fat loss.

ACES All Good and Losing Fat

Great! Don't change anything until either variable changes. We know you love seeing results, but this is where some women begin to want to cut food back or dial the exercise up to get even more results. However, this inevitably backfires, so don't give in to the temptation! Instead, experiment with new recipes to keep it fun but keep your carbs, protein, and fat intake the same so you get continued success without getting bored. Keep up with daily monitoring of your ACES and adjust as needed.

ACES All Good and Nothing Happening OR Losing Weight but Not Losing Fat

Remember, weight loss could be fat, muscle, or water. To ensure you're not losing muscle, using a body composition scale such as the InBody Body Composition Analyzer is your best bet. If you don't have access to InBody you can use a home body comp scale such as those from Tanita. While home body comp scales are typically not as accurate as professional analyzers such as InBody, if you use the same scale and be sure you're testing under the same conditions (same cycle day, well rested, not overly stressed or dehydrated due to alcohol or travel) it's still a step up from just the scale. To nudge things in the right direction, add 5–10 g more protein per day (which may mean cutting carbs or fat back a bit) in case the weight loss is muscle loss and add 5–8 g or 100 mg/kg of body weight of branched-chain amino acids (BCAAs) per day. Watch for your ACES to change unfavorably and become less balanced, and if they do, stop the BCAAs. Make sure you are managing your stress levels and getting adequate sleep. Also, consider blood work to assess nutrient deficiencies, inflammation, and thyroid function.

ACES All Good and Gaining Fat

Your hormones are happy, but your metabolism isn't yet on board. Check in with compliance to your UCT, low-inflammatory foods, and stress and sleep. Keep track of how many food items you have per week (or per day) that aren't working for you. Count individual food items such as one cocktail, one glass of wine, one dessert, or one serving of any food you know inflames you and decrease the frequency of these.

You may also want to consider whether you have additional food sensitivities or a source of inflammation you haven't tracked down. You can also try to nudge things by decreasing starch or fruit and/or fat intake, keeping protein intake the same, and boosting fiber. You may benefit here as well from 3–5 g of post-workout BCAAs. Also pay attention and make sure you are not overtraining or lacking in the sleep department. Gaining fat might be one of the first things you notice if you are overly stressed and too often triggering a cortisol response, so be sure to pay close attention to your ACES in this scenario.

ACES Out of Whack and Gaining Fat

Again, check your compliance to your UCT, and look at food sensitivities, inflammation, sleep, and any new, worsening, or unresolved sources of stress. Ensure you're getting 100 g of protein daily—possibly consider an additional 10 g, heeding all the low/high cortisol and insulin suggestions you've learned so far and making sure you are eating that pound of fibrous veggies daily.

ACES Out of Whack and Losing Fat

This is either due to an increase in some sort of stress or you've stumbled upon a "diet" where you're undereating and/or overexercising. Avoid the temptation to do a happy dance that you're losing fat and be grateful that you know enough about listening to your hormone talk to catch this early, because the hormonal backfire is just around the corner. So before this "diet" catches up with you and your willpower, check in to see if you are undercutting your UCT or increasing stress from exercise. Increase your protein by 10 g daily (or be sure you're at the 100 g daily minimum) and boost your fiber a bit. Next, take a look at how stressful your workouts are and consider dialing down the intensity, while keeping the heavy weights and walking going.

When Cortisol and Insulin Start Being Bad B*tches

One of the toughest fat-loss hormonal combos is high insulin and high cortisol. In chapter 7 we told you that short-term, immediate-release cortisol helps with fat burning. It does this by revving up the enzyme that releases fat from a fat cell called hormone-sensitive lipase (HSL). However, when cortisol is chronically elevated, it will crank up your main fat-storing enzyme, lipoprotein lipase (LPL)—and insulin does this as well. Also, when insulin is elevated to a large degree it blocks cortisol's fat-burning effect on HSL. Long biochemical story short: high stress (high cortisol) and high insulin (exceeding your UCT, overeating, or having unmanaged insulin resistance) together put you in big-time fat-storing mode.

Meditation, managing stress from all sources, and a positive mindset will all help lower elevated cortisol, but if you're prone to overexercising as means of trying to lose weight, be mindful of these hormonal interactions. This is especially important if you also have insulin resistance or for any reason you are eating excessively, which we all tend to do when we're stressed out!

There You Have It—Fine-Tuning for Female Hormones, Inflammation, and Fat Loss!

But whether or not you have any of those particular issues; this is Week 4, ladies! As such, we now have all the necessary adjustments to the Five Habits and your mindset insights for the week, so here goes.

5-4-3-2-1 5 Walks per Week Plus 5 Minutes of Breathing Work per Day

We have no specific adjustments for these habits but we hope we've made the case for walking when it comes to supporting your adrenals and thyroid, working with your insulin resistance, and especially if you're dealing with low estrogen and progesterone or inflammation. Walking remains one of your best hormone-normalizing tools! As for the breathing, at this point it has likely improved your posture and oxygen flow, which will continue to help your progress and health in the gym and has improved your digestion and your stress response overall. Both walking and restorative breathing will lead to better hormone balance and being more of a Happy Babe.

5-4-3-2-1 4 Meals per Day

By this week you should have made adjustments to this variable, whether that means moving to three meals or to five meals per day to honor your cortisol issues. We hope you're clear on your UCT by now as well and that you're armed with more information about how lower estrogen and progesterone can affect your insulin and cortisol. We also hope that if you're still struggling to find what works for you with your meal timing and carb consumption, you're able to resolve that this week.

Also, as you enter post–Hangry B*tch and new Happy Babe life, know that your UCT can change. For example, with perimenopause, as your estrogen wanes you become more insulin-resistant and less carb-tolerant so you likely need to adjust your carb intake. With this hormonal transition or with any new stress that arrives, you may also notice that your ACES change and you need to adjust both your UCT and your meal timing. Yet another challenge that can arise is a new food sensitivity—especially if it's a food you eat nearly every day or if you have an unhealthy gut or a low thyroid. So always continue to listen when your ACES get out of whack or you aren't getting the same results with your current plan. Your hormonal landscape as a woman is different throughout the month and certainly through the seasons of life. Simply don't ignore your hormone talk and you'll be just fine! Knowing exactly how to adjust your diet, exercise, and lifestyle to continue to work with your hormones and not against them is so empowering, and now you have the tools to do just that.

5-4-3-2-1 3 Strength Training Sessions per Week

If you've been doing the HB Core+Floor Recovery Template, this week you'll start the HB Hormone Reset Template and you'll be doing it three times per week for three weeks. If you decided last week to stick with the HB Hormone Reset Template for one additional week, you'll transition to the HB Strength Training Template now; see Week 3 for how to use that template. If you're a week into the HB Strength Training Template, you'll keep going, alternating between your two workouts for four to six weeks, and then you'll return to the template and create two new workouts that you'll use for four to six weeks—and on you go!

5-4-3-2-1 2 Liters (or More) of Water per Day

There are no adjustments to the amount of water this week, but we want to mention the importance of drinking out of glass or stainless steel over plastic. Plastics leach powerful estrogen-mimicking compounds, and we are literally awash in a sea of plastic these days. Be mindful of not only your drink and food containers, but also how often you grab a plastic bottle of water. These seemingly innocuous substances found in all of our plastic sources have significant hormonal impact, and they abound in our modern world. We are exposed to plastic-based estrogen mimickers and endocrine disrupters everywhere, from our plastic water bottles to our shampoo to our food supply. It really does add up, and compared to the other stuff we've asked you to do, how hard is it to get a new water bottle and food storage containers?

5-4-3-2-1 1 Daily Commitment to Rest, Recovery, and Real Self-Care

Rest and Recovery

You totally know what we're going to say, but we'll say it anyway: if you have still not managed to get a full seven to eight hours of restful sleep, bump that bedtime up by another fifteen minutes. If you've tried all of our sleep suggestions to no avail, it's time to get yourself some customized help from a qualified functional medicine practitioner, as you know by now that lack of sleep is a hormonal deal-breaker if there ever was one.

Real Self-Care

We hope that by now you are meditating at least three minutes a day, but we suspect that you've added even more. This week, add at least one more minute, and we'd suggest that for the long haul you begin to shift to a daily meditation practice no shorter than ten minutes. The benefits are too great to ignore.

As for your mantras, if you're loving the ones you're doing, there's no need to change them. If you struggle to remember to say them, be sure you get into the habit of saying them first thing in the morning, before each meal, and last thing before sleep. If you want to try out some new ones, here are our suggestions for this week:

I am enough. OR I am more than enough. (We personally like the latter!)

I am happy to be who I am.

I am proud to be who I am.

I am safe to be who I am.

I am grateful to be learning who I am.

Finally, continue to opt out of overwhelm by taking something off your plate.

Coming Home to Who You Are

All of these mantras go nicely with the last and perhaps most important pillar in lowering your stress and finding your joy: Be Who You Are. In chapter 3 we encouraged you to make a list of things you used to love but haven't made time for since life got in the way. So pull that baby out, and if you didn't make the list yet, do that now!

We understand that you might not have written that list because you can't even think of one thing to put on it. You might feel disconnected from who you are outside of your many roles—mother, teacher, daughter, wife, sister, friend, employee, boss, breadwinner, head of family, or other hats you might be wearing in your life.

Whether you remember something you used to love or have to find something new, you need to find those things that make you YOU! It may be that you love to play an instrument but haven't touched it since you were in high school or that you feel more like yourself when you spend time in nature. The answer is simple: dust off that old piano or make sure you go on hikes (or at least sip your morning tea out on your porch). This is about hobbies and play. They are not a means to an end. You may love your new washing machine and it may indeed make life easier; you may even break into a smile when you see it after living with an old, unreliable machine for so long, but the new washing machine is still a means to an end—getting the laundry done. What we really want for you here is not about getting things done; it's about doing things simply because they bring you joy, fill you up, and allow you to feel the peace that only being who you are can give.

Remember, whatever it is you love to do or think you may love to do, it has to bubble up to your Top Five priority list. It's how you live a more complete version of you, in full expression of who you so uniquely are. In the end, we believe that not living in the full experience of who you are is a cause of chronic stress and, if ignored, can result in hormonal disruption as well as depression and anxiety. However, if you're very far from who you truly are, it can also be stressful getting back to it—or finding it for the first time. It will feel like it doesn't quite fit, like you're six years old walking around in Mom's heels. It will feel disorienting and can create some pushback from the people in your life. Some of them may not like you breaking from the norm they grew to expect from you. In fact, when you choose to be more of who you truly are, this may trigger them to realize how far they are from their true selves. Please know that it's not your job to help them understand, but maybe you will be an example and inspire them to take the leap as well. Or if you rock the boat and notice that people start falling off, that's OK, too. The people you need to have in your life will hold on tight and support you as you wiggle, nudge, rock, and roll your way to being exactly who you are supposed to be. Finally, for those in your life who need a bit of a clue as to what you are up to, here's a hint: simply give them a copy of this book.

As you start finding your voice and your authenticity, use these tools to guide you:

Be Unapologetically Who You Are. Count how many times you say "sorry" in a day. We bet it nears the double digits for most of you. Save "sorry" for when it's truly warranted, and that's when you've done something you shouldn't have. You should not be sorry when you don't want to eat something with gluten in it if it doesn't work for you. You for sure shouldn't be sorry for guarding your time for self-care. No more saying "sorry" for expressing your truth. In fact, practice saying "pardon me" or "excuse me" instead of "sorry" when you bump into someone. It's such a ubiquitous part of our vocabulary that it turns many of us into a walking apology.

Take a Compliment. This comes on the heels of saying "sorry" less, as so many times we get a compliment and immediately defer the compliment by making excuses for how we should've shown up even better. Consider this: someone tells a new mom three months postpartum how great she looks. She responds with, "Really? Oh gosh, I had hoped to be back in my pre-baby jeans by now. I'm having such a hard time working out cuz I'm so tired and the baby is so fussy" . . . and on and on she goes, when the best response is simply "thank you!" How you show up—especially when it comes to how your body looks—needs absolutely no apology. Post baby or not, too often we receive a compliment and then just "sorry" all over it. Practice simply being gracious and not apologetic; this simple adjustment will help you start to shine brighter. When you deflect a compliment, you just reaffirm your own negative self-image, but when you are open to receiving kindness and compliments from others, you'll notice that what you project out into the world looks kinder and more complimentary as well, so let that light shine!

Loosen Your Attachment to What Others Think. We know, it's ingrained in women to be aware at best and paralyzed at worst by what others think. This keeps us from doing exercises at the gym we may fumble with at first, because we'll look silly. It keeps us from giving our opinion because, "Yikes, what kind of woman will they think I am if I say that?" It keeps us in a million ways from living in full expression of who we are because we fear judgment, ridicule, pain, argument, upset, or hurting someone's feelings. However, you can rest assured that if your actions come from a kind heart and respectfully being who you truly are, there's no need for you to feel guilty or manage another person's response to your truth. So be kind, compassionate, and honest, but be you. Second, while some people will give you their two cents about what you think or what you're doing, most people are actually so worried about what you're thinking about them and aren't even noticing what you're doing! It's human nature to feel concerned about what other people think, but when you wriggle away from it, you'll be much more at peace with being who you are.

This Week's Tangible Tools

Embrace the Bad to See the Good. We have all been there: an argument with a loved one, a faceoff with the kids, drama at work or with friends, a health crisis, or just a moment of total overwhelm and ensuing meltdown. When you are in the middle of the upset, we encourage you to give it some space for a moment, pause and look at it, and decide instead that what you initially perceive as a threat to your happiness and well-being may actually be an opportunity. It may feel all bad and you struggle to see the good there, but can you see even a crack of light? A chance for growth or for improvement? Usually our best lessons come from a place of pain, and we can all look back at an event that felt terrible but that in hindsight was a gift. What if we could learn to experience that in the moment instead of just when we look back?

To get the lesson in real time, we want to avoid our first inclination: avoid, distract, or react to uncomfortable or threatening situations because we are afraid. Be brave and look deeper while you're in the midst of a stressful moment and see what good can come from this thing that feels oh-so bad right now. The same goes for when you make a mistake; instead of feeling horrendously guilty and filled with shame, realize in that moment that you are still a good, loving, wonderful person and sit with the fact that even from our worst mistakes come great lessons. Next, voice your shame to someone you love and who cares for you because, as the great Brené Brown says (and as we've experienced), "Shame cannot survive empathy." Don't panic; just focus on who you are at your core. Own your mistake but don't let it define you, and be grateful for whatever the impending lesson will be.

The Power Shift. When you feel out of control or powerless in a situation, get back into your power by shifting your focus to something you can control. This stops the fearful thoughts spinning in your mind and helps you see more resources and creative solutions. If all you can control in that moment is your breathing, do it! If you can exercise, drink a glass of water, make a healthy meal, journal, meditate, make a list, pick up the phone, whatever it is: DO IT. Do one thing that puts you back in your power, one little step toward your ultimate goal. It may not solve the whole problem, but you'll be reminded you have power and that you're not always at the mercy of life. You will calm down, be able to breathe deeper, and see more opportunities and resources to help solve your problem.

Rocking Chair Test. We love each of our Twelve Tangible Tools and have seen their magic in action, but we saved the best for last: the rocking chair test. When you're in a tough situation, imagine yourself in your later years, sitting in a rocking chair, gently rocking back and forth. The rocking chair is very meditative; you can feel yourself rocking when you hold this image. You can also pull yourself back to the present with a clear sense of what matters most right now. In this rocking chair, looking back on your life, would what you're losing it over right now really matter? Would you even remember it?

Running a few minutes late, your finances, the argument you just had, your to-do list, and that pile of dirty laundry will likely feel less catastrophic after doing the rocking chair test. Hopefully the thoughts of what does matter will come to mind and, after initiating this quick meditation, you'll be able to slow things down, hug someone you love, reconnect with your own heart and soul, and let it go knowing it's never as big a deal in the long run as it feels right now.

Reminder: Check Your Hangry B*tch Scale

ACES are Balanced. Your appetite is not too high or low, your cravings are minimal and well managed, your energy is even and adequate, it's easy for you to fall asleep and stay asleep.

Tolerating Exercise Well, Not Under- or Overtraining. You are not feeling that energy is depleted after exercise or showing any signs of RAMP (reluctance to train, aches and soreness, moodiness, and puffiness; see page 83).

Feeling Positive and Peaceful Overall. You are using meditation and mantras, choosing a positive perspective more often than not (listening to best friend voice), experiencing little to no stress, anxiety, and overwhelm.

Able to Stay Present in Your Life. You are using meditation, mantras, and third pillar tools for full-engagement living, and you are feeling little to no distraction from the present moment.

Being Who You Are. You are confidently speaking your truth, engaging in activities solely because they bring you joy and help you feel more like yourself.

Aim for a score 5 or less. If you do not achieve it, pull out your tools and take care of yourself. Your health and happiness depend on it.

Welcome to Being a Happy Babe

Now What?

Congrats, you did it!

Really, you did. Even if you only managed one workout and are still trying to find your UCT, congratulations are still in order. If you have read up to this point and have yet to actually implement one habit or one minute of meditation, we are still proud of you, because you at least made it to this chapter, so let's celebrate that as a huge win. You showed up, page after page, and if you haven't implemented it all yet, you are at least armed with more info than you had before—and maybe a little more hope as well. If you have really been living this plan, we want to be sure you're prepared to keep this groove going, as we know life has a way of getting back to being all life-y again. The whole point is that your newfound lifestyle is a sustainable one and that this book will be your health bible from here on out. All you have to do is return to these pages when you need some reminding of how to stay on track.

OK, Happy Babe, Now What?

If you've been working this plan, we know you are starting to feel better than you have in a very long time, meaning you've healed or started to heal your hormones and soothe your psyche. However, we also totally understand that you may not be all the way there yet, especially if underlying stressors haven't been dealt with, thyroid levels haven't been optimized, or things like autoimmunity are lurking. The truth is, if you've been feeling bad for a very long time, one month isn't enough time to completely undo that. You must be patient with yourself if you fall into this category; you are not doing anything wrong, it just takes some time to undo all that has been done. The results that you'll walk away with once you are healed are results you can keep forever. Remember, you aren't on another bad diet; you are on a path to real health, wellness, and longevity. So no matter where you're at, it's all good because we'll walk you through your next steps regardless of the situation you find yourself in at the end of these four weeks.

While this is where most books leave you sorta "Good-bye and good luck!" not us. We know that this is not the end of your story with your hormones or your real self-care. Because your hormones will change over time, even when you're in perfect health, we want you to get comfortable with the reality and beauty of being a woman with an amazing, intricate, adaptable, and ever-changing unique hormonal landscape. Owning this reality is truly part of our Fifth Pillar: it's part of who you are. Moving forward, when you need to adjust this plan because of in-evitable hormone fluctuations, know you will always have the guidance and tools offered here in this book. Specifically, you can stay tuned in to your hormonal cues from your ACES, RAMP, and your Hangry B*tch Hormone Quiz results (which we suggest you retake every thirty days or so), as well as your Hangry B*tch Scale, which can be used daily if you like. We want you to use the Quiz and the Scale as a way to consistently check in with your nutrition, exercise, stress, sleep, and other lifestyle habits and as a way to stay committed to adjusting these habits as needed to do what works best for you.

Your new routine of doing what works for you should eventually be as ef-fortless as remembering to brush your teeth every morning, with the under-standing that what works today may need to be adjusted next week or in six months, and in the years to come. Furthermore, sometimes a few old habits might creep back in and you feel yourself getting a little more like a Hangry B*tch instead of a Happy Babe. It happens to everyone, including us—Sarah and Dr. Brooke! The difference for us is that we have years of experience living these principles, honoring our hormones, and making necessary adjustments within hours or days instead of months and years. It's part of why the mind-fulness component of this plan is so important. When you are present in your own life, it's easier to see your old patterns show up, address them, and then go back to doing what works. Our hope for you is that you can continue to show up for yourself by living the Five Pillars, following the Five Habits, and using the Twelve Tangible Tools.

However, life will throw you curveballs, there will be times of crisis, and there will be times when you decide you have to put your health and fitness on the back burner. This is when we want to encourage you to leave a solid foundation of self-care in place. For example, if you need to put workouts or walks on hold while you're handling a work or family emergency, make sure you stay committed to prioritizing two of your Five Habits: your sleep and nutrition. Holding strong to these two habits will help hold your hormones and health together while you get through the rough patch and back to implementing the rest of the Five Habits. Sometimes we simply can't do everything, but if we can at least do something, it's better than jumping off the deep end doing absolutely nothing. This is why you are doing this work, so that when life feels like it's falling apart, you don't fall apart with it. Remember, it's always going to be OK.

Keep recommitting, keep showing up, and keep simply doing the best you can, and in the hardest of times, let it be easy and keep it simple: deep breaths, nourishing food, mantras, and sleep.

Moving from the Hangry B*tch Reset to Your Five Habits Forever

5-4-3-2-1 5 Walks per Week Plus 5 Minutes of Breathing Work per Day

We hope these habits will be yours forever now! If they haven't completely taken hold, keep making them a priority. Walking and restorative breathing are both great for normalizing a stress response. Although they may be the first habits you're tempted to let go of when life takes over, they will absolutely save you during times when life feels all crazy-pants, as both of them help lower inflammation, normalize cortisol, and give you a chance to step outside, smell the flowers, be present, and literally catch your breath.

As we have said before, we know there will be times when you can't get outside for a walk due to weather, location, or other circumstances. When this is the case, walking on a track or a treadmill is another option, as is implementing some restorative yoga. When all else fails, at least do the restorative breathing, and if you're still wondering how to find the time to do the walking, we think it's a problem worth solving. What could you let go of that would give you those forty-five to sixty minutes, how could you rearrange your schedule to make it less stressful, or who could you ask for help so that this time is available for you to get in those walks? See what's possible! We truly believe this habit is one that will continue to serve you, so do what you can to build it in for the long haul. If you have children, get them involved! You can include them on your walks or workouts or wherever you feel like you can't fit something in because of them—we don't want you to use your kiddos as the excuse for not having time to take care of yourself, but instead have them be the reason you decide to make your self-care a priority. Modeling for your children what real self-care looks like will be sure to leave a lasting impression.

If walking for forty-five minutes is still out of reach because you've been struggling with fatigue and exercise tolerance, simply continue to support your system with the nutrition advice you've gleaned thus far (keep your blood sugar balanced and focus on lowering inflammation), get help from a qualified provider, and remember to add time to your walks in five- to ten-minute increments as your hormones continue to heal.

5-4-3-2-1 4 Meals per Day

This will be the habit that will likely change the most for you now. There are several things to consider as you wonder what to do now with the four-meal-per-day template and the content of those meals. However, there are a few things that should remain the same:

Adequate Protein. At a minimum, we suggest you maintain the 100 g per day recommendation and possibly slightly more if you follow a lower-carb diet (ideal for high cortisol and insulin resistance) or if you start training more intensely.

One Pound of Vegetables per Day. These hormone- and hunger-managing helpers will always be your beacon of health with their fiber and phytonutrients. Several handfuls at each of your meals, even if it's more of a snack than a full meal, will help keep your ACES in balance and your digestion on track. If for any reason you're experiencing bloating or you still don't tolerate a high veggie intake, be sure you follow our gut-healing regimen on page 385, and consider a digestive enzyme (see Supplement & Testing resources for our fave brands). You might also consider working with a functional medicine doctor to get tested for things like SIBO, candida, or dysbiosis and to get more help uncovering any underlying issues that may still be hindering your results beyond what we were able to cover in this book. See Supplement and Testing Resources on page 382 for more info or visit www.sarahand drbrooke.com.

Honoring Your UCT. We can't say this often enough: you are special! Always stay mindful of your carb tolerance changing over time as you go through things such as periods of stress, new hormonal imbalances, perimenopause, or an increase in inflammation. Remember that your ACES will help alert you to these changes as you notice them becoming unbalanced. Also you may have more longstanding issues like diabetes, metabolic syndrome, or PCOS, which means your UCT will always be on the lower side for optimal results and hormone balance. Or, instead, you may find that once you resolve stress and inflammation you tolerate more carbs and you might even need to up them to support and fuel your workouts. Again, always stay tuned in to your ACES to know if what you're doing now is still working down the line.

Possible Changes to How Often You're Eating

If you were/are low cortisol, low thyroid, or insulin-resistant, we've been suggesting you stick with eating four meals a day, roughly the same size, protein- and veggie-based. If you are dealing with high cortisol or with insulin resistance, you might have moved to just three meals per day.

As for what's in those meals, if you are low cortisol and low thyroid, you are likely eating a small amount (¼–⅓ cup, four to six bites, or what works for you per your UCT) of starch or fruit at each meal, whereas if you are higher cortisol and insulin-resistant, you are eating your carbs at dinner only (around ⅓–½ cup or eight to ten bites, or what works for you per your UCT).

Some of you might have also added some post-workout carbs in addition to this. All of this is good, as long as your ACES feel in balance and you're getting the results you want.

Eating four meals per day that are roughly the same size typically works for those with blood sugar problems of all types; however, this doesn't give us much time away from food throughout the day, which has its benefits in terms of digestion recovery, triggering growth hormone, and giving us a break from insulin. So ultimately, as your adrenals and thyroid recover, you can hopefully get back to either three meals per day or even longer periods of fasting in the morning. Strategies like intermittent fasting and ketogenic diets certainly have well-documented hormonal benefits as long as your adrenals and thyroid can handle them. This is why we saved any of this talk till the end: you need to be in a good place with your more-delicate hormones before you can try some of these strategies that may put too much heat on your adrenals and thyroid if they aren't in good working order.

Now before you go full keto or start fasting for days, know that many women can get that growth-hormone boost and other benefits by being away from food for just twelve to fourteen hours. This fasting window can easily be achieved by wrapping up dinner by 7 P.M. and not eating again until 7 or 9 A.M. the next morning. Again, and as always, watch your ACES and see if you are tolerating this well. In particular, notice if you're having a harder time falling or staying asleep or getting ravenous between meals or ravenous during the time you are fasting, causing you to overeat at your next meal. Any benefits from fasting are going to be totally thwarted if fasting means you have erratic sleep (this tanks growth hormone and will whack out your ACES fast; you know that by now!) or consume a thousand calories for lunch because you skipped breakfast. You simply can't go wrong by continuing to listen to your hormones talk to you. By now, hopefully you feel like BFFs with those ACES and you can step away from the notion that "Oh I heard this strategy is supposed to be so good!" if your hormones say, "Well, it isn't good for us!"

Possible Changes to What You're Eating

As a woman, you'll be wise to refrain from overdoing animal fat, especially as your hormones wane and become more imbalanced in your forties and beyond. But what about all the food that's been off your list during the HB Hormone Reset—the grains, gluten, processed food, and other common inflammatory or hard-for-your-hormones foods?

Some of them should stay gone, baby, gone. None of us need to be eating a lot of processed foods or using processed seed oils for cooking at any point. Sure, there will be times when these things creep in, whether for convenience or because they are part of a food you indulge in on occasion; however, try to keep these things to a minimum for the long haul. You know they increase inflammation, significantly muck up all your hormones, and, let's be honest, none of them make you feel all that great! Also, going back to old indulgent habits is worth a revisit of your relationship with food. Often we eat for comfort when we aren't staying present and dealing with our emotions, so keeping on track with your mindfulness practice and really paying attention to old patterns resurfacing will keep you clued in to why and how often you cave in to old cravings. We suggest you save these for occasional indulgences and celebrations (if it's worth it) or when you have no other options (for instance, a salad dressing when you're dining out).

But what about many of the foods you haven't had during this plan, like gluten, dairy, grains, legumes, sugar, and alcohol? Thank goodness you're now stepping away from the idea that a food is good or bad or carries a lot of emotional weight and are now looking at your food as falling into these three categories:

Food That Works for You. Included in this list are high-quality proteins, vegetables, water, high-fiber starches, or fruit, according to your UCT.

Food That Doesn't Work Well for You. You may still want to have wine, sugar, some grains, and possibly dairy from time to time. These might not be your best options, but maybe some of these choices won't totally wreck you for days, especially if you don't overdo it. We both have our "worth-it" moments, but it's usually around stuff that doesn't leave us down for the count and unable to jump back into life the very next day.

Food That Doesn't Work at All for You. These are things that just wreck you, causing joint pain or general achiness, depression or anxiety, skin flare-ups, headaches or stuffy nose, or any kind of digestive upset. These are the foods you need to make your peace with and kiss good-bye. Remember that knowing what works for you is empowering; now you have the responsibility to heed that knowledge and practice the first pillar to its fullest by committing to what works for you. Will you ever have a slip-up, momentary lapse in judgment, or accidental exposure? Yes, probably, but just do your best to avoid these foods at all costs, because at the end of the day they aren't worth the damage they can cause.

The foods that don't work for you may include gluten, dairy, soy, sugar, alcohol, or even coffee. Or they may be less common culprits, such as eggs, black beans, or even chicken. Remember, we can develop issues with nearly any food, so be honest with yourself about what's worth it and what really works for you or not. Commit to that and get your mindset right about it. Avoiding certain foods may be a necessity for you, but suffering about it is optional.

To ease the suffering, first remember that we always have the power to change how we see a situation. We can mire in the restriction and kick our feet or we can be grateful that, as hard as it is to give some foods up, at least we feel better, and these days we are lucky to have so many substitutions and alternatives for dairy, gluten, and even healthier bottled salad dressings. So find and utilize those when possible, assuming the swap works for you! For example, many women swap packaged coconut creamers for their dairy-based coffee creamer and then realize the carrageenan or guar gum in some of these products also cause issues. You're in this for the long haul; keep trying to find options that work better for you, and always remember: you are worth the effort.

If you do find yourself struggling and suffering with the avoidance of certain foods that don't work well for you, listen to your internal dialogue about those foods. Saying "I can't have this" or "I have to have this thing instead" will make you instantly feel agitated and frustrated. "Can't" and "have to" are the language of struggle. Instead, focus on the 900,007 foods you do get to eat (OK, we made that number up, but you know what we mean), review the section on "healing your relationship with food" on page 48, and, as always, simply go back to the pillars:

1. Find and commit to what works for you. Again, great power but great responsibility to commit to it once you know it, and if you haven't figured out what works, it's all good—just stay in the process, keep listening to your ACES, digestive issues, or other signs of inflammation, and get help if you need it.

2. Opt out of overwhelm. Let it be easy here. Know you have other choices that may take some getting used to but that you'll be less overwhelmed and stressed out overall when you don't feel like crap, right?

3. Full-engagement living. Part of being fully engaged is staying committed to what works for you, because when you feel like crap, it's really hard to be present and engaged with what matters. How can you show up and enjoy your amazing life when you feel bloated, have a headache, or are tired and frustrated that your skin is flared up and your joints hurt?

4. Be your best friend. Being your best friend is how you support your choices, knowing that there is zero judgment and only encouragement around eating foods that work for you.

5. Be who you are. If you are someone who can't tolerate gluten/dairy/sugar/wine/coffee/[insert food of choice here], then that Happy Babe is WHO YOU ARE! Go ahead and be her.

How Do You Know What Foods Don't Work for You?

If you've gone through the Hangry B*tch Reset and are feeling much better because of it, it may mean that foods that were no-go's were part of the problem. You might have stepped away from those foods before and felt better for it but never made peace with having to eliminate them longer term or they just slipped back into your diet somehow. So, if you're feeling better, what you can do now is systematically reintroduce those foods back in. Here's how:

Reintroduce one food at a time—for example, wheat, then cheese, then tomato rather than going right for the pizza. Then try a combo, as you may feel fine on cheese alone but when you have it combined with tomato sauce and the gluten that's in a pizza crust, it doesn't work.

Try the food in its purest form; for example, eat whole wheat cereal rather than a piece of bread.

No reaction? Great, go ahead and wait three days to watch for a delayed reaction and then try another food.

If you get a reaction, which can include digestive symptoms, headache, stuffy nose, rash, acne, racing heart, anxiety, depression, fatigue, brain fog, joint pain, or other symptoms, wait until the reaction clears to try another food. If you suspect you might have a skin reaction such as eczema or acne that cleared when you were on the Hangry B*tch Reset, know that you may need to give it three to five days before you think you're in the clear, as it often takes time for skin reactions to appear.

Also know that your food reactions can change. You may be fine with dairy now and then, but in two years you may find that it's bothering you, so come back to this plan as you need to or seek out testing. Again, the testing we suggest is available through Cyrex Labs (www.cyrexlabs.com).

For those foods you've reintroduced that were no-no's on the Hangry B*tch Reset but that actually work well for you, don't be overly attached to the dogma of this plan or any other plans, for that matter. If you've found what works for you, again, just commit to it! Finally, we don't recommend that you reintroduce foods until you are doing great and your symptoms have cleared. If you're at the end of this program and your symptoms haven't cleared and you haven't done the gut repair regimen on page 385, then complete that or find a qualified functional medicine doctor to help you.

5-4-3-2-1 3 Strength Training Sessions per Week

By this point in the program, you might be using the HB Strength Training Template from chapter 7, or you might still be doing or just beginning the HB Hormone Reset Template. Or it's possible you are still doing the HB Core+Floor Recovery Template. Again, it's all good; you need to be OK with exactly where you are, knowing you'll move on to the next phase as you're ready.

If you've been doing the HB Core+Floor Recovery Template only and you're feeling ready, move on to the HB Hormone Reset Template for two to three weeks, doing that workout three times per week. If you've been doing the HB Hormone Reset Template for two to three weeks, you are likely ready to move on to the HB Strength Training Template. The HB Strength Training Template was designed for you to be able to use forever because it will help you continue to train without getting wiped out. Remember that the initial two workouts you designed should be done for four to six weeks only—four weeks if you're hitting those three sessions per week or five or even six weeks if you only can manage two sessions per week. After that, you will create two new workouts based on the choices in the template and go through another four- to six-week rotation and on from there!

Progressing with Cardio

If you haven't yet dabbled with adding back cardio at this point and your ACES are consistently in check, you've been handling the Section B metabolic portion of the HB Strength Training Template well, and recovering well in general from your workouts, this could be a good time to try some sprints on for size. We are talking the short-duration stuff we explained earlier in the book on pages 195 and 196 that your body responds to and appreciates more than the long-duration cardio you may have done in the past. If fat loss is your goal, adding in some sprints is a great way to help move the needle on that, if your hormones are ready to handle this kind of work.

We suggest starting with just one sprint session per week as prescribed. Start out with just the minimum and build from there, and if it feels like it's too much, then dial it back. If you are recovering well from your first sprint session, consider adding in one day a week of sprints, either on days you lift or not; you'll still get the same benefits as long as your hormones are happy with this new addition. Remember, however, that sprint sessions do not take the place of your walks!

If you are a long-duration or intense cardio gal and are missing it, we suggest you make sure it's a good idea for your health, head, and hormones before you add back in the Zumba, CrossFit classes, or marathon training. Remember your commitment to doing what works for you? Was your lack of results with your old workout routine part of what got you to buy this book in the first place? Are you feeling better, injury-free, and energy-filled now that you've dialed back the intensity? It could be that these more intense and longer-duration cardio sessions no longer fit into your life. We understand that it's a loss psychologically if you loved it, but what's more important in the long run? Really assess before you leap back into the tough stuff because overdoing it with exercise on an already-delicate, healing hormonal system is a sure way to turn things back to Hangry, and quickly.

If you are missing your community, consider a class or two a month instead of four or five times a week, and then check back in with yourself after your first session back and really notice how you feel. If you decided to join in on a previously loved exercise regimen, but your ACES didn't respond well, try cutting the workout in half and staying to cheer on your friends while you foam roll, or bring them their water bottle in between sets, or work on mobility or some auxiliary lifts—this way you can still be a part of your crew while staying committed to your new better-for-your-body exercise approach.

5-4-3-2-1 2 Liters (or More) of Water per Day

Hopefully by this week you're at a minimum of two liters of water per day and have played with that amount to see if you need a bit more. Also, if you've struggled with peeing twenty times a day when you keep your water intake where it should be or know you have cortisol or insulin issues, it's important that you get enough electrolytes. As for other hydration issues, you may have realized that your tummy fares a bit better with less carbonated water, so, again, commit to what works for you.

Next up: coffee! You may have cut your caffeine intake during the Hangry B*tch Reset and likely have noticed better balanced energy and improved sleep, thanks to your now-healthier cortisol levels. So, if you feel much better with less caffeine or off of coffee all together (note: coffee can create inflammation and symptoms unrelated to caffeine), consider giving it a real go to keep this habit at bay.

Coffee and caffeine, along with sugar and alcohol, tend to be the nutritional components that creep back in over time. Little by little or when things get busy or stressful, we drift back to habits that don't work well for us overall but offer us some immediate relief. Here is where you go back to your Five Pillars and all the mindset and perspective tools you've learned.

Which brings us to the final hydration variable: booze. Wine and other alcoholic drinks may be something you've been counting down the days to welcome back (we get it; we both love a nice glass of wine), but booze often doesn't work well for women. If this applies to you, honor it and use the mindset tools and Five Pillars that we've taught you.

5-4-3-2-1 1 Daily Commitment to Rest, Recovery, and Real Self-Care

We hope that you have solved your sleep problems with the suggestions we have given thus far in this book, but, alas, you may still be struggling to get yourself in between the sheets early enough. As we've suggested all along, continue to bump up bedtime by fifteen minutes until you're getting a solid seven to eight hours of restful sleep. If you're still having trouble falling asleep or staying asleep, be sure you've implemented all the lifestyle and supplement strategies. If that still doesn't fix your sleep, by all means get some help from a professional. It is truly impossible to get your health and hormones back in line without adequate sleep.

When it comes to that real self-care we've been preaching, church stays in session. This is your torch to carry for the long haul. Life will always be pulling you away from caring for yourself and flashing something shiny and distracting in your face. Only you can be the one to prioritize your beautiful self. This is your most important job from here on out. Of course, there will be ebbs and flows where you have to let another obligation bubble to the top of your Top Five, but what you can't do is take yourself off that list completely lest you need to start this book all over again! But if it happens, remember that this plan will be here for you forever, so start over if necessary. But ideally you continue to always, and no matter what, make YOU a priority. This is your new beginning, your journey from here on out with your number one priority of putting yourself first so that you can truly show up for your big beautiful life, fully engaged and present for yourself and for the people who need you.

By this point we've encouraged you to hone each one of the Five Pillars, doling them out one per week but knowing that one little week is hardly enough time to master these big ideas! From here you can continue to work on one per week or you can simply take one and work on it until you feel ready to move on. You can start back at the top with Find and Commit to What Works for You and work your way down the list, or you can pick the one that feels right to focus on. There's no right or wrong here, but we would encourage you to tackle the one that feels either most important to you at the moment or the one that feels hardest. Gaining some ground on the one that feels the biggest and scariest may be just the thing you need to cause a greater shift overall, but again there's no right way; just stay in the process and keep showing up. In time you'll live your life from these principles and it gets easier and easier to stay in that place, feeling less pull toward things that are merely distractions and don't serve you, and no longer feeling at the mercy of stress and overwhelm. Just stay in the game. It takes time but you've already come so far. When in doubt, simply opt to be your best friend—that will make any hard spot easier.

Finally, keep using your Twelve Tangible Tools as needed for those really bad days. Keep using the ones that work for you, dabble with a few new ones from time to time to build your stress defense arsenal, and by all means if a tool doesn't jive with you let it go! And be sure you keep up with our ongoing addition of resources for you on *The Sarah & Dr. Brooke Show* and at www.sarahanddrbrooke.com.

Keeping in Touch with Yourself

We know how excited you were when you picked up this book. It held the promise of feeling better, and you felt full of hope that everything was going to change. We also know that excitement wanes as these habits become exactly what they are meant to be: part of your life. Also and inevitably, your hormones will change with natural ebbs and flows of life and normal transitions. Your job is to stay in close contact with those hormones and check in daily with your Hangry B*tch Scale and your ACES. Check in weekly or so with RAMP to be sure you're still tolerating your exercise plan well. Finally, you can retake the Hangry B*tch Hormone Quiz monthly to see how things are improving or if perhaps a new hormone is trying to tell you something.

Last but not least, remember that true self-care starts with being OK with where you are, right now. It's our passion to help women just like you lead a life filled with joy and purpose, and our goal is that you remember how important you are—you are necessary, worth it, and amazing—no matter what part of your journey you are on. We also want you to know that we always have your back. What we want more than anything else for you, the woman who trusted in us and has taken the time to read our words, is to close this last page with a sense of empowerment, deep inner peace, and the confidence to stay committed to doing what works for you, because the world needs you, especially right now, and we also all need each other.

xoxo
Sarah and Dr. Brooke

Instagram: sarah_fragoso and BetterByDrBrooke

Facebook: Sarah Fragoso, Everyday Paleo, and Better By Dr Brooke

Free, Private Facebook Group: Sarah and Dr Brooke

Twitter: Everyday Paleo and DrBrookeND

Podcast: The Sarah & Dr Brooke Show

Exercise Templates

Before beginning any new exercise program, it is recommended that you seek medical advice from your personal physician. Exercise is not without its risks, and this, like any other exercise program, comes with risks, including but not limited to the following: injury, aggravation of a preexisting condition, or adverse effects of overexertion such as muscle strain, abnormal blood pressure, fainting, disorders of heartbeat, and, in very rare instances, heart attack. The exercise instruction and advice presented in this book are in no way intended as a substitute for medical consultation. Sarah Fragoso and Dr. Brooke Kalanick and their publisher disclaim any liability from and in connection with this program. As with any exercise program, if at any point during your workout you begin to feel faint, dizzy, or have physical discomfort, you should stop immediately and consult a physician.

The Importance of Technique

If we could have it our way, you would all be in the gym with us so we could teach you firsthand how to use proper technique for all the prescribed exercises; however, we feel like what we are offering you with our instruction within this book is pretty much the next best thing. If you follow our Movement Progression Guide on page 281, pay attention to mobility issues, and honor your current fitness level, you'll be able to have longevity in the gym by avoiding injury as well as getting the results you've been hoping for.

We can't stress enough that you should carefully review the movement descriptions in this section and make sure you are using proper technique. It's extremely important that you learn how to breathe and brace as instructed on page 279 in order to protect your spine while lifting and to learn to utilize your core. We urge you to incorporate the exercise we call Forced Exhalation every day in order to help you get into proper pelvic position and to practice your daily restorative breathing, which will also help you learn how to use your diaphragm and keep you in proper alignment throughout the day.

The key to longevity with heavy lifts is learning proper technique and making sure you stay within a pain-free range. If you try one of the prescribed exercises and it's painful, then stop. Nothing we ask you to do should hurt. It might push you outside of your comfort zone. It will be hard. You might challenge your body to do things it's never done before, but you should not be in pain. For example, due to an orthopedic or mobility issue, if it's impossible for you to squat to or below parallel, then squat within the range that keeps you pain-free while maintaining proper technique. Most important, follow our Movement Progression Guide so you can be confident about how to keep moving forward from wherever you need to begin.

Finally, we are available to you online if you want more instruction on how to do the exercises as described in this book! Simply find us at www.sarahanddrbrooke.com.

Strength Training Glossary of Terms

Circuit. A system of training where you perform one set of an exercise and then move quickly on to the next exercise.

Dynamic. An active movement of a muscle or muscles that results in a stretch but where muscles are not held in that stretched position.

Rep (repetition). One complete motion of an exercise. If you lift a weight 5 times, you have done 5 reps.

Set. A group of consecutive reps. For example, if you are instructed to do 10 reps for 5 sets, that means you will lift that weight 10 times and that will be one set; then you will rest before you move on to the next set of 10 reps and repeat until you complete all 5 sets.

Static. The stretching of a muscle or a position that is held for any length of time.

Workout. A generic term for an exercise session, but for the purpose of this plan a workout is one full series of prescribed exercises.

HB Core+Floor Recovery Template

If you're injured, postpartum, or have never healed your core and floor post-partum, even if it's been years, start here. Do the following workout one time through, 5 times per week for three weeks. You will then move on to the HB Hormone Reset Template for two to three weeks and then begin using the HB Strength Training Template using the customization strategies you learned in Week 3.

Forced Exhalation

○ **Perform 2 sets of 5 breaths twice daily and, if you are lifting weights, prior to your weight lifting session.**

1. Lie down flat on your back and place your feet up on a bench so that your knees are at 90 degrees, as pictured. Pull your ribs down and tilt the front of your pelvis up toward your nose (posterior pelvic tilt).

2. Inhale deeply through your nose, filling up your belly and chest with air. Try not to breathe into your neck and shoulders; instead, visualize the air going down deep into your belly, pelvic area, and low back. As pictured, make a tight fist and bring it up to your mouth to create resistance upon exhaling, then exhale through your mouth forcefully into your hand, mimicking the feeling and effect of blowing up a balloon. As you forcefully exhale, keep your pelvis tucked, abdominals engaged, and your ribs down. This should be hard work and you should feel your abdominals working as you forcefully exhale.

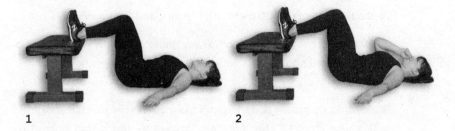

1   2

Bear Progression

○ **To begin, the goal is to attempt to hold this position up to 20 seconds.**

Bear Hold

1. Start in a quadruped position (on your hands and knees). Be sure that your knees are directly under your hips and that your hands are directly under your shoulders. Push into the ground with your hands and protract your scapula; imagine you are reaching out with your hands as far as possible as you push into the ground. Now tuck your pelvis so that you feel as if you are pulling your pubic bone toward your nose.

2. Now, holding the above position, tighten your core and raise your knees about 2 inches off the floor and hold. Keep reaching into the ground with your hands and keep your pelvis tucked. This will be very challenging, especially on your first try. Hold for at least 20 seconds or less if you are unable to maintain proper position for 20 seconds. Once you can hold this position for 45 seconds, you are ready to move on to the bear crawl.

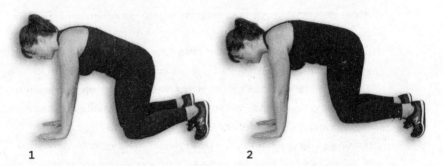

1   2

Bear Crawl

○ **Do this 2 times for 20 feet both forward and backward.**

1. Starting in the same position as the bear hold, raise your knees up off the ground about 2 inches as instructed in the bear hold. You are ready to crawl.

2. Keeping your core engaged and maintaining the reach position with your shoulders, start crawling forward by alternating limbs. Take short steps of equal distance with both hands and feet. Try to keep your knees 2 inches off the ground and your hips from swaying side to side—picture a small glass of wine on the small of your back and try not to spill it.

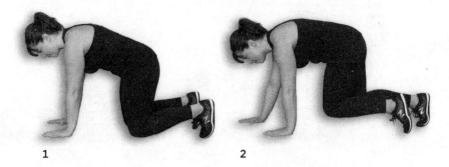

1   2

Leg Lowers

○ **Do 6–8 each leg 2 times.**

1. Lie flat on your back and bend your knees so your feet are also flat on the ground. Bring your ribs down and tilt the front of your pelvis up toward your nose (posterior pelvic tilt) so that your lower back is flat on the ground.

2. Raise your legs straight up so that the bottoms of your feet are facing the ceiling and keep your legs as straight as possible to start.

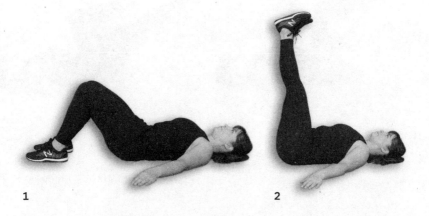

1   2

3a and 3b. Inhale through your nose into your belly. As you exhale, slowly lower one leg as far as possible, keeping your abdominals tight and engaged and without letting your lower back lose contact with the floor. If this is too challenging, then perform the modification of this movement portrayed in the next image

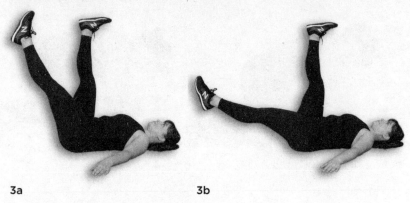

3a   3b

4a and 4b. As pictured, bend your knees into a 90-degree position, pull your ribs down, and tilt the front of your pelvis up (posterior pelvic tilt), and inhale through your nose into your belly. As you exhale through your mouth, straighten one leg out and then back in, only moving on the exhale. You can make this movement harder by straightening your leg lower to the ground and easier by straightening it higher above the ground. Again, be sure that your low back does not lose contact with the ground.

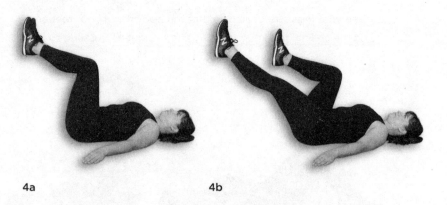

4a   4b

Bilateral Glute Bridge

◎ **Do 3 sets of 8–10 with a 5-second hold at the top.**

1. Lie flat on your back with your knees bent and your feet flat on the floor, heels between 6 and 12 inches away from your glutes. Pull your ribs down so that your back is flat on the ground underneath you and pull your pubic bone up toward your nose so that you're creating a strong abdominal contraction.

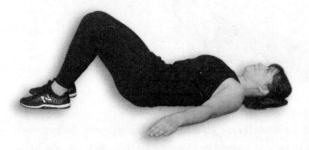

2. Pushing through your heels, drive your hips up until you are in a bridge position. Do not hyperextend your low back to get more range of motion; keep your ribs down, pelvis posteriorly tilted and abdominals contracted. Squeeze your glutes at the top and then bring your hips slowly back down to the ground, lowering one vertebra at a time back to the start position.

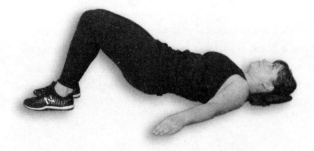

Side Plank from Knees or with Top Foot in Front

○ **Do 3 sets of 8 reps each side with a 3-second hold at the top.**

1. Lie on your side propped up on your elbow, legs straight and with your feet stacked. Be sure your elbow is directly under your shoulder and that your hips and spine are in alignment.

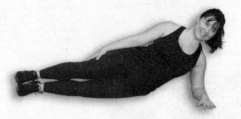

2. Tighten your core and raise your hips off the ground. Do not rock your hips forward or lean back; try to stay as straight as possible.

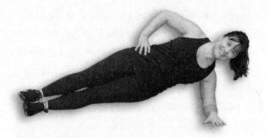

3. If you need more support, place your top foot in front of your bottom foot on the floor, creating a larger base, which will regress the movement and make it a little less challenging. Alternatively, if this movement is still too challenging, bend your legs, and leave your knees on the ground as you raise your hips.

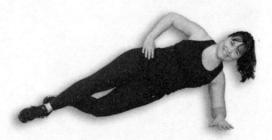

Kegels

Do sets of 10 as often as you can throughout the day—in the car, at the office, watching TV, etc. Be mindful of your pelvic position. Aim to not be anterior (low back arched, pelvis tilted forward, ribs flared), which is typically the default. Instead, try to stay neutral throughout the day. Also continually check in on your alignment to make sure your shoulders are stacked over your lower ribs and over your hips. Be especially mindful of pelvic position and keep your core tight as you do the squats of daily living, such as getting in and out of a chair, getting off the toilet, picking something up from the floor, or getting something out of a low drawer.

To do a proper Kegel, be sure you're in good alignment and posture as we just described. You may want to practice Kegels lying on your back on the ground with your knees bent and feet flat on the floor before you start doing them in a seated position. A Kegel is simply a contraction of the pelvic floor muscles, but you may not know how to isolate them and give a strong contraction and a full relaxation. To connect with them imagine picking up a blueberry with your vagina or imagine pulling your clitoris toward your vagina. This is better practice than common advice to isolate your pelvic floor muscles by stopping your urine stream midstream, but if that's the only way you can connect to them and get a feel for what you're contracting, try it. Once you've isolated your pelvic floor muscles and you are in proper alignment as described above, you're ready to do a Kegel. Take a deep breath in and imagine inflating your pelvic floor with air (this is the relaxation phase) and then, as you exhale, contract the pelvic floor (feeling your vagina and anus lift up) to about 30 percent of your max contraction. Continue breathing in and out following this relaxation and contraction for the full set of ten. If you find that the relaxation is hard for you, continue to practice just the relaxation phase without a full contraction as you may (as many women do) have a tight but weak pelvic floor, and once you properly learn to relax it you can move back to this full Kegel practice and improve your strength. Once you've mastered your Kegel technique, do sets of 10 as often as you can throughout the day—in the car, at the office, watching TV, etc. Be sure to go to full contraction and then full relaxation.

#1 Dynamic Warm Up

The Dynamic Warm Up is what you will do to warm up your body prior to performing either the HB Hormone Reset Template or the HB Strength Training Template. Before you start your workout, do the following movements in order in a continuous fashion and repeat the entire warm up in order 1 to 2 times. Finish your Dynamic Warm Up with 1 set of 3–5 Forced Exhalation breaths (page 251), and then you'll be ready to start your workout.

Knee Hugs

As pictured, lie down flat on your back, raise one knee up to your chest (or as close as you can get), grab your knee, and give a gentle squeeze into your chest. Repeat with the other leg and alternate back and forth in a dynamic fashion for 8–10 reps each leg.

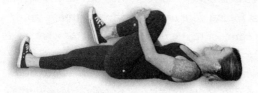

Windshield Wipers

1. Still lying on your back, place your feet shoulder-width apart flat on the floor with your knees bent.

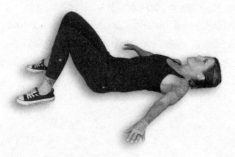

2. Internally and externally rotate your hips by moving your knees from side to side, keeping your feet in contact with the ground, as pictured, for 8–10 reps each side.

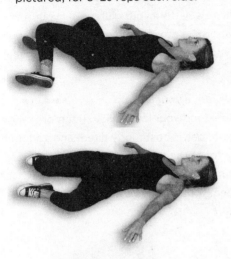

Dynamic Leg Lowers

1. Keep one knee bent with your foot flat on the ground and straighten the other leg, as pictured.

2. Keeping your leg as straight as possible, kick your leg up toward your head and back down (start out gently) and perform 8–10 consecutive reps in a dynamic fashion so that you feel this active stretch in your hamstrings. Switch and do the same thing with the other leg.

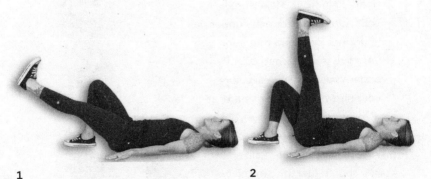

1   2

Bilateral Glute Bridge

1. Lie flat on your back with your knees bent and feet flat on the floor, heels between 6 and 12 inches away from your glutes. Pull your ribs down so that your back is flat on the ground underneath you and pull your pubic bone up toward your nose so that you're creating a strong abdominal contraction.

2. Pushing through your heels, drive your hips up until you are in a bridge position. Do not hyperextend your low back to get more range of motion; keep your ribs down, pelvis posteriorly tilted, and abdominals contracted. Squeeze your glutes at the top and then bring your hips slowly back down to the ground, lowering one vertebra at a time back to the start position, and repeat for 15–20 reps.

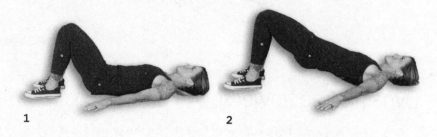

1   2

Half-Kneeling True Hip Flexor Stretch

As pictured, begin in a half-kneeling position, with your right leg in front. Make sure your right foot is directly under your right knee and that your left knee is positioned directly under your left hip. Make sure your hips are square, ribs are down, and then squeeze your left glute and posteriorly tilt your pelvis on the left side. You should feel this stretch in front of your left hip. Hold for 20 seconds, switch legs, and repeat

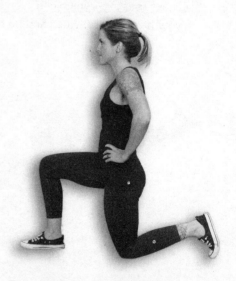

Adductor Rockbacks

1. Start in a quadruped position (on your hands and knees) with your hands directly under your shoulders and your knees directly under your hips.

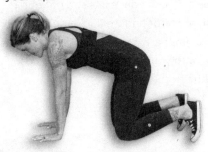

2. As pictured, move your left leg straight out to the side with your toes pointed toward the sky.

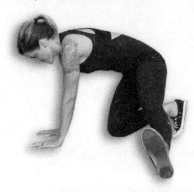

3. Rock your hips backward and forward for 8–10 reps while maintaining your left foot position. Switch legs and repeat.

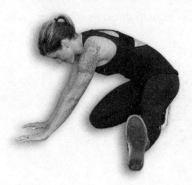

Child's Pose

1. Start in a quadruped position (on your hands and knees).

2. As pictured, bring your knees shoulder-width apart as you rest your buttocks back on your heels. Reach your arms straight out in front of you with your hands on the floor and walk your fingers out in front of you as far as possible to emphasize the stretch. Hold for 20–30 seconds. Breathe deeply into your belly through your nose; breathe out through your mouth.

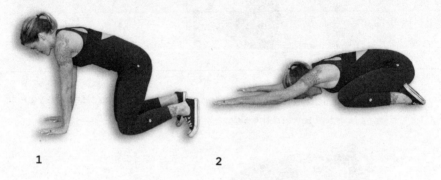

1   2

Child's Pose Lat Stretch

While still in child's pose, slowly walk your fingers over to the right side so that your torso starts to follow, keeping your arms as long as possible to feel the stretch in your lats and making sure to keep your hips back on your heels. Hold for 20–30 seconds. Breathe deeply here in through your nose, out through your mouth. Walk your fingers slowly over as far as you can to the right side and hold for 20–30 seconds. Breathe deeply here in through your nose, out through your mouth.

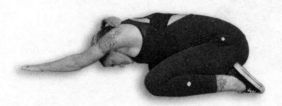

Thoracic Rotation

1. Start in child's pose.

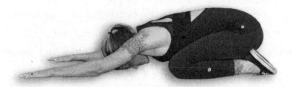

2. Place your left hand on the back of your neck and bring your left elbow down towards your right knee.

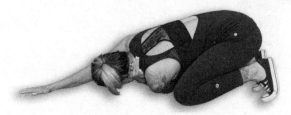

3. Inhale through your nose and as you exhale through your mouth, move your elbow up toward the sky, allowing your gaze to follow where your elbow is pointing. Be sure to move on the exhale. Inhale again back at the bottom position and repeat for 6 reps. Switch arms and repeat on the opposite side.

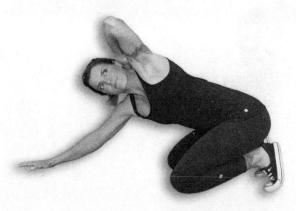

Bear Hold

1. Start in a quadruped position (on your hands and knees). Be sure that your knees are directly under your hips and your hands are directly under your shoulders. Push into the ground with your hands and protract your scapula; imagine you are reaching out with your hands as far as possible as you push into the ground. Now tuck your pelvis so that you feel as if you are pulling your pubic bone toward your nose.

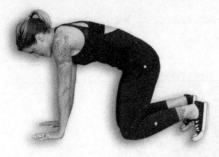

2. Now, holding the above position, tighten your core and raise your knees about 2 inches off the floor and hold. Keep reaching into the ground with your hands and keep your pelvis tucked. Hold this position for 20–30 seconds.

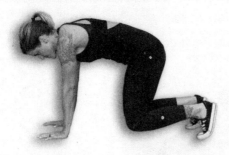

HB Hormone Reset Template

If you've determined that you do not need to start with the HB Core+Floor Recovery Template, you'll start here with the HB Hormone Reset Template. Or, if you have completed three weeks of the HB Core+Floor Recovery Template, this is the workout you'll be doing for the next two weeks. This workout targets common areas of weakness in women such as lower lats, glutes, and hamstrings as well as normalizing cortisol for all women. Do this workout three times per week for two weeks, and then move on to the customizable HB Strength Training Template that we introduced you to during Week 3.

You will do 8–10 reps of each exercise, resting as much as you need to before moving on to the next exercise. You will complete this entire circuit 3–5 times through. If you are brand-new to strength training, we suggest you start with only three times through, maybe even two times through. Listen to your body, and if your muscles are feeling super fatigued and you are not fully recovered after your second time through, it's OK to stop there. Soon you'll be able to get through the workout three to five times, but it's so important to start where you are and not overdo it!

For strength training veterans, unless you are feeling totally wiped out, you are fine to go through this circuit five times, but remember to rest as much as you need to; this is not intended to be metabolic.

Start first with the Dynamic Warm Up on page 258 and/or any unique rehab exercises that might already be prescribed for you.

#1 Squats

○ Perform these at your level as either bodyweight or goblet squats.

Bodyweight Squat

1. Start with your feet placed underneath your shoulders or slightly wider with your toes just slightly turned out. Pull your lower ribs down over your pelvis to maintain neutral spine and hold your arms out in front of you for balance.

2. Squat your hips slightly back and down to parallel if possible or just below if mobility allows. Throughout your squat, your weight should be distributed through midfoot and heel; do not come forward onto your toes. At the bottom of your squat, it might be helpful to drive your knees out as you stand up in order to keep your knees in line with your toes and to activate your glutes.

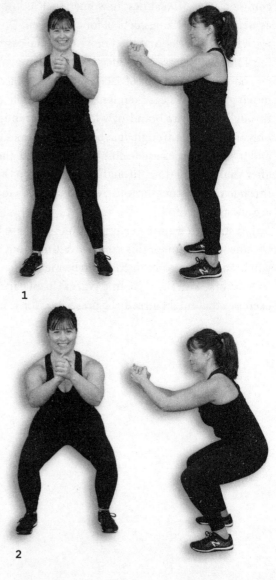

1

2

Goblet Squat

1. Start in your squat stance as described in the bodyweight squat. Hold a kettlebell or dumbbell in front of you with your elbows tight to your body but with the weight held out about 6 inches in front of your chest.

2. Pull your lower ribs down over your pelvis to maintain neutral spine and then follow the instruction as described for the bodyweight squat.

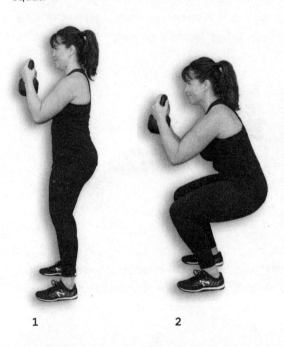

1   2

#2 Push-Ups at Your Level

○ **If the full push-up is too challenging, choose from the following regressions and follow the same directions for the full push-up.**

1. As pictured, start with your hands directly under your shoulders and your feet together up on your toes in a plank position. Rotate the pits of your elbows forward (externally rotating the shoulder) and reach long into the ground, protracting your shoulder blades. Create tension in your entire body, tightening your abdominals, glutes, and quads.

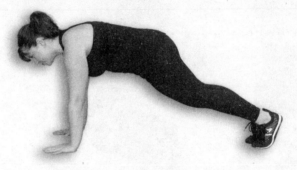

2. Lower yourself to the ground, keeping your arms in close to your side or at least at a 45-degree angle. Full range of motion should occur here. At the bottom, your thighs and chest should be on the floor and, at the top, your arms should be fully extended.

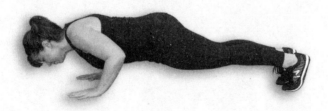

Regression #1: On Knees

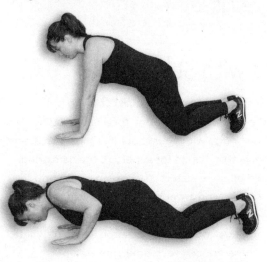

Regression #2: Up Against a Rack or Wall

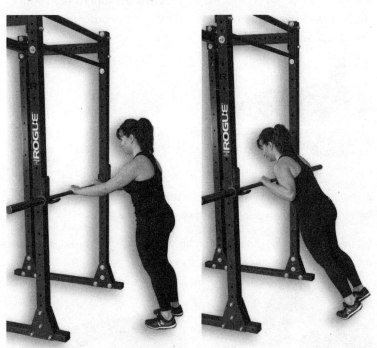

#3 Hamstring Curls

Hamstring Curls with Stability Ball

This movement will be very challenging if you are just starting out. Alternatively, you can do the bilateral glute bridge for a 5-second hold at the top or you can do a glute bridge with your shoulders raised on a bench (hip thrust). Other movements to exhange for variety to the hamstring curls with stability ball would be the unilateral (single-leg) glute bridges (10 each leg) with shoulders raised on a weight bench, or you could simply add weight to the glute bridge either on the floor or with the shoulders raised. When you are working through the HB Hormone Reset Template, feel free to pick any one of these options each time you work out.

1. Start by lying flat on your back with your feet up on the ball and calves resting on the ball. Push your feet and calves into the ball, raising your hips up off the ground and making sure to keep your rib cage down and your abdominals engaged in order to maintain a neutral spine position.

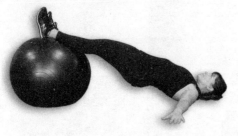

2. Pull your heels in toward your buttocks to activate the hamstrings rather than pulling your knees toward your chest.

3. Maintain neutral spine, straighten your legs as pictured, and repeat the movement, keeping your hips elevated.

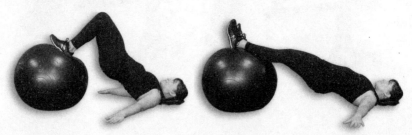

Alternatives to Hamstring Curls

Unilateral Glute Bridge

Begin in the same position as a bilateral glute bridge. Raise one leg up off the ground and, driving through the heel of the foot that's on the ground, raise your hips up, maintaining a strong posterior pelvic tilt. Slowly lower back to the ground one vertebra at a time.

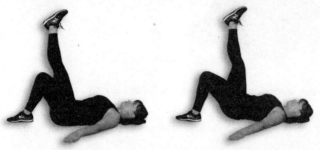

Hip Thrust (Shoulder-Raised Glute Bridge)

1. As pictured, sit with your back up against a weight bench or other solid structure. The bench should be positioned at the base of your shoulder blades. Make sure the bench is stabilized so that it cannot move (for example, up against a wall). Bend your knees so that your feet are flat on the ground about hip-width apart and your heels are about 1 foot away from your buttocks.

2. Bring your ribs down and maintain a posterior pelvic tilt as you push through your heels and raise your hips, maintaining a neutral spine. As pictured, keep your gaze forward; do not lay your head back down on the bench as your hips rise. At the top of this position, make sure your shins are vertical; adjust your foot position as needed. Hold at the top for 3–5 seconds, then slowly lower down and repeat.

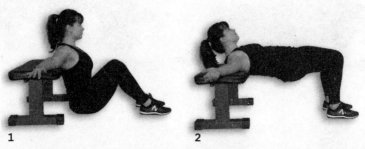

1   2

Glute Bridge with Weight and Hip Thrust with Weight

1. Start in the bilateral glute bridge position with a padded barbell or by holding a dumbbell or weight plate over the crease of your hips. If using a barbell, hold on to the barbell with your arms extended to keep it in place as you raise your hips.

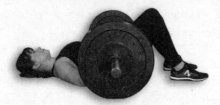

2. Follow the directions for the regular bilateral glute bridge, breathing into your belly and low back to brace your core as you drive your heels into the floor and lift the weight off the ground.

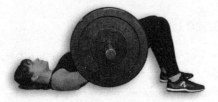

3. To increase the difficulty of this movement, perform the hip thrust with a barbell or other weight option as mentioned in the glute bridge with weight. Be sure to maintain a strong posterior pelvic tilt and tight abdominals throughout this movement, holding the bar or weight tightly over the crease of your hips, as pictured.

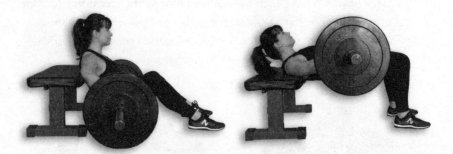

#4 Lat Pull-Down *or* Body Row *or* Pull-Up (assisted or not)

Lat Pulldown

○ **Standing with band or machine.**

1. Stand arm's length away from either the cable machine or bands; make sure your arms are fully extended when you reach out. Hold on to the bands or cable machine and make sure your lower ribs are down and positioned over your hips. Maintain a neutral pelvic position.

2. Bend your knees slightly and, while keeping your core tight, pull the bands or handle on the cable machine down to your thighs while engaging your lats. Control the movement on the way back up.

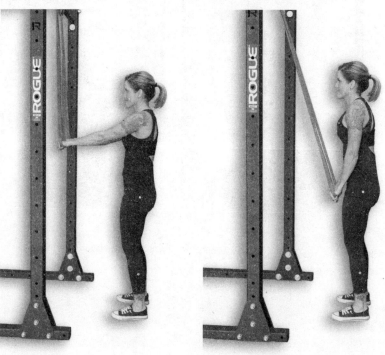

1   2

○ **Seated, using bands or machine.**

1. Sit in the machine and lock your legs into place by adjusting the thigh pad tight enough so that it will hold you seated as you pull the bar down. If using bands, sit on the floor directly under the bands with the bands attached to a stable bar above you and reach up to grab the bands so that your arms are fully extended. Make sure your pelvis is directly under your ribs and that your spine is neutral. Reach up to the bar or the bands and grip the bar or bands with your palms facing forward and hands placed just slightly wider than your shoulders.

2. Take a breath in and tighten your core, pull the bands or bar down to midchest, making sure you do not hyperextend your low back, and exhale as you let the bands or bar come back up.

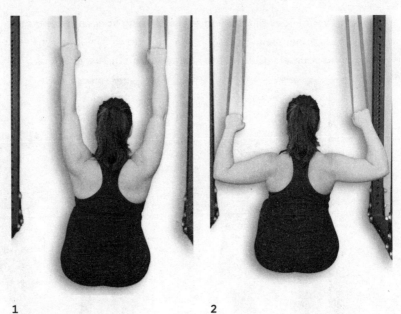

1   2

Body Row with Rings or TRX

1. Start by standing directly between the rings or TRX handles, making sure they are at armpit-height.

2. Holding the rings or handles tight, slowly lower yourself back until your arms are fully extended. Maintain a plank position, tight throughout the core, neck in neutral, and shoulder blades protracted, as pictured. You can keep your feet flat or go onto your heels.

3. Pull your chest toward the rings by first retracting your shoulder blades and then pulling your chest all the way up to the rings. Slowly lower back down and repeat. Do not drop quickly from the top of the movement into full arm extension; maintain control throughout the entirety of this movement.

You can create less resistance by walking your feet back away from the rings and more resistance by walking your feet forward so that your body is closer to parallel with the floor.

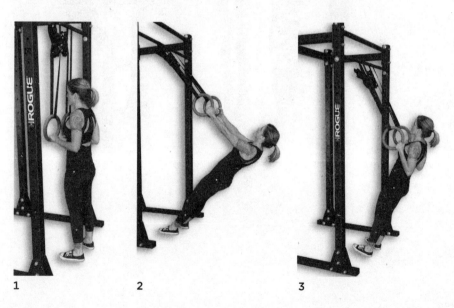

1   2   3

Pull-Up (regular or assisted)

1. With your hands pronated (facing out away from your body), grab the bar with your hands placed slightly wider than your shoulders. Pull your ribs down so that you are in a hollow position with your pelvis tilted posteriorly (pulled forward, not anteriorly; make sure you are not hyperextending your low back).

2. As pictured, pull yourself up until your chin is over the bar, maintaining a hollow position. Lower yourself down in a controlled fashion.

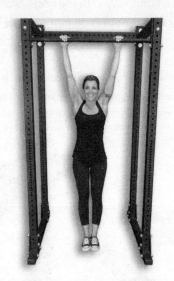

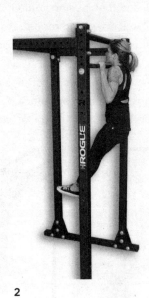

1   2

3. For an assisted pull-up either with bands or with an assisted pull-up machine, follow the same instructions as you would for a regular pull-up. When using a band, place one foot in the band and step straight down; then take the opposite foot and cross it over the foot in the band so that the band is secured as pictured. Now you are ready to pull.

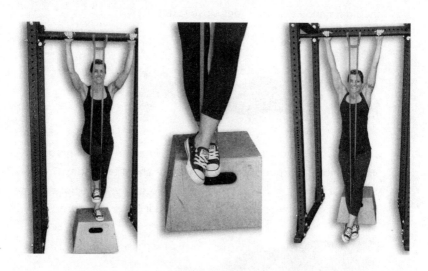

#5 Hold an Active Plank for Up to 20 Seconds or Longer, If Able

1. Lie on your stomach. Position your elbows directly under your shoulders and keep your feet close together.

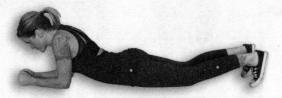

2. Push up onto your forearms and toes; imagine reaching your elbows into the ground and protract your shoulder blades. Tighten your abdominals, glutes, and quads. Make sure you are not pushing your buttocks up into the air or letting your lower back sag.

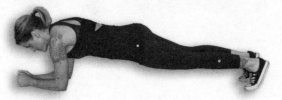

3. If you are unable to maintain this position, perform the same movement but with your knees on the ground for further support, as pictured.

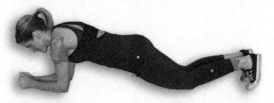

Hold for up to 20 seconds or longer. If you start to feel any discomfort in your lower back, it's time to stop. This might be 15 seconds, or it might be a minute.

HB Strength Training Template Exercise Descriptions

Start here before moving on to the exercise descriptions.

How to Breathe and Brace Your Core While Lifting

As you go through the explanations of how to do the prescribed exercises, you'll see us talk a lot about rib and pelvic position as well as cues to keep a neutral spine. You'll also see us remind you to breathe and to brace. These two concepts—neutral spine and breathing to brace your core—are potentially the most important aspects of weight lifting. Before we go any further into the "how to do it" part, we think it's important for you to understand what your core *really* is. Most of us think only about our abdominal muscles when we think "core," but in reality our core is anything that is a part of our trunk—so basically from our neck down to below our hips. The list below illustrates what is commonly considered core musculature.

- Rectus abdominus
- Transverse abdominus
- Internal and external obliques
- Spinal erectors
- Multifidus
- Hip flexors
- Hip rotators
- Pelvic floor
- Diaphragm

In reality, however, the core musculature includes any muscle that attaches to the low back or pelvis that can affect stability or movement of the trunk. In other words, overall core function is not just dependent on your "abs."

Breathing properly in order to brace is not something we always just "do" naturally. It's a learned process, but through practice you will master it, and practice you must. This is why we want you to make this such a huge priority; learning how to use your core properly ensures your ability to create pressure within your trunk, which allows you to avoid overextension in your lower back.

It also gives you the ability to function properly while lifting, thus avoiding the all-too-common "oh no, I hurt my back in the gym" problem.

We pride ourselves on helping women recover from low back pain due to having a weak core and lifting improperly, so we urge you not to skip this work. Lifting heavy is way more effective than hours of crunches and sit-ups, because, remember, your core is not just those tummy muscles, it's neck to pelvis, and a strong core equals less pain, better mobility from head to toe, and, as we mentioned before, longevity in the gym.

OK, here's how it's done:

The demand of the load will determine when you'll need to breathe and brace. Essentially, when you're "under load," such as with the deadlift or weighted squat of any kind (goblet, dumbbell, back squat), or when you bench press, do a hip thrust or weighted glute bridge, or press overhead, these are the movements in which you'll need to be intently focused on breathing and bracing. Of course, with ALL the prescribed movements you'll want to tighten your core; however, it's the "big lifts" such as those you'll find in the 5×5 Section A of the HB Strength Training Template in which you'll be moving a substantial enough amount of weight that you will absolutely need to breathe and brace in order to protect your spine.

Step one: No matter the lift, be sure you are in a neutral spine position with lower ribs down over your pelvis. (Each movement description below will have instructions for how to do so.)

Step two: Engage your abdominals and obliques in order to tighten up your entire core.

Step three: Take a strong breath in and send that air down into your lower chest and belly. Try to imagine the air is expanding into your diaphragm, obliques, and low back; in other words, get super tight all the way around your midsection as if you are creating the same support as a weight belt. You should be able to feel expansion all the way around; you're not just tightening your tummy but creating pressure circumferentially.

Step four: Now you are ready to lift. Be sure to stay tight throughout the entire lift, and reset and take another breath where you need to. You'll find over time that you will create your own rhythmic breathing pattern with each lift. The most important thing is that you remain in neutral spine and stay tight and engaged throughout each movement. In other words, do not "loosen up" under load.

For video instruction on how to do this, visit us at www.sarahanddrbrooke.com.

Movement Progression Guide

SQUATS

Air Squat   ⟶   Goblet Squat

- Spine in neutral
- Knees in line with toes
- Weight distribution through heel and midfoot

When you are ready to add weight, begin first with the goblet squat, holding the weight 6 inches in front of your body. This will allow you to experience what it's like to engage your anterior core and will assist with pulling your lower ribs down and maintaining neutral spine.
- Spine in neutral
- Knees in line with toes
- Weight distribution through heel and midfoot

Dumbbell Squat   ⟶   Barbell Back Squat

- Spine in neutral
- Knees in line with toes
- Weight distribution through heel and midfoot
- Able to keep lower ribs down over pelvis with dumbbells held up on shoulders as pictured

When determining if you are ready to squat with a barbell on your back, here's what you need to look for:
- Once you have mastered the progressions above, you are ready to move on to attempting the barbell back squat with the following consideration.
- Hand placement on the bar: This may vary based on shoulder mobility. What we're looking for here is the ability to maintain neutral spine position and keep your lower ribs down over your pelvis while holding the bar on your back, no matter where your grip might be.

DEADLIFT

Kettlebell ⟶ Dumbbell Deadlift

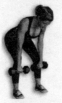

- Spine in neutral
- Shins vertical
- Knees in line with toes
- Hip height between knees and shoulders

If you're unable to get into proper position, the correction for this would be to raise the kettlebell up in order to achieve correct form.

- Spine in neutral
- Shins vertical
- Knees in line with toes
- Hip height between knees and shoulders

The dumbbell deadlift differs from the kettlebell stance, as this will have you assume a traditional deadlift position as opposed to the sumo stance with the kettlebell. All the same rules apply, but you will start in the top position, not the bottom. If you can maintain neutral spine throughout this movement, you are ready to move on to the barbell deadlift.

Barbell Deadlift

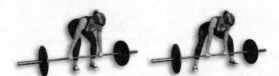

- Spine in neutral
- Shins vertical
- Knees in line with toes
- Hip height between knees and shoulders

If you have trouble achieving the above requirements with a traditional stance deadlift, sumo stance will most likely be a better option for you, as this allows you to get into the bottom position with more ease, with the hips being opened up. If in sumo stance you are still unable to maintain neutral spine at the bottom position, you can raise the barbell up onto blocks or plates.

BENCH PRESS

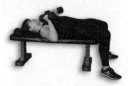

Dumbbell and Barbell

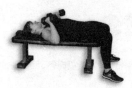 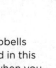 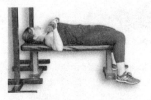

We suggest starting with dumbbells to get used to being under load in this position and then graduating when you are ready to the barbell during Section A of your workout. If you do have a shoulder injury or issue, dumbbells will be a better option and you can do this movement lying on the floor with knees bent and feet flat on the floor to keep your shoulders in a safe range of motion.

OVERHEAD PRESS

Dumbbell Press ⟶ Barbell Press

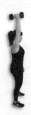 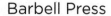

- Neutral spine—lower ribs down over pelvis throughout the entire movement
- Proper shoulder mobility—top position with dumbbells held directly over shoulders while able to keep neutral spine

- Neutral spine—lower ribs down over pelvis throughout the entire movement
- Proper shoulder mobility—top position with barbell held directly over shoulders while able to keep neutral spine

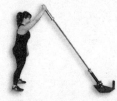

If you lack the shoulder mobility to perform this movement as pictured with the barbell or dumbbells directly overhead—the modification is the landmine press.

WEIGHTED GLUTE BRIDGE/
WEIGHTED HIP THRUST

The progression with these movements is more about level of strength than mobility or position. Start in order with the following movements. When you are able to efficiently perform these movements, you can move on to adding weight.

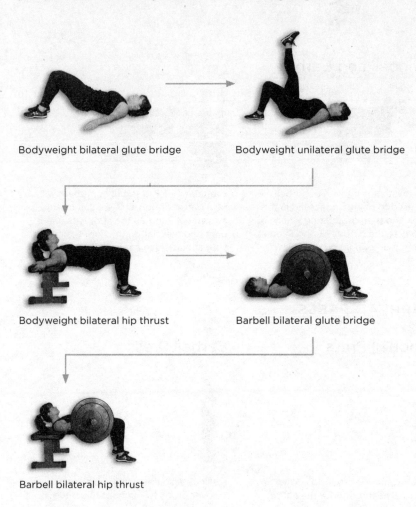

Bodyweight bilateral glute bridge

Bodyweight unilateral glute bridge

Bodyweight bilateral hip thrust

Barbell bilateral glute bridge

Barbell bilateral hip thrust

❱ Exercise Descriptions from the HB Strength Training Template

Always begin your workout with our Dynamic Warm Up (page 258) and 4 or 5 breaths of Forced Exhalation (page 251). Always end your workout with at least 3–5 minutes of restorative breathing (see page 103). Be sure to refer to chapter 9, page 180, to learn how to use the HB Strength Training Template and how to design your workouts. Don't forget to customize the template based on your Hangry B*tch Quiz Result and to change your workouts every four to six weeks.

Section A1 Exercise Descriptions

Squat Variations

Goblet Squat

See page 267.

Dumbbell Squat

1. Start by standing with your feet shoulder-width apart or slightly wider, holding the dumbbells in your hands. As pictured, hold the dumbbells up so that one end is resting on your shoulders, your elbows are straight out in front, and the heads of the dumbbells are facing out over your elbows.

2. Make sure your lower ribs are pulled down and positioned over your pelvis. Breathe and brace and then push your hips back slightly as you squat down to parallel or just below, depending on your mobility.

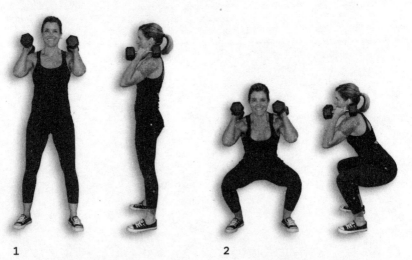

1   2

Barbell Squat

1. As pictured, make sure the rack is adjusted so that the barbell is at clavicle height, stand with your hips underneath the barbell, and position the bar on your traps, the "meatier" part of your upper back. Avoid placing the bar on your neck (cervical spine). Make sure your hands are slightly wider than shoulder-width as you evenly grip the bar with your elbows slightly back, in order to create tension and a stable shelf for the weight. If shoulder mobility does not allow for you to grab the bar just outside of shoulder width, it's OK to widen your grip position on the bar.

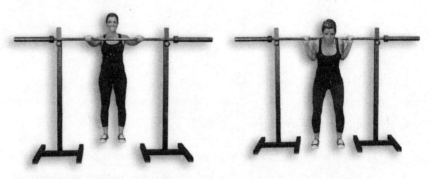

2. Make sure to create tension under the bar by tightening your core and pulling the bar into your back before you stand up. Now, stand up with the bar on your back and take two steps back, away from the rack. Position your feet in your normal squat stance and then make sure your pelvis is positioned under your lower ribs by pulling your ribs down.

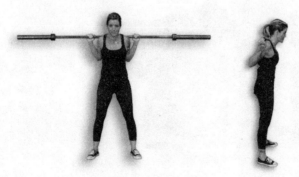

3. Before you initiate the squat, be sure to breathe and brace. Now, squat down as usual, keeping your core as tight as possible during the entire movement.

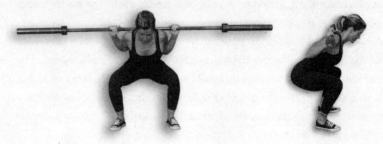

Deadlift Variations

Kettlebell Deadlift

1. Assume a wide "sumo" stance, with feet more than shoulder-width apart and toes slightly turned out. Have the kettlebell positioned so that it's at midline of your body or bisecting your feet, as pictured. Bring your lower ribs down over your pelvis, which should be posteriorly tilted, with no excessive curve in your low back. Hinge at your hips, reaching your buttocks back toward the wall behind you and, once you feel your hamstrings engage, bend at the knees until you can grab the kettlebell, as pictured.

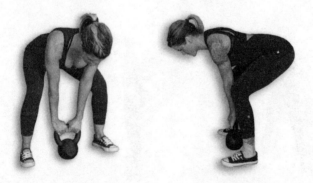

2. As pictured, in the bottom position you should have a neutral spine and vertical shins with knees in line with toes (not caving in), and be sure you are looking down at the ground about 4 feet in front of you. Now, engage your lats by pulling your shoulder blades down. Breathe and brace and then, driving your feet into the ground, stand up, holding the kettlebell. Return the kettlebell to the ground while keeping the kettlebell close to your body/midline as you return to the bottom position.

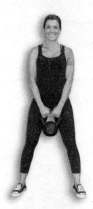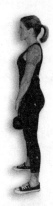

Dumbbell Deadlift

1. Start with your feet under your hips or just outside. Hold the dumbbells in your palms, palms facing the fronts of your thighs so that the dumbbell position mimics how it would look if you were holding a barbell.

2. Make sure your spine is neutral, with your pelvis under your lower ribs. Breathe and brace and hinge your hips back to lower the weights, keeping your spine neutral and keeping the dumbbells close to your body, as pictured, as you lower them just to mid-shin. Return to standing.

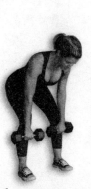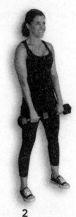

1   2

Traditional Stance Barbell Deadlift

1. Stand with your feet under your hips or slightly outside with your shins touching the barbell. The barbell should be at mid-shin height, so if your plates are not large enough to raise the bar to the appropriate height, be sure you set the bar up on blocks. Make sure that you have a neutral spine, your lower ribs are pulled down over your pelvis, and you do not have any anterior tilt in your pelvis (no excessive curve in your low back). Hinge your hips back toward the wall behind you until you can go no further (you can feel your hamstrings engage) and then bend your knees until you can grab the bar.

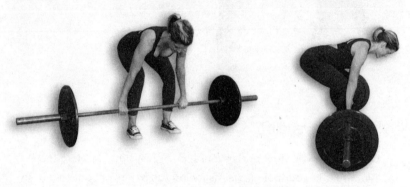

2. Grip the bar right outside your shins, making sure the barbell is snug in the crease of your palm. Your hip height should be in between your shoulders and your knees. Tighten your core, make sure your lats are engaged by squeezing your shoulder blades down, breathe and brace, and drive your feet into the ground to stand with the bar, "shaving your legs" with the barbell on the way up. It's very important that you keep the weight in close to your body; do not let it swing out in front of you. At the top of your deadlift,

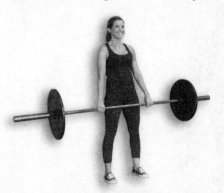
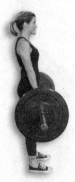

squeeze your glutes to open your hips all the way, keeping a neutral spine. Reverse the movement by hinging at your hips as you pull the bar in toward your legs on the descent.

Sumo Stance Barbell Deadlift

1. Stand with a wide sumo stance, with your feet wider than shoulder-width and turned out slightly, your shins vertical, and your knees pointing over your toes (not caved in). Your shins should be touching the bar. Follow the instructions for the traditional deadlift to reach down to the bar, but this time your grip will be directly under your shoulders and inside of your shins, as pictured.

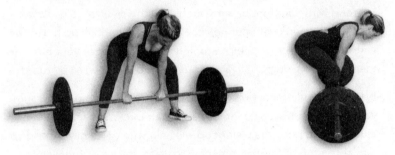

2. Follow the instructions in the traditional deadlift to pick the bar up off the ground and do the same for the return; be sure to keep the bar close to your body for the ascent and descent of the bar.

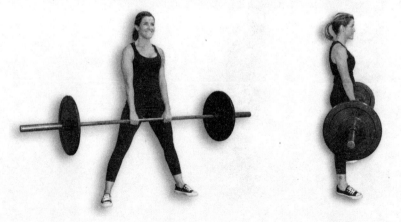

Weighted Glute Bridge or Weighted Hip Thrust

See pages 271–72.

Section A2 Exercise Descriptions

Overhead Press Variations

If you do not have the shoulder range of motion to press overhead without arching your back, please do a landmine press instead until your shoulder mobility improves.

Dumbbell Overhead Press

1. Stand with your feet under your hips with a neutral spine, lower ribs pulled down over your pelvis. Raise one dumbbell up to rest on your shoulder with your elbow pointing out in front of your body and the head of the dumbbell facing out over your elbow, as pictured.

2. Breathe and brace, pushing the dumbbell straight up. Make sure you keep a neutral spine; do not arch your back. Squeezing your glutes as you push the weight up will help with this. Fully extend your arm at the top of this movement. Exhale as you lower the weight back down to your shoulder in a controlled fashion.

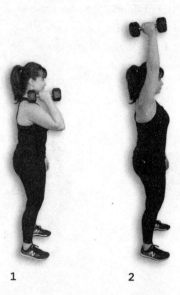

1   2

Landmine Press

1. Stand with your feet under your hips and hold the barbell in one hand with your elbow out in front and the end of the barbell near the front of your shoulder, as pictured. Make sure you have a neutral spine position as described in the dumbbell press.

2. Take in a breath to breathe and brace, and then push the barbell up, keeping the bar at midline as pictured until you reach full arm extension. Exhale as you lower the bar back to your shoulder in a controlled fashion.

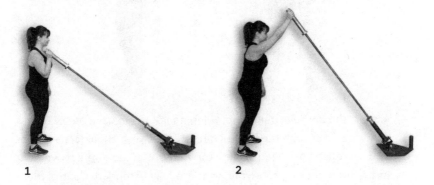

1   2

Barbell Overhead Press

1. Place the barbell in the rack at clavicle height. Stand directly in front of the bar, as pictured, with your hands on the barbell right outside of shoulder-width.

2. Step forward so that you can get under the bar, as pictured, with the barbell resting on your delts. Your elbows should be pointed out in front of you, as pictured, and the barbell should rest in your fingers, with your delts supporting the majority of the weight of the bar.

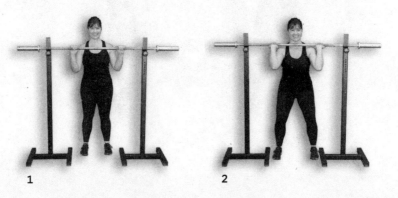

1   2

3. Stand up tall with the bar and take two steps away from the rack, roll the barbell into the crease of your palm, and move your elbows down so they are still slightly in front of the barbell, as pictured. Make sure your feet are directly under your hips, pull your lower ribs down over your pelvis, and breathe and brace.

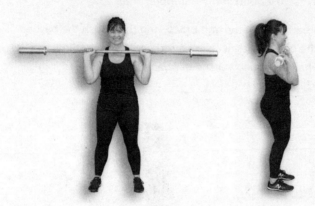

4. Push the barbell straight up, bringing your chin back out of the way, and finish with the barbell directly over your shoulders and hips. You can push your head slightly forward at the top of the movement, as pictured, making sure your arms are fully extended. Control the barbell back down to your start position, bringing your head back out of the way of the bar path. Breathe and brace again and repeat the movement.

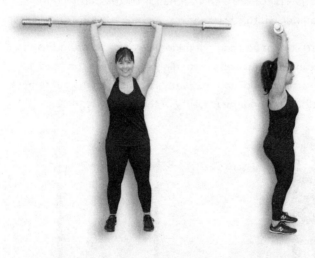

Bench Press Variations

Dumbbell Flat Bench Press

1. Lie on your back on a flat bench with your knees bent and feet flat on the floor, as pictured, holding a dumbbell in each hand.

2. Breathe and brace, press the dumbbells straight up, keeping the weights over the shoulders, and return the dumbbells back down to the start position in a controlled fashion. Your elbow position during the bench press should be between 45 degrees and 70 degrees; avoid pressing at a 90-degree angle to maintain shoulder health.

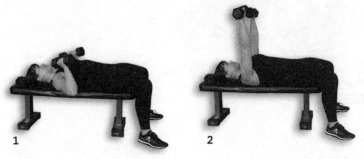

Barbell Flat Bench Press

1. Lie on your back on a flat bench with the bar racked directly above your eyes. Lift your chest up and squeeze your shoulder blades together, and create an arch in your back with your buttocks and shoulder blades on the bench. Grab the bar just outside your shoulders with the bar held tight in the crease of your palms without overextending the wrists.

2. Take a deep breath in (breathe and brace) and unrack the bar by simply straightening your arms. Then move the bar slightly forward over your shoulders, keeping your elbows locked.

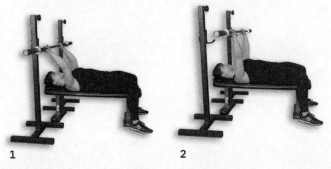

3. Lower the bar to mid-chest, keeping your elbows at approximately a 45-degree angle until the bar touches your mid-chest. Press the bar up and back so it finishes again directly over your shoulders, exhale at the top, breathe and brace again, and repeat the movement. To rack the bar, simply lock your arms as you bring the bar back until it hits the rack and lower back down into position.

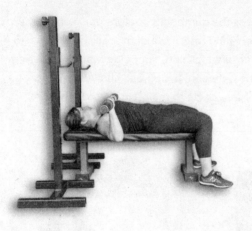

Pull-Up and Body Row Variations

See pages 275–77.

Section A3 Exercise Descriptions

Step-Ups onto Box

○ **Weighted or unweighted**

Unweighted Step-Ups

1. Stand a few inches in front of the box. Place one foot in the center of the box with your shin vertical, as pictured.

2. As you step up onto the box, hinge slightly forward and push through your heel, squeezing your glutes as you stand.

3. Open your hips fully at the top, to stand on the box with both feet. To reverse the movement, pick up the foot that was originally on the ground, hinge at the hips as you step back, and return to the start position, all the while making sure that the foot on the box maintains heel contact and that the shin remains as vertical as possible on the descent. Try to avoid letting your knee cave inward. Repeat with the opposite foot.

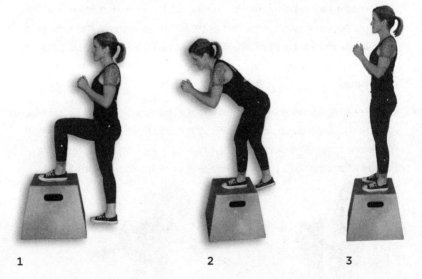

1   2   3

Weighted Step-Ups

Holding a dumbbell in each hand, follow the directions for the unweighted step-ups.

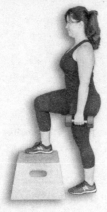

Bent-Over Row Variations

Barbell Bent-Over Row

1. Holding a barbell with your hands under your shoulders and your palms facing down (pronated grip), hinge forward at the hips with your knees slightly bent, making sure you keep your back flat and your core tight until your torso is just above parallel to the floor, as pictured.

2. Breathe and brace and then initiate the row by pulling your elbows back toward your body, retracting the shoulder blades as you pull the bar toward your belly until it touches your body. Control the movement back to the start position as you exhale. Repeat.

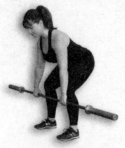

1

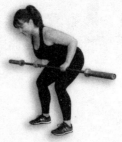

2

Single-Arm Dumbbell Row

1. Using a flat bench, place your right knee on the bench with your left foot on the floor next to the bench for support and lean forward onto your right hand placed directly under your shoulder. Your back should be flat, with no arch in your lower back. Pick the dumbbell up off the floor with your left hand keeping your back straight. Your palm should be facing the bench.

2. Start the movement by retracting your left shoulder blade and pulling the dumbbell up toward your chest, focusing on using the muscles in your mid-back to pull the weight. Stop the range of motion just below the chest; do not pull past the chest or twist the torso. Return the dumbbell to the start position and repeat and then switch sides.

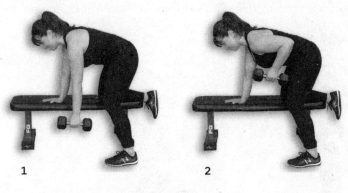

1   2

Lunge Variations

Unweighted Reverse Lunges

1. Begin in a standing position. Make sure your lower ribs are pulled down over your pelvis and your hips are squared.

2. Step straight back with your left foot, bring your left knee straight down toward the ground, and stop about an inch before your knee touches, as pictured. Make sure your torso remains upright, your hips are squared, and your spine is in neutral. The front shin should be vertical with your right knee over your right heel. Push straight up through your right heel to stand, maintaining a vertical shin (do not let your front knee drive forward over your toes or cave inward). Repeat the same movement, now stepping back with your right foot.

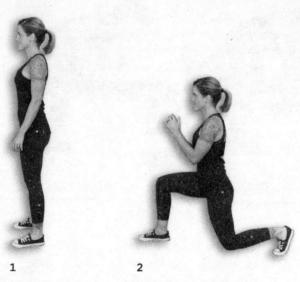

1   2

Weighted Reverse Lunges

⊙ If you are not ready to do reverse lunges because you lack core strength and balance, please start with static lunges and, if needed, hold onto a bench or rack for support while you perform the static lunge.

Perform this movement exactly the same as unweighted lunges while holding dumbbells in both hands down by your sides, as pictured. Or hold one kettlebell or dumbbell in front of your chest, elbows in tight and with the weight 6–8 inches in front of your body, as you would in a goblet squat.

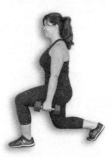

Unweighted Static Lunges

1. Start in a half-kneeling position, as pictured, with your right leg in front. Place your left knee directly under your left hip and your right foot directly under your right knee so that your shin is vertical.

2a and 2b. Push straight up through your right heel, being sure to avoid transfering your weight forward as you rise. Do not come back up to stand with your feet together but rather stay in the lunge position as you extend both legs and open your hips fully at the top of this movement. Repeat by simply lowering your left knee back down to the ground and then back up again, as pictured. Finish your reps on that leg and then switch sides. (Do not let your front knee drive forward over your toes or cave inward.)

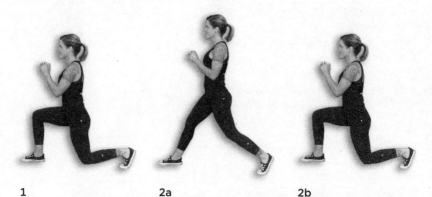

1   2a   2b

Weighted Static Lunges

Perform this movement exactly the same as the unweighted static lunges while holding dumbbells in both hands down by your sides, as pictured. Or hold one kettlebell or dumbbell in front of your chest, elbows in tight and with the weight 6–8 inches out in front of your body.

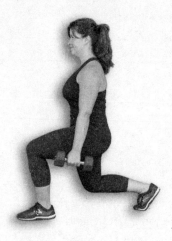

Section B Exercise Descriptions

Lunges

See pages 300–02.

Glute Bridges

See page 260.

Hamstring Curls

See page 270.

Dumbbell Bench Press

See page 295.

Push-Ups

See pages 268–69.

Parallel Bar Dips

○ **Assisted or not**

1. As pictured, place your hands on the parallel, or dip, bars that are set to shoulder-width apart.

2. Slightly tilt your torso forward and slowly lower yourself down until your upper arms are parallel with the floor. Be sure not to let yourself drop lower than this in order to stay in a safe range of motion. Push yourself up until your arms are almost fully extended. It's OK to maintain a slight bend in the elbow at the top of this movement, but you want to come close to achieving full range of motion.

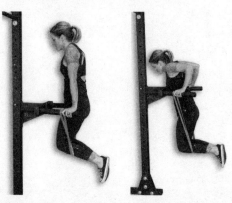

Assisted Dips

⊙ **The setup and execution of this movement are the same as unassisted dips; however, you will be using a dip-resistant machine, if available, in which you adjust the amount of help you receive on the way up out of your dip.**

Skull Crushers

1. Lie on your back on a flat bench with your back flat on the bench and your feet flat on the floor. Or lie on the floor with your knees bent and feet on the floor so that your lower back is supported. Hold two dumbbells in your palms with your palms facing each other directly over your shoulders.

2. Bending only at the elbow and keeping your shoulders at 90 degrees and your elbows tucked in, as pictured (not pointed out), control the dumbbells down toward the sides of your head as you lengthen the triceps until the dumbbells are down next to your head. Extend your arms back up to the start position and repeat.

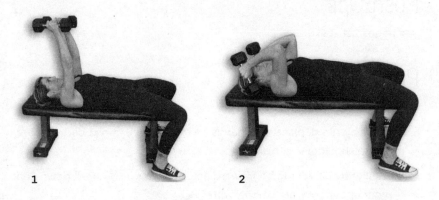

1   2

Bicep Curls

1. Stand up straight with your feet under your hips, with your ribs pulled down over your pelvis in order to create a neutral spine. Hold the dumbbells at your sides and rotate them so that your palms are facing forward, as pictured.

2. Keeping your elbows in close to your torso and your upper arms stationary, curl the weights up toward your shoulders while contracting your biceps. Control the weights back down to the start position and repeat the movement.

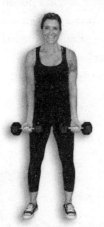 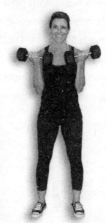

Lat Pull-Down

See page 273.

Single-Arm Dumbbell Row

See page 299.

Seated Cable Row

○ **This movement can also be performed with resistance bands, as pictured.**

1. Sit on the bench on your sit bones with a slight knee bend and your feet flat on the platform in front of you. Lean forward, grab the handle, and pull it out until your arms are fully extended and let your shoulder blades protract. (A V-shaped handle is preferred so that your palms are facing each other.)

2. Make sure that your back is straight and your lower ribs are pulled down to create a neutral spine. Keep your torso stationary as you pull the cable toward your chest, first by retracting your shoulder blades, keeping elbows in as you pull and squeeze your back muscles to execute the movement. Control the handle back to the start position, maintaining an upright posture, and repeat the movement.

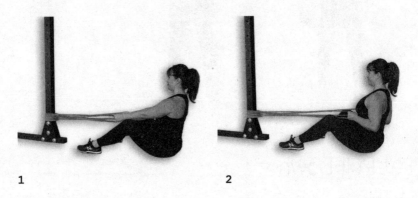

1   2

Standing Cable Row

○ **This movement can also be performed with resistance bands, as pictured.**

1. Use the V-shaped handle and make sure the cable is set at approximately chest height. Stand in front of the cable machine with your feet shoulder-width apart and with a slight knee bend. Grab the cable and pull it toward you until you're in your starting position, as pictured. Make sure you maintain a neutral spine by pulling your lower ribs down over your pelvis.

2. Let your shoulder blades protract and then, as you pull, retract your shoulder blades to start the movement and squeeze your back muscles as you pull the cable to your sternum. Keep your torso stationary during the movement.

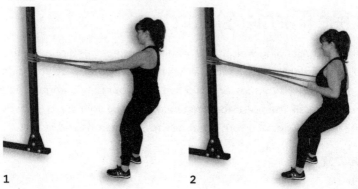

1   2

Plank

See page 278.

Side Plank

See page 256.

Superwoman

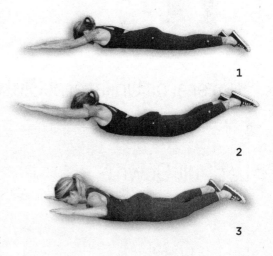

1

2

3

1. Lie flat on your stomach with your arms outstretched in front of you, as pictured.

2. Simultaneously lift your arms, chest, and legs up off of the floor and hold for 1–2 seconds. Focus on squeezing your lower back as you do this movement.

3. If you have limited range of motion and are unable to outstretch your arms, keep your arms at 90 degrees, as pictured, and perform the same movement as described.

Section C Exercise Descriptions

Suitcase (Farmer's) Carry

Select a challenging weight with either a kettlebell or a dumbbell.
Hold the weight in one hand, palm facing your body in by your side
as pictured. Pull your lower ribs down over your pelvis, engage your
core, and walk the prescribed distance, keeping your torso long; do
not let the weight pull your chest down. Switch arms and repeat.

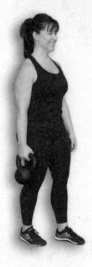

Bilateral or Unilateral Glute Bridges

See pages 260 and 271.

Lat Pull-Down

See page 273.

Plank Hold

See page 278.

How to Outfit a Home Gym

For those of you who want to know how to outfit a basic home gym, we've got you covered here. We've broken up what you'll need based on our three workout templates and have created categories of what's absolutely necessary for each template, what would be optimal, and finally an "above and beyond" category if you really want to get fancy. In other words, you can start with the bare-bones basics if you need to and then work up from there!

HB Core+Floor Equipment

Necessary:

Nothing!! Such good news here, right? The only thing we would recommend is maybe a yoga mat if you have hard wood or tile flooring, since basically all of your exercises will require you to be down on the floor. How's that for easy?

HB Hormone Reset Equipment

Necessary:

Good news again: there's no equipment that is absolutely necessary to do this workout, although we do suggest goblet or dumbbell squats if you are strong enough to progress from the air squat. The hamstring curls in this workout do require some equipment, but again, we offer alternatives to this movement that only require YOU!

Optimal:

5- to 35-pound dumbbells and/or 15- to 35-pound kettlebells

Exercise ball

Above and Beyond:

Glute ham developer (This is quite the investment, and an exercise ball works just fine, but if you really want to get fancy, this is the machine to have on hand.)

HB Strength Training Template Equipment

Necessary:

5- to 35-pound dumbbells and/or 15- to 65-pound kettlebells

Step-up box 12 to 24 inches

Exercise ball

Pull-up bar (You can use one that can easily be installed in a doorway or a more advanced system that can be secured into studs in the ceiling or wall.)

Pull-up assistance bands, gymnastics rings, or a TRX system (Choose one of these three items to suspend from the pull-up bar.)

Resistance bands for lat pull-downs, standing rows, and seated rows

Optimal:

You'll need everything listed above plus the following:

35- or 45-pound barbells

10-, 25-, and 45-pound Olympic lifting plates

2.5-, 5-, and 10-pound metal plates

Barbell collars

Flat bench

Freestanding rack

Barbell pad (for weighted glute bridges and hip thrusts)

Above and Beyond:

Cable machine

Glute ham developer

Assisted dip and pull-up machine

How to Interview a Personal Trainer

To begin, we want you to get one thing straight. We know it can be intimidating to go into a gym, period, and even more intimidating to try to find the right personal trainer to work with. But we want you to remember that *you* are the one with the power in this situation. It doesn't matter if you are interviewing a doctor, lawyer, lawn-care-service provider, piano instructor, or personal trainer—you are giving that person your hard-earned money, so even if that person has a few more certifications or letters behind their name than you do, it doesn't mean they are in charge.

Our intuition is powerful, and if we listened to it more often, we could probably save ourselves from a lot of "holy guacamole, I should have done that differently" situations. So our first bit of advice in interviewing a personal trainer is this: if it doesn't feel right, it's not, so don't walk away—run. Our second bit of advice when hiring a personal trainer is to make sure they first ask *you* all the right questions. A trainer who knows what they are doing should do a consultation with you before they ever even bring you out to the gym floor. They should ask you about your history and what your goals are. They should ask about everything from previous and current injuries to orthopedic issues to medications to what your past gym or fitness experience might be. They should also ask you about your current lifestyle and express interest in your stress level, how well you're sleeping, what you are currently doing for exercise, and what your nutrition is like. Finally, they should ask to see what your movement looks like. They should assess at the very least your shoulder and hip mobility and preferably your ability to perform basic movement, such as your squat, lunge/step-up, and push-up.

If the trainer you are meeting with does none of these things, then there is no need for you to even ask any questions—this is not the right trainer for you. If your potential trainer does do at least most of these things and your intuition is telling you this could be a good fit, now it's time for you to ask your questions. First, ask if this trainer has any testimonials and if any of their current or past clients would be willing to tell you about their experience with this trainer. Next, ask what their take is on nutrition and lifestyle. If they dive into wanting to put you on a calorie-restrictive and/or low-fat diet and say that you should come to the gym as many days as possible, this is not the trainer for you. If the answer is reasonable, well-rounded, and biased toward balance and overall health with an emphasis on recovery and efficient time spent in the gym rather than the "more is best" philosophy, then you can keep going with your interview. Your most important question now would be to ask if your trainer is familiar with the lifts we prescribe in our template, specifically the deadlift, back squat, bench press, and overhead press. Most personal trainer certification programs, even the highly accredited ones, do not teach these important lifts, and these are secondary skills that trainers must go out and seek on their own. If they are familiar with these lifts, ask them about their experience coaching them. If they say this is the foundation of how they train their clients, hooray, you are getting closer to finding the right person for you!

You'll need to be brave now; ask your potential trainer if they would be willing to follow a template designed by other fitness professionals that is tailored to fit your own unique hormonal profile. Explain that you are following a program designed to help you heal and that you want guidance and technique coaching for the prescribed lifts but that you are pretty much hell-bent on following the program that has been customized just for you! A good trainer will be eager, excited, and interested to learn more; see what you are up to; or at least agree to explore this option further. There are good trainers out there and, as in any other profession, there are bad ones. Don't be shy, and remember, just because this person might know more than you, it does NOT mean they know what's right for you. We have given you the tools to know what's right for you, so you are walking in armed with knowledge that few people have. Most important, let your amazing, powerful, awesome-sauce intuition be your guide.

Finally, don't forget: we've got your back. We've left no stones unturned, and even if you strike out finding a trainer, we are certain that between the lifting instructions in the pages of this book and the coaching we offer online (available to you at www.sarahanddrbrooke.com, we'll get you to where you feel confident walking into any gym!

The Hangry B*tch Food Fix

Recipes

In this section, you'll find recipes for breakfast, lunch and snacks, and dinner, as well as staples. We suggest that you make enough of each recipe to last a few days, and if you have a big family, you can double most of the recipes.

Almost all of the recipes include instructions and suggestions for how to turn leftovers into another meal, which is an incredible time-saver! We are also huge advocates of eating dinner leftovers for breakfast, lunch, or snacks—because who has the time to spend half the day in the kitchen?

Ingredient Reminder

Grass-fed and pasture-raised meat, and eggs from pasture-raised chickens are preferred and so, too, are organic vegetables. Also, if a recipe calls for something like store-bought bone broth or deli meat that is prepackaged, look for organic, gluten-free, and free-range options.

Breakfast doesn't always have to look like our preconceived notions of the first meal of the day, and getting over hang-ups about meal number one will make your life much easier. The most important thing is that you get enough protein and fibrous veggies, that you hone in on your UCT, and that you are doing what works for *you* every time you feed yourself.

This "keep it simple" perspective doesn't mean you can't enjoy your food, or love to cook, or that this section is full of what looks like "diet fare"—because that's for sure not what we are aiming for. We simply want you to nourish your body in a doable, tangible fashion that stays in line with the first pillar, and we hope this section leaves you feeling inspired rather than worried about the logistics or how-to's.

When you're making a huge lifestyle change, what you perceive to be the hardest part can become easy when you have a plan and are prepared and, most important, when you have a positive perspective—which is why we have taken the guesswork out of meal planning for you. Enjoy!

The Hangry B*tch
BREAKFAST FIX

Breakfast Soups

We love soup for breakfast. It's a nutrient-dense powerhouse, it's simple to make a big pot and have leftovers for the week, and it's an easy way to get in plenty of protein and veggies first thing in the morning without slogging through a pile of eggs. We suggest having plenty of already-cooked protein like our Basic Chicken (page 373) on hand so you're ready to go in the morning, or, while you are making dinner, we suggest you prepare your breakfast soup at the same time. This way you'll have several meals ready for the week ahead.

Planning ahead for the first meal of the day is paramount to your success and a sure way to keep your blood sugar balanced. Plus, soup is delicious!

Basic Breakfast Soup

- Keeps well in the refrigerator up to four days or in the freezer up to three months.
- Prep time: 10 minutes
- Cook time: 10 minutes
- Serves 2

4 cups Beef or Chicken Bone Broth (page 374) or store-bought beef or chicken broth

2 pounds cooked meat, such as diced or shredded chicken (see page 373); ground bison, turkey or lean beef; or leftover steak cut into bite-size pieces

1–2 tablespoons extra virgin olive oil or avocado oil

3–5 large handfuls baby spinach, baby kale, or other tender greens

1–2 garlic cloves, minced

Juice of ½ lemon

Sea salt and freshly ground pepper
Chopped fresh cilantro or flat-leaf parsley (optional)

1. Combine the broth and meat in a large saucepan and bring to a simmer.
2. In a large skillet, heat the oil over medium heat; add the greens and garlic and cook, stirring, until the greens are tender. Add the greens to the broth, stir, and season with the lemon juice and salt and pepper to taste. Sprinkle with cilantro and serve.

Breakfast Soup Five Ways

Start with the base recipe of the broth, your choice of protein, and the greens and consider the following options to switch up your breakfast soup!

1. Change the veggies up! You can use other vegetables along with the greens. Good choices include diced zucchini, cauliflower "rice," chopped green beans, quartered Brussels sprouts, diced red bell pepper, and/or shredded cabbage. Cook the vegetables in the oil until tender before adding the greens and garlic.
2. To make an Asian-inspired soup, substitute 4 teaspoons tamari or coconut aminos for the lemon juice and add 1 teaspoon grated fresh ginger (or more to taste) and a few drops of sesame oil. Sprinkle with chopped green onion along with the cilantro.
3. Make a mock tortilla soup by adding 1 cup salsa verde or other salsa of your choice, ½–1 tablespoon of chili powder, and ½–1 tablespoon ground cumin to the broth. Top each bowl with diced fresh jicama and sliced radishes along with fresh cilantro.
4. Make it like a minestrone by adding one (14.5-ounce) can diced tomatoes, 2 tablespoons dried basil, and 1 tablespoon dried oregano to the broth. Sprinkle with chopped fresh flat-leaf parsley.
5. Top each bowl of soup with a poached or fried egg for some extra protein.

Breakfast Skillets

Herbed Cauliflower Rice Breakfast Skillet

You can double or triple this recipe on the day you make it and then on busy mornings all you'll need to do is add leftover protein to the cauliflower rice, reheat, and eat!

Second meal idea: Simply add your leftovers to some bone broth (page 374) along with leftover protein to whip up a quick soup for any meal of the day.

- Keeps well in the refrigerator for up to five days or in the freezer for up to twelve months.
- Prep time: 15 minutes
- Cook time: 10 minutes
- Serves 3

1 tablespoon coconut oil or avocado oil
½ small red onion, finely chopped
1 garlic clove, minced
2 zucchini, diced
1 pound bagged riced cauliflower or 1 small head cauliflower, chopped in a
    food processor to a rice-like consistency
5–6 large handfuls of tender greens such as spinach, baby kale, or arugula
1 tablespoon Italian seasoning
1 tablespoon balsamic vinegar
Sea salt and freshly ground pepper
Eggs or other protein of your choice

1. In a large skillet, heat the oil over medium heat. Add the onion and cook, stir-ring, until it starts to brown. Add the garlic and sauté for just a few seconds. Then add the zucchini and sauté for 2 minutes. Add the cauliflower rice and continue to cook until the vegetables are tender, 5 to 7 minutes.
2. Add the greens and cook until wilted, then add the Italian seasoning and vinegar. Season with salt and pepper to taste. Serve with eggs.

Chop-Chop Chicken and Veggie Hash Skillet

This is an awesome make-ahead meal that you can have on hand for quick reheat, grab-and-go breakfast, or any other meal. Make this on the weekend, portion it out into separate food storage containers, and in the morning rush all you have to do is heat and eat! You can replace the jicama with cauliflower florets, quartered Brussels sprouts, sliced fennel, diced red bell pepper, sliced water chestnuts, or any vegetable (or combination of vegetables) you like.

Second meal idea: Combine leftover hash with your favorite salsa, heat, and make tacos by using either lettuce wraps or Siete Foods Cassava Flour tortillas. Top your taco filling with Zesty Cabbage Slaw (page 335) for another layer of delicious flavor.

- Keeps well in the refrigerator up to five days or in the freezer up to three months.
- Prep time: 20 minutes
- Cook time: 15 minutes
- Serves 4

2–3 tablespoons coconut oil, avocado oil, or extra virgin olive oil

1 small yellow onion, diced

1½ pounds chicken sausage, casings removed, or 1½ pounds leftover shredded chicken or chopped Basic Chicken (page 373)

2 cups diced jicama

2 small zucchini, grated

5 large handfuls baby spinach, kale, or other braising greens

1½ teaspoons dried oregano

1½ teaspoons dried basil

1½ teaspoons dried parsley

Sea salt and freshly ground pepper

Juice of ½ lemon

1. In a large skillet, heat the oil over medium heat. Add the onion and cook until translucent. If using sausage, crumble it into the pan and cook until browned. Add the jicama and continue to cook until the jicama becomes tender but still has a slight crunch.
2. Add the zucchini and greens and cook until tender. Add the oregano, basil, parsley, and lemon juice and season with salt and pepper to taste. Serve.

Tip: If you are using already-cooked chicken, add the jicama in after the onions are translucent, and cook as instructed and then add the cooked chicken with the zucchini and greens and cook until the chicken is warmed through and the zucchini and greens are tender.

Italian Eggs

This is a fancy, fun, and easy way to eat your eggs. You can easily make this meal several different ways by simply subbing in different vegetables. For example, try cauliflower or quartered Brussels sprouts instead of the zucchini.

Second meal idea: Double all the ingredients (except for the eggs) and cook the vegetables as directed. Before adding the eggs, transfer half of the vegetable mixture to a container and refrigerate. Reheat and serve over grilled or baked chicken.

- Keeps well in the refrigerator up to four days; do not freeze.
- Prep time: 15 minutes
- Cook time: 10 minutes
- Serves 3 or 4

1–2 tablespoons extra virgin olive oil or avocado oil
1 small yellow onion, halved and sliced
2–3 small zucchini, halved lengthwise and sliced
4–5 large tomatoes, diced
3 garlic cloves, minced
4–5 large handfuls baby spinach, kale, or other tender cooking greens
⅓ cup chopped fresh basil
Sea salt and freshly ground pepper
12 eggs
¼ cup finely chopped fresh chives

1. In a large skillet, heat the oil over medium heat and sauté the onion until translucent. Add the zucchini, tomatoes, and garlic and bring to a simmer. Add the spinach and stir into the sauce until wilted. Let the mixture simmer, stirring occasionally, until it begins to thicken, about 5 to 6 minutes. Add the basil and season with salt and pepper to taste.
2. Make 12 golf ball size holes in the sauce with your spoon and crack an egg into each hole. Sprinkle the whole dish with chives, turn the heat to low or medium-low, cover, and cook until the egg whites are done but the yolks are still runny, 5 to 8 minutes. Cook longer if you want your eggs cooked all the way through.
3. Scoop out desired amount of eggs for each person and serve.

Snappy Salmon Patties

We love these easy and portable protein patties. They're fantastic on the day they are made and just as tasty for leftovers, so make enough for lunch or breakfast for the next couple of days during your busy weeks and simply serve with your favorite veggies! You can serve them on top of salad greens or quickly sauté five large handfuls of baby spinach or baby kale in the same pan used for the patties and serve together.

Second meal idea: Use leftover salmon patties as the protein option for Two-Minute Lettuce Wraps (page 332) or your "Bowl Fix" meal (page 325) for a quick snack or lunch. Add a little avocado mayo or HB Ranch Dressing (page 379) and you'll be good to go!

- Keeps well in the refrigerator up to four days or in the freezer up to three months.
- Prep time: 20 minutes
- Cook time: 8 minutes
- Serves 4

2 (6-ounce) cans wild-caught salmon
3 green onions, chopped
2 eggs or 2 flax eggs (see tip below)
1 tablespoon dried dill
2 garlic cloves, minced
1 teaspoon grated fresh ginger or ½ teaspoon ground ginger
Sea salt and freshly ground pepper
2 tablespoons coconut oil or avocado oil
Lemon wedges

1. Mix the drained salmon, onions, eggs, dill, garlic, and ginger together in a bowl; season with salt and pepper to taste. Form into 6 equal patties about ½ inch thick.
2. Heat the oil in a large skillet over medium- to medium-high heat. Once the pan is hot enough for the salmon patties to sizzle, add them to the hot oil and cook until they are browned on the bottom and are easy to flip, 3 to 4 minutes. Cook until browned on the second side, 3 to 4 minutes. Serve with lemon wedges.

Tip: Flax eggs are an egg replacement—simply combine 1 tablespoon ground flax meal with 2 tablespoons water to make 1 egg. Let the mixture sit for at least 5 minutes, stir again, and then add to the salmon cake mixture.

Breakfast Casseroles

Fabulous Frittata

This is such a delicious way to start your day, and when you make a giant frittata on the weekend, it will literally take you seconds to grab and go in the busy A.M.! We suggest cooking up a bunch of Sautéed Greens (page 340) to eat along with this Fabulous Frittata for an extra veggie kick.

Second meal idea: Reheat leftovers and serve with the Basic Green Salad (page 333) for a fast lunch or snack.

- Keeps well in the refrigerator up to five days or in the freezer up to three months.
- Prep time: 30 minutes
- Cook time: 45 minutes
- Serves 6

1 pound Italian chicken sausage, casings removed, or ground turkey

1 (12-ounce) jar roasted red peppers, drained and roughly chopped (do not chop too fine or the frittata will be watery)

4–6 cups chopped baby kale

12 eggs, beaten

¼ cup coconut milk

2 tablespoons minced fresh chives

1 tablespoon dried basil

1 teaspoon sea salt

1 teaspoon freshly ground pepper

1. Preheat the oven to 450°F.
2. Crumble the sausage into a large skillet and brown over medium heat. Spread the cooked meat on the bottom of a 9 x 13-inch baking dish. Spread the red peppers on top of the sausage, followed by the kale.
3. In a large mixing bowl, whisk the eggs and coconut milk together. Add the chives, basil, salt, and pepper and mix together. Pour the egg mixture evenly over the sausage and vegetables.
4. Cover the dish tightly with foil and bake for 35 to 40 minutes. Remove the foil and bake for an additional 10 to 15 minutes, or until the frittata is cooked all the way through and is slightly browned on top. Cut into squares and serve.

Unstuffed Breakfast Bell Pepper Casserole

This protein- and veggie-packed casserole is a fun twist on the classic stuffed bell pepper and is super yummy topped with a poached or fried egg.

Second meal idea: Reheat leftovers and serve with the Quick Kale Salad (page 334) or Basic Green Salad (page 333) and a side of mashed sweet potatoes for dinner or lunch.

- Keeps well in the refrigerator up to four days or in the freezer up to three months.
- Prep time: 20 minutes
- Cook time: 30 minutes
- Serves 5 or 6

4 red or yellow bell peppers (or a combination)

1 tablespoon extra virgin olive oil or avocado oil

1 small yellow onion, diced

1 pound ground bison, turkey, or beef

1 pound mild Italian chicken sausage, casings removed

3 garlic cloves, minced

1 (15-ounce) can tomato sauce

2 small zucchini, grated (about 2 cups)

5–6 handfuls tender baby greens such as baby spinach or baby kale

½ cup coarsely chopped fresh basil

2 tablespoons balsamic vinegar

1 tablespoon dried oregano

Sea salt and freshly ground pepper

Chopped fresh flat-leaf parsley, for garnish

1. Preheat the oven to 500°F.
2. Place the bell peppers on a baking sheet and roast, turning often until the peppers are tender and the skin starts to blacken, 15 to 20 minutes. Remove the peppers from the oven and reduce the oven temperature to 350°F.
3. Let the peppers cool until they are cool enough to handle and then cut them in half, scrape the seeds out, and slice lengthwise into 1-inch-wide strips; set aside.
4. In a large oven-safe skillet, heat the oil over medium heat. Add the onion and cook until soft; add the ground meat and sausage and cook until brown. Add the garlic and cook for another minute. Add the tomato sauce, zucchini, greens, and basil and stir well; bring to a simmer. Add the vinegar and

oregano and season with salt and pepper to taste; simmer until the zucchini and greens are soft, 3 to 5 minutes.

5. Layer the sliced roasted bell peppers on top of the meat mixture and transfer the skillet to the oven. Cook for 10 minutes or until bubbling around the edges. Sprinkle with parsley, if desired, and serve.

Smoked Salmon Casserole

This casserole reminds us of Easter brunch, but why wait for a holiday to have a decadent breakfast when you can feel like you are at a fancy-pants big-hat-wearing party even on a Monday?

Second meal idea: Reheat leftovers and pair with Summer Spinach Salad (page 334) for a quick lunch.

- Keeps well in the refrigerator up to four days or in the freezer up to two months.
- Prep time: 15 minutes
- Cook time: 35–40 minutes
- Serves 4

12 ounces cauliflower florets, cut into bite-size pieces (4 cups)
6 ounces asparagus, trimmed and cut into ½-inch pieces (1 cup)
4 ounces smoked salmon, finely chopped
10 eggs
¼ cup coconut milk
⅓ cup finely chopped fresh chives
1 tablespoon finely chopped fresh dill
Freshly ground pepper

1. Preheat the oven to 350°F.
2. Steam the cauliflower for 4 to 6 minutes or until the cauliflower florets are tender but not mushy. Spread the cauliflower evenly in a 9 x 13-inch baking dish and layer the asparagus on top, followed by the salmon.
3. In a bowl, whisk together the eggs, coconut milk, chives, and dill and season with pepper. Pour the egg mixture evenly over the salmon. Bake for 35 to 40 minutes or until the eggs are set all the way through. Cut into squares and serve.

The Hangry B*tch
BOWL FIX

Fast Food Fixes for Any Meal of the Day

These bowls can be eaten for any meal of the day. We recommend making one of the bowl options for dinner and preparing enough to have for leftover bowls for breakfast and lunch the next day!

This is your chance to get creative and have fun—and, most important, keep it simple! We have given you four different protein options so all you have to do is pick which protein to prepare, and then choose one starch from the Hangry B*tch Carb Fix section on page 343, pick as many veggies as you like from the list below and then one of the dressings (page 377), and then you are ready to build your bowl!

We suggest setting aside some time on the weekend to make two of the protein options along with two carb choices and prepping all the veggies you want for your bowls ahead of time so you can have plenty of bowl ingredients ready to go for the entire week.

How to Build a Bowl

Step 1: Pick a protein option from pages 326–28.

Step 2: Pick your carb from pages 343–47.

Step 3: Pick your vegetables from the list provided.

Step 4: Pick a dressing from pages 377–79.

Step 5: Prepare the protein, carb, vegetables, and dressing as directed.

Step 6: Place the carb choice in the bottom of a bowl, add the veggies, pile high with the protein, top with the dressing, and enjoy!

Step 7: Use leftovers for bowls for your next meal or two!

Protein Options for Your Bowls

Herb-Baked Salmon

- Keeps well in the refrigerator up to four days or
  in the freezer up to six months.
- Prep time: 15 minutes
- Cook time: 20–30 minutes
- Serves 3 to 4

2 pounds wild-caught salmon fillet, cut into 4 equal-size pieces

2–3 tablespoons avocado oil or extra virgin olive oil

1–2 tablespoons dried dill

3 garlic cloves, minced

Sea salt and freshly ground pepper

2 lemons, sliced into rounds

Handful fresh basil leaves (optional)

1. Preheat the oven to 350°F.
2. Place the salmon skin side down in a 9 x 13-inch baking dish. Drizzle with the
   oil and top each piece evenly with the dill and garlic. Season with salt and
   pepper and lay the lemon slices over the salmon. Sprinkle the basil, if using,
   on top.
3. Cover tightly with foil and bake for 20 to 30 minutes or until the fish easily
   flakes apart with a fork.

Rosemary Chicken

- Keeps well in the refrigerator up to four days or
  in the freezer up to six months.
- Prep time: 15 minutes
- Cook time: 20 minutes
- Serves 4

3 tablespoons coconut oil or avocado oil

3 pounds bone-in, skin on chicken thighs

Sea salt and freshly ground pepper

1 yellow onion, sliced

5–6 garlic cloves, coarsely chopped

4 rosemary sprigs

½ cup chicken broth

Juice of ½ lemon

1. In a large skillet, heat the oil over medium-high heat. Season the chicken pieces on both sides with salt and pepper.
2. When the oil is hot, add the chicken and sear for 5 minutes on each side or until golden brown. Add the onion, garlic, and rosemary sprigs on top of the chicken. Pour the broth and lemon juice over the chicken, cover, and reduce the heat to medium-low.
3. Cook for 10 to 15 minutes or until the chicken is tender and no longer pink in the middle.

Ginger Beef

◎ Keeps well in the refrigerator up to four days or in the freezer up to two months.

◎ Prep time: 20 minutes (plus 1 hour or up to overnight to marinate the meat)

◎ Cook time: 5 minutes

◎ Serves 4

¼ cup orange juice

¼ cup tamari or coconut aminos

2 garlic cloves, minced

1 teaspoon grated fresh ginger

1 teaspoon ground black pepper

2 pounds rib eye, top sirloin, or tri-tip steak, thinly sliced

1 tablespoon coconut oil or avocado oil

1. Combine the orange juice, tamari, garlic, ginger, and pepper in a medium bowl. Add the beef and toss to coat. Marinate for 1 hour (or overnight).
2. Heat the oil in a large skillet over medium-high heat. Remove the steak from the marinade and add to the hot oil. Stir-fry for 4 to 5 minutes or until done to your liking.

Lamb Sliders

- Keeps well in the refrigerator up to four days or in the freezer up to three months.
- Prep time: 15 minutes
- Cook time: 10 minutes
- Serves 4

2 pounds ground lamb or other lean ground meat
1 teaspoon sea salt
1 teaspoon freshly ground pepper
2 garlic cloves, minced
1 tablespoon extra virgin olive oil or avocado oil

1. Mix the lamb, salt, pepper, and garlic in a bowl with your hands. Form into 8–10 small patties, or "sliders," about ½ inch thick and 4 inches across.
2. Heat the oil in a large skillet over medium-high heat. Cook the sliders for 3 to 5 minutes on each side, until the meat is rare to medium-rare. Watch them closely, as lamb cooks quickly and will taste gamey if overdone.

Veggie Options for Your Bowls

Mixed salad greens

Shredded purple or green cabbage

Baby spinach or kale leaves

Green Bean Fries (page 337)

Roasted Brussels Sprouts (page 336)

Chopped jicama

Grated carrots

Grated or diced cucumbers

Sprouts

Diced red bell pepper

Fresh chopped herbs, such as flat-leaf parsley or cilantro

The Hangry B*tch
LUNCH AND SNACK FIX

As previously mentioned, we suggest doubling recipes for your dinners if necessary and relying on leftovers for lunches and snacks as well. However, sometimes we need some easy go-to lunch and snack ideas for the days we don't have leftovers handy. These recipes can also be doubled, of course, so you'll have lunch ready for at least a couple of days. When eating four meals a day, it's much easier to have two of your meals be very similar or even the same.

We also suggest you stock up on fast protein options such as Diestel Farms deli meat, Applegate Farms deli meat, or other lunch meat options that are organic and minimally processed without added preservatives or fillers. Keeping these on hand will make your Two-Minute Lettuce Wraps a breeze when you do not have any other leftover protein. Finally, if you tolerate eggs well, you can simply hard cook some eggs so they're ready for a quick protein boost.

Chicken Broccoli Salad

The addition of fresh herbs really makes this standard chicken salad pop. You can use any vegetables that you have on hand—but we love the crunch of the cabbage and broccoli, and it's simple! Make enough for at least three days of lunches; you can dress this salad ahead of time and it will keep just fine. In fact, it will taste even better the next day, as the flavors have a chance to all meld together.

Second meal idea: Make this salad into a lettuce wrap or use a Siete Foods tortilla for another wrap option.

- Keeps well in the refrigerator up to five days; do not freeze.
- Prep time: 20 minutes
- Serves 3 or 4

4 cooked chicken breasts or thighs, shredded or chopped (see page 373)

4–5 cups chopped or shredded purple cabbage

1 large cucumber, diced

3–4 cups chopped broccoli florets

¼ cup chopped fresh flat-leaf parsley

1 apple, diced (optional)
Handful of sliced almonds (optional)
Balsamic Vinaigrette (page 378)

Combine the chicken, cabbage, cucumber, broccoli, and parsley in a large bowl and add the apple and almonds, if using. Drizzle the desired amount of vinaigrette over the salad, toss, and serve.

Smoky Chicken-Jicama Slaw

This is a delicious twist on the standard chicken salad—so tangy, smoky, and delicious! Eat it as is or make a lettuce wrap out of it. Most grocery stores offer prepackaged shredded broccoli, or "broccoli slaw"—just make sure you find an option that does not include dressing, as you'll be making your own for this recipe!

Second meal idea: Scoop up leftovers of this salad with sliced cucumbers and bell peppers for a quick lunch or snack.

- Keeps well in the refrigerator up to five days; do not freeze.
- Prep time: 20 minutes
- Serves 3 or 4

½ cup HB Ranch Dressing (page 379)
1 tablespoon balsamic vinegar
1 teaspoon paprika
½ teaspoon chili powder
Pinch of cayenne pepper
4 cooked chicken breasts or thighs, shredded or chopped (see page 373)
4 cups broccoli slaw or shredded purple cabbage
2 cups diced jicama
1 red bell pepper, diced
½ small red onion, finely diced

Place the dressing, vinegar, paprika, chili powder, and cayenne in a large bowl and whisk to combine. Add the chicken, broccoli slaw, jicama, bell pepper, and onion. Mix well and serve.

Arugula Chicken Salad

The peppery goodness of arugula makes this chicken salad one you'll go back to again and again, and it's so fast to make when you have leftover chicken on hand!

- Keeps well in the refrigerator up to five days without the dressing; do not freeze.
- Prep time: 10 minutes
- Serves 3 or 4

4 cooked chicken breasts or thighs, shredded or chopped (see page 373)
6–8 ounces baby arugula
1 apple, diced
½ cup chopped pecans or almonds
¼ cup pitted kalamata olives
Lemony or Balsamic Vinaigrette (pages 377–78) or HB Ranch Dressing
(page 379)

Combine the chicken, arugula, apple, pecans, and olives in a large bowl. Toss with the desired amount of Lemony or Balsamic Vinaigrette or HB Ranch Dressing and serve.

Two-Minute Tuna or Salmon Salad

OK, so maybe this will take you a bit longer than two minutes, but this is a fast and delicious way to get your lunchtime salad fix on! You can make it ahead of time and dress it just before you serve it.

- Keeps well in the refrigerator up to two days without the dressing; do not freeze.
- Prep time: 2–10 minutes
- Serves 4

4 (6-ounce) cans wild-caught tuna or salmon
1 large head red or green leaf lettuce, washed and torn
2 big handfuls baby spinach
5 celery stalks, chopped

4 hard-cooked eggs, chopped (optional)
3 tablespoons capers, rinsed (optional)
Lemony Vinaigrette (page 377)

Combine the fish, lettuce, spinach, and celery in a large bowl and add the eggs
and capers, if using. Add the desired amount of vinaigrette, toss, and serve.

Two-Minute Lettuce Wraps

Some days, a quick lettuce wrap might be all you have time for, and that's OK!
Make sure you have your fridge stocked with the Two-Minute Lettuce Wrap
essentials, and you'll be so glad you did because even when all heck goes haywire, you still need to eat. You are worth it!

- Prep Time: 2–10 minutes
- Serves as many as you like

3–4 romaine lettuce leaves per serving
Mayonnaise (see page 375)
Mustard
Salad dressing (pages 377–79)
Leftover cooked protein, such as chopped or shredded chicken (see page 373),
    burgers, fish, steak, or high quality lunch meat
Raw vegetables, such as baby arugula, shredded cabbage, grated carrots,
    cucumber slices, sprouts, and/or tomato slices

For each serving, place two or three lettuce leaves on a plate and spread some
mayonnaise and mustard on them, or drizzle some salad dressing on them.
Add your choice of protein and veggies, wrap, and enjoy!

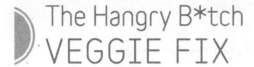

The Hangry B*tch
VEGGIE FIX

Salad Options

A quick salad is about the easiest way to get in some veggies, but it's hard to find dressings that aren't filled with nasty oils or a ton of sugar. Don't worry; we've got you covered! The salads in this section all use dressings from our Hangry B*tch Staples Fix section on pages 377–79. You can use our suggestions or pair your salad with whichever dressing recipe looks good to you. Make any of these salads into a complete meal by adding leftover protein and serving with a starchy side from our Carb Fix section on page 343. *Enjoy!*

- All salads will keep well in the refrigerator up to three days without dressing; do not freeze.
- Prep time for each salad is about 10 minutes.
- All salads serve 2 to 4

Basic Green Salad

6–8 ounces mixed baby greens (buying bagged and prewashed is easiest)
Shredded carrots (optional)
Diced cucumber (optional)
Diced apple (optional)
Chopped fresh herbs such as flat-leaf parsley or cilantro (optional)
Lemony Vinaigrette (page 377) or Balsamic Vinaigrette (page 378)

Place the baby greens in a large bowl. Add the carrots, cucumber, apple, and/ or herbs, if using. Add the desired amount of vinaigrette, toss, and serve.

Quick Kale Salad

6–8 ounces baby kale (buying bagged and prewashed is easiest)
1 cup cherry tomatoes, halved
1 small cucumber, thinly sliced
½ cup shelled pistachios or chopped walnuts
Lemony Vinaigrette (page 377) or HB Ranch Dressing (page 379)

Combine the kale, tomatoes, cucumber, and pistachios in a large bowl. Add the desired amount of dressing, toss, and serve.

Summer Spinach Salad

6–8 ounces baby spinach (buying bagged and prewashed is easiest)
1–2 cups thinly sliced strawberries
½ small red onion, thinly sliced
½ cup chopped pecans or ¼ cup toasted pine nuts
Lemony Vinaigrette (page 377) or Balsamic Vinaigrette (page 378)

Combine the spinach, strawberries, onion, and pecans in a large bowl. Add the desired amount of vinaigrette, toss, and serve.

Crunchy Cucumber Salad

3 small cucumbers, halved and thinly sliced
½ cup halved cherry tomatoes
¼ cup chopped cashews
¼ cup chopped fresh cilantro
Asian Vinaigrette (page 379)

Combine the cucumbers, tomatoes, cashews, and cilantro in a large bowl. Add the desired amount of vinaigrette, toss, and serve.

Zesty Cabbage Slaw

4 cups chopped or shredded purple or green cabbage
2 green onions, chopped
1 small cucumber, diced
4 radishes, cut in half and sliced or 1 cup diced jicama
1 cup chopped fresh cilantro
Cumin and Lime Dressing (page 378)

Combine the cabbage, green onions, cucumber, radishes, and cilantro in a large bowl. Add the desired amount of dressing, toss, and serve.

Quick Ranch Slaw

4 cups chopped or shredded purple or green cabbage
1 cup shredded carrots
1 cucumber, diced
2 green onions, chopped
HB Ranch Dressing (page 379)

Combine the cabbage, carrots, cucumber, and green onions in a large bowl. Add the desired amount of dressing, toss, and serve.

Sriracha Broccoli Slaw

3 cups broccoli slaw mix
½ cup HB Ranch Dressing (page 379)
1–2 teaspoons sriracha
1 tablespoon honey (optional)

Mix all the ingredients together well in a large bowl.

Roasted Veggies

Roasted veggies are simply the best. Roasting is super easy and brings out an abundance of flavor that helps make those vegetables disappear—even kids love them! We offer a few jazzed-up roasted vegetable options, but most are pretty much the same because, why mess with delicious? And remember: good food should be EASY!

Second meal idea: With all of the roasted veggies, if you make them as a side dish with your dinner, you can add any leftovers to your breakfast soup in the morning, to your Bowl Fixes on page 325, to the Two-Minute Lettuce Wraps on page 332, or as an addition to the Basic Green Salad page 333.

Roasted Brussels Sprouts

- Keeps well in the refrigerator up to four days or in the freezer up to three months.
- Prep time: 15 minutes
- Cook time: 20–30 minutes
- Serves 4

1 pound Brussels sprouts, quartered
2–3 tablespoons avocado oil or extra virgin olive oil
4 garlic cloves, thinly sliced
Sea salt
Juice of ½ lemon

1. Preheat the oven to 400°F.
2. Toss the Brussels sprouts with the oil and garlic, and season generously with sea salt. Spread evenly on a baking sheet and roast for 20 to 30 minutes or until crisp but tender. Toss with the lemon juice and serve.

Green Bean Fries

- Keeps well in the refrigerator up to four days or in the freezer up to three months.
- Prep time: 5 minutes
- Cook time: 15–20 minutes
- Serves 4

1 pound green beans, trimmed
2–3 tablespoons avocado oil or extra virgin olive oil
Sea salt

1. Preheat the oven to 400°F.
2. Toss the green beans with the oil and season generously with salt. Spread evenly on a baking sheet and roast for 15 to 20 minutes, or until the beans start to brown, stirring about halfway through the cooking time. Serve.

Roasted Broccoli

- Keeps well in the refrigerator up to four days or in the freezer up to three months.
- Prep time: 5 minutes
- Cook time: 15–20 minutes
- Serves 4

1 pound broccoli florets
2–3 tablespoons avocado oil or extra virgin olive oil
Sea salt
Lemon juice

1. Preheat the oven to 400°F.
2. Make sure the broccoli is dry. Toss the broccoli with the oil and season generously with salt. Spread evenly on a baking sheet and roast for 15 to 20 minutes, or until crisp-tender and beginning to brown, stirring about halfway through the cooking time. Finish with a squeeze of fresh lemon juice and serve.

Roasted Cabbage Wedges

- Keeps well in the refrigerator up to four days or
  in the freezer up to three months.
- Prep time: 5 minutes
- Cook time: 30–40 minutes
- Serves 4

1 head cabbage, cut into 10 to 12 wedges
Avocado oil or extra virgin olive oil
Sea salt

1. Preheat the oven to 400°F.
2. Place the cabbage wedges on a baking sheet, drizzle with avocado oil, and sprinkle with salt. Flip the wedges over; drizzle with oil and sprinkle with sea salt on the other side.
3. Roast for 15 to 20 minutes, flip the wedges over, and roast for an additional 15 to 20 minutes, or until the cabbage is fork-tender and browned and crispy on the outside.

Roasted Summer Squash

- Keeps well in the refrigerator up to four days or
  in the freezer up to three months.
- Prep time: 5 minutes
- Cook time: 15–20 minutes
- Serves 4

1 pound zucchini or yellow squash or a mixture of both, cut in half and then into
  3-inch pieces
2–3 tablespoons avocado oil or extra virgin olive oil
Sea salt

1. Preheat the oven to 400°F.
2. Toss the squash with the oil and season generously with salt. Spread evenly on a baking sheet and roast for 15 to 20 minutes or until the squash is crisp-tender and beginning to brown, stirring about halfway through the cooking time. Serve.

Roasted Curried Cauliflower

- ⊙ Keeps well in the refrigerator up to four days or in the freezer up to three months.
- ⊙ Prep time: 10 minutes
- ⊙ Cook time: 30–40 minutes
- ⊙ Serves 4

3 tablespoons coconut oil or avocado oil
1 tablespoon curry powder
2 garlic cloves, minced or grated
¼ teaspoon ground turmeric
Sea salt
1 head cauliflower, cut into bite-size florets

1. Preheat the oven to 350°F.
2. Melt the coconut oil and pour into a small bowl (if using avocado oil, just pour it into the bowl). Add the curry powder, garlic, and turmeric and whisk; season with salt.
3. Place the cauliflower in a medium bowl, drizzle the oil mixture over it, and toss until all the pieces are coated. Spread the seasoned cauliflower onto a parchment paper–lined baking sheet and roast for 30 to 40 minutes or until crisp yet tender, stirring halfway through the cooking time. Serve.

Sautéed Greens

We suggest you always have tender greens on hand for a super fast Hangry B*tch Veggie Fix. Tender cooking greens are nutrient-dense powerhouses, take just minutes to cook, and can accompany any meal.

Here's our go-to greens recipe. Feel free to keep it as simple as a little cooking oil and salt or add the lemon juice and garlic for a yummy addition to your quick greens.

- Keeps well in the refrigerator up to three days; do not freeze.
- Prep time: 10 minutes
- Cook time: 3–5 minutes
- Serves 3 to 4

2–3 tablespoons coconut oil, avocado oil, or extra virgin olive oil
6–8 ounces tender greens (see tip below)
2–3 garlic cloves, minced (optional)
Lemon juice (optional)
Sea salt and freshly ground pepper

Heat the oil in a large skillet over medium heat. Add the greens and garlic and sauté until the greens are tender. Remove from heat and season with lemon juice, salt, and pepper to taste. Serve.

Tip: You can sauté any of the following greens or a combination. Wash and dry them well and, if needed, chop them into bite-size pieces.

Arugula	Endive
Beet greens	Kale (all varieties; baby kale is simplest because there is zero prep work)
Bok choy	
Broccoli raab	
Cabbage	Mustard greens (these are very bitter and best mixed with a milder green)
Chard	
Collards	Napa cabbage
Dandelion greens (these are very bitter and best mixed with a milder green)	Radicchio
	Spinach

Veggie Noodles

You can have your sauce and eat it, too—just replace the pasta with veggie noodles! Our two favorite and easiest go-to's for this option are zucchini and spaghetti squash. Spaghetti squash is often thought of as a starchy carb but is actually very low in carbs and should be considered a fibrous veggie.

Roasted Spaghetti Squash

Serve this squash with Sun-Dried Tomato Chicken Bake (page 351) or Easy Meat Sauce (page 354), or any other protein you choose.

- Keeps well in the refrigerator up to four days or in the freezer up to three months.
- Prep time: 10 minutes
- Cook time: 35–45 minutes
- Serves 3 or 4

1 spaghetti squash
2 tablespoons extra virgin olive oil
Sea salt and freshly ground pepper

1. Preheat the oven to 375°F.
2. Cut the squash in half lengthwise and scrape out the seeds. Drizzle the inside with oil and season with salt and pepper. Place the squash, cut-side down, in a 9 x 13-inch glass baking dish. Bake for 35 to 45 minutes or until tender.
3. Let the squash rest until cool enough to handle. Using a fork, scrape out the flesh to create long strands. Serve.

Tip: We love the flavor of roasted spaghetti squash, but sometimes there just isn't enough time. For a quick fix for your noodle needs, take a whole spaghetti squash, poke several times with a sharp knife, and microwave for 8 to 10 minutes, or until fork-tender. Carefully cut the hot cooked squash in half, scoop out the seeds, and scrape out the cooked flesh with a fork. Serve seasoned with extra virgin olive oil, salt, and pepper; top with Easy Meat Sauce (page 354); or serve as a side with any protein of your choice.

Zucchini Noodles

- Keeps well in the refrigerator up to four days or
  in the freezer up to three months.
- Prep time: 10 minutes
- Cook time: 1–2 minutes
- Serves 3 or 4

1 pound zucchini squash, spiralized or thinly sliced

Bring a large pot of water to a boil. Add the zucchini and cook for 1 to 2 minutes. Remove immediately from the hot water and serve.

The Hangry B*tch
CARB FIX (UCT)

These are your UCT recipes. Having some of these starchy recipes prepped and ready for your week ahead of time makes meal prep and planning so much easier. We suggest you pick two that sound good from this list and make them ahead of time so you can reheat them for your meals throughout the week.

Roasted Carbs

Roasted Mashed Sweet Taters

- Keeps well in the refrigerator for three to four days or in the freezer for two to three months.
- Prep time: 15 minutes
- Cook time: 1 hour
- Serves 4 or 5

4 sweet potatoes, scrubbed and dried
Coconut oil
Sea salt
Ground cinnamon (optional)

1. Preheat the oven to 400°F.
2. Rub the skin of each sweet potato with a thin layer of coconut oil. Place the sweet potatoes on a baking sheet and roast for 1 hour, or until very soft.
3. Let the sweet potatoes cool until you can handle them and peel the skins off (they should come off easily if the potatoes are cool enough).
4. Transfer them to a large bowl, add ½ teaspoon coconut oil if desired, and, using either a hand-held immersion blender or a hand mixer, mix until smooth. Season to taste with salt and a little bit of cinnamon if desired. Serve.

Garlic Roasted Potatoes (White or Sweet)

- Keeps well in the refrigerator up to four days or in the freezer up to three months.
- Prep time: 20 minutes
- Cook time: 35–40 minutes
- Serves 4

2 pounds (about 2 medium) white potatoes or sweet potatoes, peeled and chopped into 1-inch cubes
12–15 garlic cloves, peeled and cut in half lengthwise
3 tablespoons coconut oil, avocado oil, or extra virgin olive oil
1 tablespoon dried basil
Sea salt and freshly ground pepper

1. Preheat the oven to 400°F.
2. In a large bowl, toss the potatoes with the oil, sliced garlic, dried basil, and a generous sprinkle of salt and pepper.
3. Spread the potatoes evenly on a baking sheet and roast for 35 to 40 minutes, or until the potatoes are crispy on the outside and fork-tender, stirring halfway through the cooking time.

Roasted Root Veggies and/or Winter Squash

You can use any root veggie or winter squash of your liking, or a combination. We suggest a mixture of three of these root vegetables: beets, parsnips, sweet potatoes, carrots, rutabagas, or turnips. As for winter squash, our favorites are butternut, delicata, and acorn.

- Keeps well in the refrigerator up to four days or in the freezer up to three months.
- Prep time: 20 minutes
- Cook time: 35–40 minutes
- Serves 4

2 pounds root vegetables and/or winter squash, peeled and cut into 1-inch cubes
3 tablespoons coconut oil, avocado oil, or extra virgin olive oil
Sea salt

1. Preheat the oven to 400°F.
2. In a large bowl, toss the vegetables with the oil and a generous sprinkle of salt.
3. Spread the vegetables evenly on a baking sheet and roast for 35 to 40 minutes, or until the veggies are crispy on the outside and fork-tender, stirring halfway through the cooking time.

Crispy Plantains (Tostones)

These are delicious paired with Slow-Cooker Beef Barbacoa (page 358).

- Keeps well in the refrigerator up to four days or in the freezer up to three months.
- Prep time: 10 minutes
- Cook time: 5–8 minutes
- Serves 4

1 cup coconut oil for frying

2 or 3 green plantains, peeled and cut into 2-inch-long pieces

1. In a deep frying pan, melt the coconut oil over medium-high heat. Once the oil is hot, add the plantains, standing the pieces upright (on one of their cut ends). Fry until the plantains are golden brown on one side, then flip and fry the other side until golden brown.
2. Carefully remove the plantains from the hot oil and place cut-side down on a large cutting board or other flat surface. Using the bottom of a dinner plate, flatten the plantains.
3. Return the flattened plantains to the hot oil and fry until crispy, 30 to 60 seconds per side. Watch carefully as they will go from browned to burned rather quickly! Remove the tostones from the oil and serve.

Slow-Cooker or Instant Pot Carbs

Sweet Potatoes or White Potatoes

- Keeps well in the refrigerator up to four days or in the freezer up to three months.
- Prep time: 10 minutes
- Cook time: 3½–7 hours (slow cooker) or 1 hour (Instant Pot)
- Serves 8

4 or 5 potatoes, washed and scrubbed but not dried

SLOW-COOKER INSTRUCTIONS

Place the wet potatoes in the slow cooker, cover, and cook on high for 3½ to 4 hours or on low for 6 to 7 hours, until fork-tender. Serve.

INSTANT POT INSTRUCTIONS

1. Place the steamer basket in the Instant Pot and add 1 cup water. Place the potatoes in the steamer basket and lock the lid.
2. Set the vent on "sealed" and press the "steam" button and set for 12 minutes. (It will take 15 to 20 minutes for the cooker to come up to pressure before the 12-minute cooking time begins.)
3. Once the Instant Pot alerts you that it is done, allow the pressure to release naturally, which will take another 25 to 30 minutes. Serve.

Root Veggies and/or Winter Squash

We suggest a mixture of three of these root vegetables: beets, parsnips, sweet potatoes, carrots, rutabagas, or turnips. You can also use winter squash; our favorites are butternut, delicata, and acorn.

- Keeps well in the refrigerator up to four days or in the freezer up to three months.
- Prep time: 30 minutes
- Cook time: 3–7 hours (slow cooker) or 1 hour (Instant Pot)
- Serves 6

2 pounds root vegetables, or winter squash peeled and cut into large segments of equal size.

SLOW-COOKER INSTRUCTIONS

Place the vegetables in the slow cooker, pour in 1 cup water, cover, and cook on high for 3 to 4 hours or on low for 6 to 7 hours. Serve.

INSTANT POT INSTRUCTIONS

1. Place the steamer basket in the Instant Pot and add 1 cup water. Place the vegetables in the steamer basket and lock the lid.
2. Set the vent on "sealed" and press the "steam" button and set for 12 minutes. (It will take 15 to 20 minutes for the cooker to come up to pressure before the 12-minute cooking time begins.)
3. Once the Instant Pot alerts you that it is done, allow the pressure to release naturally, which will take another 25 to 30 minutes. Serve.

Salad Carbs

Mom's Potato Salad

- Keeps well in the refrigerator up to five days; do not freeze.
- Prep time: 30 minutes
- Serves 10

2 pounds Yukon gold or red potatoes

1 dozen eggs

6–8 celery stalks, diced

3 cups diced dill pickles (we love fermented dill pickles like Bubbies brand or Sonoma Brinery)

½ medium red onion, finely diced

1½ cups Homemade HB Mayonnaise (page 375), or more to taste, or an avocado oil–based store-bought mayo

2 tablespoons dried dill

1 tablespoon apple cider vinegar, or more to taste

2 teaspoons yellow mustard, or more to taste

Sea salt and freshly ground pepper

1. Place the potatoes in a large pot and cover with cold water. Bring to a boil, reduce the heat to a simmer, and cook for 15 to 20 minutes or until fork-tender; drain and set aside to cool.

2. While the potatoes cool, place the eggs in a large saucepan, cover with cold water, and bring to a boil. Reduce the heat to a simmer and set the timer for 8 minutes. When the timer is up, drain the eggs and transfer to a bowl of ice water to cool.

3. Once the potatoes are cool enough to handle, cut into bite-size pieces and transfer to a large bowl. Peel and dice the cooked eggs and add to the potatoes.

4. Add the celery, pickles, onion, mayonnaise, dill, vinegar, and mustard and mix well. Season to taste with salt and pepper and add more vinegar and mustard if desired. Serve.

Warm Spinach and Sweet Potato Salad

- Keeps well in the refrigerator for one to two days; do not freeze.
- Prep time: 20 minutes
- Cook time: 10 minutes
- Serves: 5 or 6

8 strips bacon or turkey bacon, chopped

2 leeks, cut in half lengthwise and sliced

6 ounces baby spinach leaves

3 cups Roasted Sweet Potatoes (page 344)

1 small apple, diced

¼ cup sliced almonds

Apple Cider Vinaigrette (page 377)

1. Cook the bacon in a medium skillet over medium heat until beginning to brown and crisp. Drain all but about 1 tablespoon of the grease from the pan, add the leeks, and cook with the bacon for another 3 to 4 minutes. Then remove from the heat. If using turkey bacon, you'll need to add 1 tablespoon avocado or coconut oil.
2. Put the spinach in a large bowl, add the warm bacon and leeks, and toss together until the spinach is just slightly wilted. Add the sweet potatoes, apple, and almonds and toss.
3. Add the desired amount of dressing, toss to coat the salad, and serve.

Moroccan Beet Salad

- Keeps well in the refrigerator up to four days; do not freeze.
- Prep time: 20 minutes
- Serves: 3 or 4

2 medium beets, peeled and grated

2 carrots, grated

1 apple, grated

¼ cup thinly sliced red onion

1–2 teaspoons ground cumin

Lemony Vinaigrette (page 377)

¼ cup chopped fresh flat-leaf parsley

Sea salt and freshly ground pepper

Combine the beets, carrots, apple, onion, and cumin in a medium bowl and mix well. Add the desired amount of dressing and toss to combine. Sprinkle with the chopped parsley and season with salt and pepper to taste. Serve.

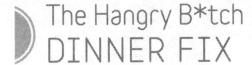

The Hangry B*tch
DINNER FIX

Family Favorite Fixes

The first few recipes you'll find here are family favorites—easy but timeless and a whole lot of comfort. Yes, we will keep reminding you: make sure you rely on leftovers from these meals to get you through breakfast and/or lunch for the following day! It's really the best thing ever to be prepared—we promise.

Sun-Dried Tomato Chicken Bake

This is a super delicious way to make a family-friendly dinner, and for those "oh shoot, I have only a few minutes to prep dinner" moments, this meal is sure to become a staple. We suggest serving this with Roasted Spaghetti Squash (page 341) and Roasted Broccoli (page 337).

Second meal idea: Use leftovers for one of your Bowl Fixes (page 325) or for a Two-Minute Lettuce Wrap (page 332) or simply add to a Basic Green Salad (page 333) for lunch the next day.

- Keeps well in the refrigerator up to four days or in the freezer for up to three months.
- Prep time: 20 minutes
- Cook time: 35 minutes
- Serves 4

2 pounds boneless, skinless chicken breasts, sliced into 2-inch pieces

2 tablespoons dried basil

Sea salt and freshly ground pepper

8 garlic cloves, thinly sliced

1 (8.5-ounce) jar julienne-cut sun-dried tomatoes packed in olive oil

2 tablespoons balsamic vinegar

1. Preheat the oven to 375°F.
2. Place the chicken in a 9 x 13-inch baking dish. Sprinkle with the basil, add the balsamic vinegar, season with salt and pepper, and mix well. Sprinkle the sliced garlic on top and spread the sun-dried tomatoes with their oil over the entire dish.
3. Seal the dish tightly with foil and bake for 20 minutes. Remove the foil and bake for another 15 minutes or until the chicken is no longer pink in the middle. Serve.

Ginger Chicken Stir-Fry

Simple and satisfying, this stir-fry can be made a few different ways simply by mixing up the veggies. Try it with broccoli, carrots, and bok choy for a whole new twist!

- Keeps well in the refrigerator up to four days; do not freeze.
- Prep time: 30 minutes
- Cook time: 15 minutes
- Serves 4

¼ cup coconut oil or avocado oil
2 pounds boneless, skinless chicken thighs or breasts, cut into bite-size pieces
1 cup sliced mushrooms
1 red bell pepper, thinly sliced
4 green onions, chopped
Juice of 1 orange (about ½ cup)
¼ cup chicken broth
1 tablespoon dried basil or ¼ cup chopped fresh basil leaves
1 teaspoon grated fresh ginger
1 small jalapeño, seeds removed, minced (optional)
5–6 big handfuls tender cooking greens such as baby kale, spinach, or chard
Tamari or coconut aminos
Sea salt and freshly ground pepper
¼ cup sliced almonds

1. Heat the oil in a large skillet or wok over medium heat. Add the chicken and stir-fry for 5 to 7 minutes. Add the mushrooms, bell pepper, and green onions and stir-fry for another 2 minutes.

2. Add the orange juice, broth, basil, ginger, and jalapeño, if using, and bring to a simmer. Cook for 1 to 2 minutes. Add the greens and stir until wilted.

3. Season with tamari, salt, and pepper to taste. Sprinkle with the almonds and serve.

Southwestern Chicken Bake

We love the versatility of this recipe; you can create totally different recipes simply by changing up the spices. We've given one variation, but you can also make up your own.

- Keeps well in the refrigerator up to four days or in the freezer up to three months.
- Prep time: 30 minutes
- Cook time: 40 minutes
- Serves 4 or 5

2 medium zucchini, cut into 1-inch pieces
1 medium sweet potato, grated or 3 cups cauliflower rice (see tip next page)
4–5 large handfuls tender greens, such as baby spinach, kale, arugula, chopped
1 small yellow onion, diced
1 red or yellow bell pepper, chopped
1 (12-ounce) jar salsa verde
2 tablespoons ground cumin
1 tablespoon smoked paprika
1 tablespoon dried oregano
1 tablespoon sea salt
2 garlic cloves, minced
Freshly ground pepper
2 lbs boneless, skinless chicken breasts, cut into bite-size pieces
Chopped fresh cilantro for garnish

1. Preheat the oven to 375°F.
2. Combine the zucchini, sweet potato, greens, onion, bell pepper, salsa, cumin, paprika, oregano, salt, garlic, and pepper to taste, and mix well. Add the chicken and fold into the mixture.
3. Spread evenly in a 9 x 13-inch baking dish, cover with foil, and cook for 30 minutes. Uncover and cook for another 10 minutes or until the chicken is no longer pink in the middle.

4. Top with cilantro and serve.

Italian Chicken Bake

Replace the salsa verde with 1 (14.5-ounce) can diced tomatoes, omit the paprika and cumin, and add 2 tablespoons dried basil.

Tip: To make your own cauliflower rice, simply place raw cauliflower florets in your Vitamix or food processor and process until the cauliflower is chopped to the consistency and size of rice.

Easy Meat Sauce

"Easy" is an understatement. You'll love this sauce as a quick go-to on busy nights. Served with either Roasted Spaghetti Squash (page 341) or Zucchini Noodles (page 342), it's a meal your whole family is sure to enjoy.

Second meal idea: Sauté some tender greens, add them to leftover sauce, and top with a fried or poached egg for breakfast.

- Keeps well in the refrigerator up to four days or in the freezer up to four months.
- Prep time: 10 minutes
- Cook time: 20 minutes
- Serves 4 or 5

1–2 tablespoons extra virgin olive oil

1 yellow onion, diced

2 pounds ground beef, bison, or turkey

Sea salt and freshly ground pepper

2 tablespoons red wine or balsamic vinegar

2–3 garlic cloves, minced

1 (16-ounce) jar or can diced tomatoes

2 tablespoons dried basil

1. Heat the oil in a large saucepan over medium heat. Add the onion and sauté until translucent. Add the ground meat and cook until brown; season with 2 teaspoons salt.

2. Add the vinegar, stir well, and simmer for 3 to 4 minutes. Add the garlic and cook for another minute or two. Add the tomatoes and basil, bring to a simmer, reduce the heat to low, and simmer for 10 to 15 minutes.
3. Season with more salt and pepper to taste. Serve.

Mini Meatloaves

This is not your mom's meatloaf! We love these mini and portable protein powerhouses. Make sure you prepare enough to have on hand for quick grab-and-go meals for your busy week. If you're including the optional ketchup, buy an organic brand that contains no corn syrup; this is available at most natural food stores.

Second meal idea: Add these to your Bowl Fixes or serve alongside any of the salad options for a quick leftover lunch!

- Keeps well in the refrigerator up to four days or in the freezer up to four months.
- Prep time: 30 minutes
- Cook time: 15–20 minutes
- Serves 4 or 5

1 pound ground beef, bison, lamb, or turkey

1 pound ground pork

1 cup finely diced carrot or sweet potato

1 cup finely chopped spinach leaves

¼ cup yellow onion, minced or 1 teaspoon onion powder

2 garlic cloves, minced

1½ teaspoons sea salt

1 teaspoon dried parsley

½ teaspoon freshly ground pepper

Coconut oil

Ketchup (optional)

1. Preheat the oven to 350°F.
2. In a large bowl, mix the beef, pork, carrot, spinach, onion, garlic, salt, parsley, and pepper until well combined.
3. Grease a muffin tin with coconut oil. Measure ⅓ cup of the meat mixture into each muffin cup. Spread a generous amount of ketchup, if desired, on top of each meatloaf.

4. Bake for 15 to 20 minutes or until the meatloaves are no longer pink in the middle. Serve.

Tip: Double this recipe for super easy breakfast and lunch leftovers. Serve with the recipe for Roasted Curried Cauliflower (page 339; both bake at the same temperature, the cauliflower just takes longer—so start that first), a green salad, and baked sweet potatoes.

Spanish Meatballs

These meatballs are a bit more labor-intensive than some of our other recipes, but holy guacamole they are the BOMB. So if you are feeling inspired and want to make something special, we promise these are not your average meatballs, baby. Serve with Basic Green Salad (page 333) and one of the carb options on page 343.

Second meal idea: Add leftover meatballs to your Bowl Fixes or serve with any of the salad options for a quick leftover lunch.

- Keeps well in the refrigerator up to four days or in the freezer up to four months.
- Prep time: 45 minutes
- Cook time: 20 minutes
- Serves 6

FOR THE MEATBALLS

2 pounds ground beef

1 pound ground pork

1 egg

¼ cup minced fresh flat-leaf parsley

4 garlic cloves, minced

2½ teaspoons sea salt

2 teaspoons ground cumin

1½ teaspoons smoked paprika

1 teaspoon freshly ground pepper

FOR THE SAUCE

¼ teaspoon saffron threads

¼ cup hot water

1 tablespoon extra virgin olive oil

1 yellow onion, cut in half and sliced

3–4 garlic cloves, minced

½ cup white wine

1 (28-ounce) can diced tomatoes

1 cup pimento-stuffed Spanish olives

2 tablespoons minced fresh parsley

1 teaspoon smoked paprika

¼ teaspoon cayenne pepper

Salt and freshly ground pepper

Juice of 1 lemon

1. To make the meatballs: Combine all the ingredients in a large bowl and mix with your hands. Using a ⅓-cup measuring cup, measure out the meat and roll into meatballs (you should have about 15 meatballs).
2. To make the sauce: Toast the saffron threads in a warm skillet over low heat for 1 minute. Crumble the toasted saffron threads into the hot water and set aside.
3. Heat the oil in a large skillet over medium heat, add the onion, and sauté for 5 to 7 minutes or until translucent. Add the garlic and sauté just until fragrant.
4. Turn the heat up to high and add the wine. Cook until reduced by half, stirring occasionally. Add the saffron water and tomatoes and bring to a simmer. Add the olives, parsley, paprika, and cayenne and season to taste with salt, pepper, and lemon juice.
5. Gently nestle the meatballs into the sauce, turn down to low or medium-low, and simmer, covered, for 15 to 20 minutes until the meatballs are cooked through and tender. Serve.

One-Pot / Slow-Cooker / Instant Pot Fixes

It's so convenient to have your entire meal in one pot or to be able to rely on your slow cooker or Instant Pot on the crazy days that you know would normally leave you relying on the drive-through or takeout. These recipes will make you so happy you'll want to cry and will give you time to be exactly where we want you to be: Present. Focused. Happy. Authentically you. Joyful. Fed. Nourished. Overcoming the overwhelm.

Slow-Cooker Beef Barbacoa

Filled with flavor and so versatile, this is sure to be a big hit! Serve this simply in bowls topped with Zesty Cabbage Slaw (page 335) or make into tacos with Siete Foods Tortillas topped with chopped cilantro, onions, avocado, and lime wedges.

Second meal idea: Add leftovers to your Bowl Fix, to your breakfast soup, serve with eggs and greens for breakfast, or make into Two-Minute Lettuce Wraps (page 332). The possibilities for a second meal with leftovers are endless!

- Keeps well in the refrigerator up to four days or in the freezer up to four months.
- Prep time: 45 minutes
- Cook time: 7–8 hours
- Serves 5

3–4 pounds chuck roast, cut into 2 or 3 big pieces
Sea salt
1 tablespoon coconut oil
1 yellow onion, diced
2 jalapeños, halved lengthwise, seeded, and cut into matchstick strips
4 garlic cloves, minced
1 (6-ounce) can tomato paste
½ cup beef broth
¼ cup white wine vinegar
Juice of 2 limes
2 tablespoons ground cumin

2 tablespoons dried oregano

2 teaspoons chipotle powder

1 teaspoon freshly ground pepper

¼ teaspoon ground cloves

2 bay leaves

1. Pat the meat dry with paper towels and sprinkle on all sides with 1 table-spoon salt.
2. Heat the oil in a large skillet over medium-high heat. When the oil is hot enough for the meat to sizzle, add the meat and sear until it easily releases from the pan; continue to cook until the meat is seared on all sides.
3. Transfer the meat to the slow cooker and add the onion, jalapeños and garlic.
4. In a large bowl, whisk together the tomato paste, broth, vinegar, lime juice, cumin, oregano, chipotle powder, pepper, and cloves. Pour over the meat and add the bay leaves. Stir together with the peppers, onions, and garlic to coat the top of the roast.
5. Cook on low for 7 to 8 hours or until the meat easily shreds apart with a fork. Shred the meat and mix with the liquid in the slow cooker; taste and season with more salt if needed. Let the meat sit in the liquid for 10 to 20 minutes to soak up all the delicious juices before serving.

Asian Beef Stew

This comforting and satisfying stew is delicious paired with the Basic Green Salad (page 333) tossed with the Asian Vinaigrette (page 379). It also pairs well with the Garlic Roasted Potatoes (page 344) or any of the Roasted Root Veggies (page 344).

- Keeps well in the refrigerator up to four days or in the freezer up to four months.
- Prep time: 30 minutes
- Cook time: 6–8 hours (slow cooker) or 30–45 minutes (Instant Pot)
- Serves 5

2½ pounds beef chuck roast, cut into 2-inch pieces

1½ tablespoons Chinese five-spice powder

1 tablespoon coconut oil, avocado oil, or extra virgin olive oil

6 ounces white mushrooms or shiitake mushrooms, sliced

5 carrots, cut in half lengthwise and cut into 3-inch pieces

5 celery stalks, cut into 3-inch pieces

1 yellow onion, sliced

½ cup orange juice

¼–½ cup beef broth

2 tablespoons tamari or coconut aminos

1 tablespoon fish sauce

1 tablespoon rice vinegar

4 garlic cloves, minced

1 teaspoon grated fresh ginger

OPTIONAL GARNISHES

Chopped green onions

Bean sprouts

Chopped fresh cilantro

Sesame seeds

Sriracha

SLOW-COOKER INSTRUCTIONS

1. Place the beef in a large bowl and add the five-spice powder; stir to coat.
2. Heat the oil in a large skillet over medium-high heat, add the beef, and cook until browned. Transfer the beef to the slow cooker. Add the mushrooms, carrots, celery, onion, orange juice, broth, tamari, fish sauce, vinegar, garlic, and ginger. Mix well, cover, and cook on low for 6 to 8 hours.
3. Top with any of the optional garnishes and serve.

INSTANT POT INSTRUCTIONS

Place the beef in a large bowl and add the five-spice powder; stir to coat. Heat the oil in the Instant Pot and turn it to the sauté setting. Once the pot is hot, brown the meat right in the Instant Pot. Add the mushrooms, carrots, celery, onion, orange juice, broth, tamari, fish sauce, vinegar, garlic, and ginger. Mix well, seal the lid, and either cook on the slow-cooker setting on low for 6–8 hours or cook for 1 hour under high pressure.

Creamy Pumpkin Curry with Seafood

This recipe has starchy carbs included in the ingredients, so be mindful of your UCT when dishing up this luscious one-pot meal. Look for already peeled and cubed winter squash at your grocery store! Serve with Roasted Curried Cauliflower (page 339) and a Basic Green Salad (page 333).

- Keeps well in the refrigerator up to three days or in the freezer up to two months.
- Prep time: 45 minutes
- Cook time: 1½ hours
- Serves 4

1 small sugar pumpkin or butternut squash, peeled and cubed (6 cups)

4 tablespoons coconut oil

1 medium yellow onion, diced

2 carrots, sliced

1 (14-ounce) can coconut milk, chilled

1 cup chicken broth

2 garlic cloves, minced

1½ teaspoons ground turmeric

1 teaspoon grated fresh ginger

1 teaspoon ground coriander

4 small zucchini, diced

2 pounds medium shrimp, peeled and deveined, or solid white fish such as cod or halibut, cut into 2-inch cubes

Chopped fresh cilantro

1. Preheat the oven to 400°F.
2. Toss the pumpkin with 2 tablespoons of the coconut oil, spread evenly on a baking sheet, and roast for 20 to 30 minutes or until fork-tender.
3. While the pumpkin is cooking, heat the remaining 2 tablespoons coconut oil in a large soup pot over medium heat. Add the onion and carrots and cook until the onion becomes translucent.
4. Increase the heat to medium-high, scoop out just the cream from the can of chilled coconut milk, and add it to the pot. Let it sizzle, and stir until the cream is melted and mixed well with the onion and carrots. Reduce the heat to medium-low and let it simmer.
5. While the vegetables and coconut cream simmer, transfer the roasted pumpkin to a food processor or blender along with the remaining coconut

milk from the can, the broth, garlic, turmeric, ginger, and coriander. Process until completely smooth.

6. Add the zucchini and the pumpkin mixture to the pot. Mix well and bring to a simmer. Add the shrimp to the soup and cook until the shrimp are pink and firm, 3 to 4 minutes (or, if using fish, until the pieces flake easily).

7. Sprinkle with cilantro and serve.

Seafood and Veggie Chowder

This is so fantastic left over for breakfast or lunch, there's no need for a "second meal idea"—this is a second meal ready to go all on its own! It's packed with nutrient-dense veggies and protein-powered seafood. We know you'll love this delicious chowder just as much as we do.

- Keeps well in the refrigerator up to three days or in the freezer up to two months.
- Prep time: 30 minutes
- Cook time: 30 minutes
- Serves 4

6 strips bacon or turkey bacon, chopped
1 small yellow onion, diced
3 celery stalks, chopped
2 garlic cloves, minced
4 cups chicken broth
1 cup canned coconut milk
1 pound Brussels sprouts, quartered
2 carrots, chopped
2 pounds wild-caught salmon, cod, or other fish, cut into bite-size pieces, or whole medium shrimp, peeled and deveined
1 small red bell pepper, diced
1 tablespoon dried dill
½ teaspoon crushed red pepper or to taste (optional)
Sea salt and freshly ground pepper

1. Cook the bacon in a large pot over medium to medium-high heat until beginning to brown and crisp. Drain all but about 1 tablespoon of the grease from the pot, add the onions to the bacon, and sauté until the onions become

translucent. If using turkey bacon, you'll want to add 1 tablespoon avocado or coconut oil to the pan before you add the onions.

2. Add the celery and garlic and sauté until the garlic is fragrant. Add the broth and coconut milk and bring to a boil. Add the Brussels sprouts and carrots and simmer until the vegetables are tender but not mushy.

3. Add the seafood and bell pepper and cook just until the fish flakes apart easily or, if using shrimp, until they turn pink. Add the dill and crushed red pepper, if using, and season with salt and pepper to taste. Serve immediately.

Ginger-Carrot Chicken Soup

We suggest having bone broth (page 374) on hand and our Basic Chicken (page 373) ready to pull out of the freezer to make delicious one-pot meals like this one. Serve with any salad you choose. This soup also has starchy carbs included, so watch your serving size according to your UCT when eating a bowl.

- Keeps well in the refrigerator up to four days or in the freezer up to three months.
- Prep time: 30 minutes
- Cook time: 20 minutes
- Serves: 4 or 5

2 tablespoons olive oil

4 cups Chicken Bone Broth (page 374) or store-bought

2 cooked chicken breasts, shredded or chopped (see page 373)

1–2 teaspoons grated fresh ginger

3 garlic cloves, minced

6 small carrots, sliced

6 small celery stalks, sliced

1 small white sweet potato, diced (about 1½ cups)

Pinch of cayenne pepper

Chopped fresh parsley

1 tablespoon honey or monk fruit

Lemon juice

Sea salt and freshly ground pepper

1. Heat the oil in a large pot over medium heat. Add the onions and sauté until tender. Add the garlic and sauté until fragrant, 1 to 2 minutes. Add the

celery, carrots, and sweet potato, sprinkle with a big pinch of sea salt, and
sauté for 2 to 3 minutes. Add the chicken broth and bring to a simmer; cook
until the carrots and sweet potatoes are tender.

2. Add the chicken, honey or monk fruit, a squeeze of lemon juice, and the cayenne and simmer for another 3 to 5 minutes. Season with salt and pepper to
taste and garnish with a little chopped fresh parsley. Serve.

Bison Chili

We suggest serving this scrumptious chili with Roasted Broccoli (page 337) or
Green Bean Fries (page 337) and any of the Carb Fixes you choose (page 343).
If you can't find bison, you can use lean ground beef, turkey, or a combination
of the two.

Second meal idea: Use as the protein for a Bowl Fix (page 325) or eat the
leftovers for breakfast with some sautéed greens.

- Keeps well in the refrigerator for up to four days or
  in the freezer up to four months.
- Prep time: 45 minutes
- Cook time: 45 minutes
- Serves 5 or 6

2 tablespoons coconut oil, avocado oil, or extra virgin olive oil

1 small yellow onion, diced

2 pounds ground bison

4 celery stalks, diced

4 carrots, diced

3 garlic cloves, minced

3 tablespoons chili powder

3 tablespoons Italian seasoning

2 tablespoons ground cumin

2 teaspoons crushed red pepper

1 cup chicken broth

28 ounces canned diced or crushed tomatoes

1 bay leaf

Sea salt

1. In a large pot, heat the oil over medium heat. Add the onion and sauté until
   translucent. Add the ground meat and cook just until browned.

2. Add the celery, carrots, garlic, chili powder, Italian seasoning, cumin, and crushed pepper and mix well.
3. Add the chicken broth and tomatoes and stir; bring to a simmer and add the bay leaf. Turn the heat to low and let simmer for 25 to 30 minutes or until the carrots and celery are tender. Season with salt to taste. Serve.

The Hangry B*tch
TWO-FOR-ONE FIX

The following recipes will give you two different options for two meals in one; that is, directions to turn night one's dinner into night two. How fantastic is that! Two-for-one night makes life so much easier because the planning is already done for the next day. Hurray for #lettingitbeeasy!

First Two-for-One Dinner

NIGHT ONE DINNER:
Easy Roast Chicken, Roasted Mashed Sweet Taters, and Basic Green Salad

The Dinner Setup and Prep for Tomorrow's Lunch and Dinner

1. Prepare the Easy Roast Chicken (page 367) and the Roasted Mashed Sweet Taters (page 343). Both the chicken and the sweet potatoes can be roasted at the same time.

2. While the chicken and potatoes are roasting, prepare the Basic Green Salad (page 333) and the dressing of your choice. Cover and refrigerate separately. (Remember to set aside some greens and dressing for your lunch tomorrow in a separate container!)

3. After you make your salad, prep the Seasonal Soup Base (page 368) that you will use for tomorrow night's dinner. Place all the ingredients in the slow cooker except for the water and the chicken carcass, the rest you will complete after you eat dinner.

4. Once the chicken and sweet potatoes are done, let the chicken rest while you mash the sweet potatoes as directed on page 343. Take the salad out of the fridge and toss with the dressing.

5. Once the chicken has rested, carve all the meat off the bones and cut off the drumsticks and wings. At this point you can place the carcass in the slow cooker, but come back to finish the Seasonal Soup Base after you eat dinner!

6. After dinner, store any leftover chicken in the fridge for tomorrow night's soup and for an easy lunch tomorrow of leftover chicken on top of your leftover Basic Green Salad. You might not have enough chicken left over for your soup, so you will want to make sure you have additional chicken on hand to make the Basic Chicken Recipe on page 373 to add to tomorrow's soup.

7. Now, finish prepping the Seasonal Soup Base by following the rest of the directions on page 368.

Easy Roast Chicken

We realize that this chicken sounds super simple, almost too simple to even be good (come on, just salt and chicken?). But trust us, this will be one of the absolute BEST roast chickens you will ever eat. Tender, juicy deliciousness awaits—we promise.

- Keeps well in the refrigerator up to four days or in the freezer up to six months.
- Prep time: 15 minutes
- Cook time: 1 hour
- Serves: 4 or 5

1 (5- to 7-pound) whole chicken, rinsed and dried
Sea salt

1. Preheat the oven to 450°F.
2. Place the chicken in a roasting pan with a rack and generously sprinkle the entire chicken with sea salt (inside the cavity as well).
3. Roast the chicken, breast side up, for 1 hour, or until the skin is golden brown and crispy and the breast registers 165°F. Let the chicken rest for 10 minutes before carving so that you don't lose all the delicious juices.

Seasonal Soup Base for Night Two

1 yellow onion, cut in half and then quartered

4 carrots, cut into 3- to 5-inch pieces

6 celery stalks, cut into 3- to 4-inch pieces (do not trim any leaves from the stalks)

1 whole bunch fresh parsley

3–4 garlic cloves, smashed with the flat side of your knife and peeled

3–6 slices fresh ginger (optional)

2 tablespoons apple cider vinegar

1 tablespoon black peppercorns

2 bay leaves

Place all the veggies in the bottom of your slow cooker; add the apple cider vinegar, peppercorns, and bay leaves. Place the chicken carcass on top of the veggies, add enough cold water to cover the carcass and fill your slow cooker, and cook on low for 24 hours.

NIGHT TWO DINNER:
Simple Seasonal Soup

This is an example of a summer soup; if it's winter, we recommend replacing the zucchini with cubed winter squash or sweet potatoes. All the soup toppings are optional, but at the very least try the jicama, cilantro, and lime!

- Keeps well in the refrigerator up to four days or in the freezer up to three months.
- Prep time: 45 minutes
- Cook time: 10–15 minutes
- Serves 4 or 5

FOR THE SOUP

Seasonal Soup Base that's been cooked overnight

¼ cup extra virgin olive oil

1 small yellow onion, diced

1 red bell pepper, diced

Sea salt and freshly ground pepper

2–4 garlic cloves, minced

3 ears sweet corn (optional)

2 yellow summer squash or zucchini

2 pounds shredded cooked chicken

5–6 ounces tender greens, such as baby spinach or baby kale

Juice 1–2 limes, to taste

1 tablespoon ground cumin or more, if desired

1 tablespoon dried oregano or more, if desired

½–1 teaspoon chipotle chile powder or ancho chile powder (we suggest
  chipotle for the smoky flavor)

FOR THE TOPPINGS

1 small jicama, peeled and diced

1 bunch fresh cilantro, chopped

5 radishes, halved and thinly sliced

4 green onions, chopped

2 avocados, peeled and diced

1 lime, sliced

1. To make the soup: Strain the broth through a fine-mesh strainer from your slow cooker into a large saucepan and set aside. Let the chicken carcass cool until you are able to handle the meat and bones. Pick out all the delicious edible meat that's still left on the chicken, pulling what you can from the bones, and set the meat aside to be added to your soup later. Discard the bones.
2. Heat the oil in a large pot over medium heat. Add the onion and bell pepper, season with a little sea salt, and sauté until the onion and peppers are soft. Add the garlic and sauté just until the garlic is fragrant. Slowly pour in the strained chicken broth and bring to a simmer.
3. While the broth comes to a simmer, cut the kernels off the ears of corn, if using. Add the corn and the summer squash to the broth and cook for 5 to 7 minutes. Add the cooked, shredded chicken, greens, lime juice, cumin, oregano, and chile powder and season with salt and pepper to taste. Simmer another 5 to 7 minutes. Taste and add more cumin, oregano, salt, pepper, and/or lime juice if desired. This soup should be bursting with flavor!
4. To top and serve: Ladle the soup into individual bowls and add generous amounts of the toppings. Enjoy and eat the leftovers for breakfast and/or lunch the next day.

Second Two-for-One Dinner

NIGHT ONE DINNER:
Ginger-Cilantro Burgers and Sriracha Broccoli Slaw

The Dinner Setup and Prep for Tomorrow Night's Dinner

This two-for-one meal is so simple. All you need to do to be prepared for night two is to store half of your ground beef mixture in the fridge, and you'll be ready to rock!

Ginger-Cilantro Burgers

- Keeps well in the refrigerator up to four days or in the freezer up to four months.
- Prep time: 45 minutes
- Cook time: 15 minutes
- Serves 5 or 6

2–3 tablespoons extra virgin olive oil

1 small yellow onion, diced

4 garlic cloves, minced

Sea salt

4 pounds ground beef, bison, or turkey

¼ cup tamari or coconut aminos

¼ cup minced fresh cilantro leaves and steams, plus cilantro leaves for garnish

2 teaspoons grated fresh ginger

1–2 tablespoons honey or monk fruit (optional)

2 teaspoons sriracha, or to taste (optional)

Cucumber slices (optional)

1. Heat the oil in a small skillet over medium heat, add the onion, and sauté until translucent. Add the garlic and a generous pinch of salt and sauté just until the garlic is fragrant. Set aside to cool.

2. Combine the ground beef, tamari, cilantro, and ginger in a medium bowl and add the honey and sriracha, if using. Add the cooled onions and garlic and mix together with your hands. Transfer half of the mixture to a container, cover, and refrigerate. Form the remaining mixture into 5 or 6 patties, 1 to 1½ inches thick, and set aside.

3. Prepare the Sriracha Broccoli Slaw as instructed on page 335, cover, and refrigerate.

4. Heat a grill pan over medium-high heat (or heat an outdoor grill to medium-high). Once it's hot enough for the meat to sizzle, place the burgers on the grill pan or grill.

5. Cook for 3 to 5 minutes each side, for medium burgers. (Do not press on the burgers while cooking; this will release the juices and leave you with a dry, crumbly burger.) Top with cucumber slices, if using, and serve with a side of the Sriracha Broccoli Slaw.

NIGHT TWO DINNER:
Thai Basil Lettuce Wraps

- The cooked ground beef will keep well in the refrigerator for three to four days or in the freezer for three to four months.
- Prep time: 20 minutes
- Cook time: 10 minutes
- Serves 5

Seasoned ground meat from Night One
1–2 teaspoons rice vinegar
Tamari or coconut aminos to taste
Sriracha (optional)
Fish sauce (optional)
1 head Bibb or romaine lettuce, leaves separated
4 green onions, chopped

1 cup chopped cilantro

1 cup torn or chopped fresh Thai basil or sweet basil leaves

1 cup fresh mint leaves

1 red bell pepper, chopped

½ cup chopped cashews or almonds

1. In a large skillet brown the ground beef mixture over medium heat. Add 1 teaspoon of rice vinegar, and add the sriracha, tamari or coconut aminos to taste, fish sauce to taste, if desired, and the remaining teaspoon of rice vinegar, if desired.

2. To assemble the lettuce wraps, add a scoop of the meat mixture to the lettuce leaves and top with green onions, cilantro, basil, mint, bell pepper, and cashews or almonds. Serve.

The Hangry B*tch
STAPLES FIX

Although you can easily buy a few of these staples, such as the avocado oil mayo and bone broth, we LOVE our homemade versions, and they are money savers. Plus, it's not as hard as it sounds—we promise! The other staples you'll find in this section include basic cooked chicken to have on hand for quick meal fixes throughout the week and our salad dressings.

Slow-Cooker or Instant Pot Basic Chicken

- Prep time: 5 minutes
- Cook time: 2–7 hours (slow cooker) or 10–15 minutes (Instant Pot)
- Serves 6 or 7

3 pounds boneless, skinless chicken breasts or thighs
1 cup water or chicken broth
Sea salt and freshly ground pepper

SLOW-COOKER INSTRUCTIONS

1. Season the chicken generously on both sides with salt and pepper and place in the slow cooker. Add the water or broth.
2. For chicken breasts, cook on low for 4 to 5 hours or on high for 2 to 3 hours. For chicken thighs, cook on low for 6 to 7 hours or on high for 3 to 4 hours.

INSTANT POT INSTRUCTIONS

1. Add 1 cup water to the Instant Pot and place the trivet in the bottom.
2. Season the chicken generously on both sides with salt and pepper.
3. Place the chicken on the trivet in the Instant Pot. Lock on the cover and make sure the vent is sealed.
4. For chicken breasts, set the pressure cooker to cook for 6 minutes on high pressure and let it release pressure naturally for 5 minutes and then open the steam valve to release the rest of the pressure if necessary.
5. For chicken thighs, follow the same instructions as for the breasts but set to cook on high pressure for 13 minutes.

Beef or Chicken Bone Broth

- Keeps well in the refrigerator up to four days or in the freezer up to three months.
- Prep time: 30 minutes
- Cook time: 24 hours (slow cooker) or 1½ hours (Instant Pot)
- Makes 2 to 3 quarts

FOR BEEF BONE BROTH

2–4 beef shanks, marrow bones, knuckle bones, or any combination thereof

FOR CHICKEN BONE BROTH

1 leftover chicken carcass from Easy Roast Chicken (page 367)

FOR BOTH RECIPES

Sea salt

1 yellow onion, cut in half and quartered

4 carrots, cut into 3- to 4-inch pieces

6 celery stalks, cut into 3- to 4-inch pieces (do not trim any leaves from the stalks)

1 whole bunch fresh parsley

3 or 4 garlic cloves, smashed and peeled

3–6 thin slices fresh ginger (no need to peel)

2 tablespoons apple cider vinegar

1 tablespoon black peppercorns

2 bay leaves

SLOW-COOKER INSTRUCTIONS

1. To make the beef bone broth: Preheat the oven to 400°F.
2. Line a baking sheet with parchment paper. Place the beef shanks and/or bones on the paper, season with salt, and roast until browned and the marrow is bubbling, about 30 minutes.
3. Transfer the shanks and/or bones to the slow cooker and add the onions, carrots, celery, parsley, garlic, ginger, vinegar, peppercorns, and bay leaves.
4. Add enough cold water to fill the slow cooker, cover, and cook on low for 24 hours.
5. Strain through a fine-mesh strainer and serve or transfer to glass storage jars, cover, and refrigerate.

6. To make the chicken bone broth: Place the chicken carcass in the slow cooker and add the onions, carrots, celery, parsley, garlic, ginger, vinegar, peppercorns, and bay leaves.

7. Add enough cold water to fill the slow cooker, cover, and cook on low for 24 hours.

8. Strain through a fine-mesh strainer and serve or transfer to glass storage jars, cover, and refrigerate.

INSTANT POT INSTRUCTIONS

Follow all of the instructions for the slow-cooker beef or chicken bone broth but only add enough water to reach the pressure cooker fill line. Once everything is in the pot, simply close and lock the lid, set the vent to sealed, and cook on high pressure for 1½ hours. Use the "natural release" method; strain and store as described in the slow-cooker method.

Homemade HB Mayonnaise

You can use a hand-held mixer, immersion blender, food processor, or a blender that does not get too hot to make this mayonnaise. Do not use a Vitamix blender because it will make the mayonnaise too hot and it will not emulsify.

- Keeps well in the refrigerator for one to two weeks; do not freeze.
- Prep time: 15 minutes
- Makes about 2 cups

2 egg yolks
2 tablespoons apple cider vinegar
1 teaspoon yellow mustard
1 teaspoon sea salt
¼ teaspoon cayenne pepper
2 cups avocado oil

1. Combine the egg yolks, vinegar, mustard, salt, and cayenne in a food processor, blender, or mixing bowl. Process, blend, or use a hand-held mixer or immersion blender to mix for 5 seconds.

2. Leave the processor, blender, mixer, or immersion blender running and slowly, slowly, slowly, drop by drop or in a very slow drizzle, add the oil. Be patient. Do not dump all the oil in quickly and give up!

3. When the mixture begins to emulsify, or thicken, only then can you be a bit faster about pouring in the oil, but still take your time. Turn the machine off once all the oil is in and the mayonnaise is thickened to your desired consistency. (You can also make mayonnaise by hand using a whisk; it's a great way to get in a quick workout and fun to do with a partner or child.)

Tip: Do not throw away your mayonnaise mixture if it doesn't work or if the oil separates from too much blending. Simply take another egg yolk and tablespoon of vinegar, whisk those two ingredients together, and slowly whisk or blend into the original "messed-up" mayonnaise. Remember that a slow pour is the secret to success and stop blending once you reach your desired mayo consistency.

HB Salad Dressings

Lemony Vinaigrette

- Keeps well in the refrigerator for up to six months; do not freeze.
- Prep time: 10 minutes
- Makes approximately ½ cup

⅓ cup extra virgin olive oil

Juice of 1 lemon

1 tablespoon honey or monkfruit (optional)

2 teaspoons dried dill

2 teaspoons dried parsley

2 teaspoons Dijon mustard

1 teaspoon apple cider vinegar, or more to taste

Sea salt and freshly ground pepper

Whisk all the ingredients, including salt and pepper to taste, in a small bowl until well blended. Taste, and add more vinegar if desired.

Apple Cider Vinaigrette

- Keeps well in the refrigerator for up to six months; do not freeze.
- Prep time: 10 minutes
- Makes approximately ½ cup

⅓ cup extra virgin olive oil

2 tablespoons apple cider vinegar, or more to taste

2 tablespoons dried basil

2 teaspoons brown mustard

Pinch of cayenne pepper

Sea salt and freshly ground pepper

Whisk all the ingredients, including salt and pepper to taste, in a small bowl until well blended.

Balsamic Vinaigrette

- Keeps well in the refrigerator for up to one week or up to six months if you omit the garlic; do not freeze.
- Prep time: 10 minutes
- Makes approximately ½ cup

⅓ cup extra virgin olive oil

2 tablespoons balsamic vinegar, or more to taste

1 tablespoon dried parsley

1 teaspoon Dijon mustard, plus more if desired

1 garlic clove, minced

Sea salt and freshly ground pepper

Whisk all the ingredients, including salt and pepper to taste, in a small bowl until well blended.

Cumin and Lime Dressing

- Keeps well in the refrigerator up to two weeks; do not freeze.
- Prep time: 10 minutes
- Makes approximately ½ cup

½ cup finely chopped fresh cilantro

⅓ cup avocado oil

Juice of 1 lime, or more to taste

1½ teaspoons ground cumin

¼ teaspoon smoked paprika

Pinch of cayenne pepper

Sea salt and freshly ground pepper

Whisk all the ingredients, including salt and pepper to taste, in a small bowl until well blended.

Asian Vinaigrette

- Keeps well in the refrigerator up to two weeks; do not freeze.
- Prep time: 10 minutes
- Makes approximately ½ cup

⅓ **cup avocado oil**

1–2 tablespoons toasted sesame oil, or more to taste

2–4 tablespoons fresh lime juice

1 tablespoon maple syrup or 1½ teaspoons xylitol or monk fruit

1 tablespoon rice vinegar

1 teaspoon fish sauce, or more if desired

Whisk all the ingredients in a small bowl until well blended.

HB Ranch Dressing

- Keeps well in the refrigerator up to one week; do not freeze.
- Prep time: 10 minutes
- Makes approximately 1½ cups

1 cup avocado oil mayonnaise, see (page 375) to make your own

¼ **cup canned coconut milk**

1–2 tablespoons lemon juice, or more to taste

1 tablespoon dried dill

1 tablespoon dried parsley

1 tablespoon dried basil

1 or 2 garlic cloves, minced

Sea salt and freshly ground pepper

Whisk all the ingredients, including salt and pepper to taste and 1 tablespoon of the lemon juice, in a small bowl until well blended. Taste and add more lemon juice if desired.

Sample Week Meal PLAN

Day 1

Breakfast: Breakfast Soup (page 316)

Lunch: Two-Minute Lettuce Wraps (page 332)

Third Meal: Leftover Breakfast Soup

Dinner: Ginger-Cilantro Burgers and Sriracha Broccoli Slaw (page 370), Roasted Root Veggies (page 344)

Day 2

Breakfast: Leftover Breakfast Soup

Lunch: Leftover Ginger-Cilantro Burgers

Third Meal: Two-Minute Tuna or Salmon Salad (page 331)

Dinner: Thai Basil Lettuce Wraps (page 371), Leftover Roasted Root Veggies

Day 3

Breakfast: Leftover Breakfast Soup

Lunch: Leftover Thai Basil Lettuce Wraps

Third Meal: Leftover Two-Minute Tuna or Salmon Salad

Dinner: Southwestern Chicken Bake (page 353), Quick Kale Salad (page 334), Slow-Cooker Sweet Potatoes (page 346)

Day 4

Breakfast: Snappy Salmon Patties (page 321) with Sautéed Greens (page 340)

Lunch: Leftover chicken bake, kale salad, and sweet potatoes

Third Meal: Leftover salmon patties or other protein of your choice made into Two-Minute Lettuce Wraps (page 332)

Dinner: Easy Meat Sauce (page 354) with Zucchini Noodles (page 342), Quick Kale Salad (page 334) with HB Ranch Dressing (page 379), and Garlic Roasted Sweet Potatoes (page 344)

Day 5

Breakfast: Leftover salmon patties and sautéed greens

Lunch: Leftover Easy Meat Sauce, salad, and potatoes

Third Meal: Cucumber and carrot slices with HB Ranch and turkey deli meat

Dinner: Easy Roast Chicken Two-for-One Meal (page 366), leftover Slow-Cooker Sweet Potatoes.

Day 6

Breakfast: Italian Eggs (page 320)

Lunch: Two-Minute Lettuce Wraps (page 332) using leftover roast chicken

Third Meal: Cucumber and carrot slices with HB Ranch Dressing and turkey deli meat

Dinner: Simple Seasonal Soup from Two-for-One Meal (page 368)

Day 7

Breakfast: Leftover Simple Seasonal Soup

Lunch: Chicken Broccoli Salad (page 329)

Third Meal: Leftover Chicken Broccoli Salad made into Two-Minute Lettuce Wraps (page 332)

Dinner: Lamb Slider Bowls (page 328)

Supplement and Testing Resources

For multivitamins, choose a formula that includes methylated forms of folate (avoid folic acid) and B12, contains a wide array of minerals, and does not contain sugar, artificial dyes, or excessive additives.

For herbs, consider brands with standardized extracts instead of simply powdered whole herbs. For example, you can purchase capsules with powdered rhodiola or capsules with rhodiola extract standardized to 3 percent total rosavins. We prefer the latter.

For fish oils, be sure you are buying high-quality oil that has been processed to prevent rancidity. Taking bad fish oil is worse than not taking any at all! Be sure your product is tested for heavy metals and pesticides as well as preserved properly.

Brands we trust and recommend are all available at www.sarahanddr brooke.com:

Hangry B*tches

Better by Dr. Brooke

Designs for Health

Apex Energetics

Pure Encapsulations

Vital Nutrients

Seeking Health

Nordic Naturals (omega-3 fish oil)

Chapter 2

General Nutrient Suggestions for Women

Multivitamin: Choose one with methylated forms of folate 800 mcg per day (avoid folic acid) and 1000 mcg per day B12, a wide array of minerals, and no sugar, artificial dyes, or excessive additives. Consider Hangry B*tch Basic Multi 2 caps (take 1 capsule 2 times per day).

Zinc: Take 30 mg per day minimum. (This may be in your multivitamin.)

Magnesium: Take 300–1200 mg per day in divided doses (i.e., 300 mg 1 to 4 times per day). (Consider glycinate, citrate, or chelated forms.)

Omega-3 fatty acids from fish oil: Take 1–2 g per day (typically 850 mg EPA and 200 mg DHA per serving).

Selenium: Take 200 mcg per day. (This is the total amount; there will likely be 50–100 mcg in your multi.)

Antioxidant and anti-inflammatory nutrients include resveratrol (100–400 mg per day), turmeric (1–3 g per day), boswellia, ginger, and bromelain. These are important for high cortisol, insulin resistance, Hashimoto's disease, or other autoimmune or inflammation issues.

For mitochondrial and antioxidant support, use liposomal glutathione (100–500 mg per day or more) or n-acetyl cysteine (300 mg 1 to 3 times per day; doses of NAC range typically from 600–2400 mg per day). Glutathione is ideal for PCOS, Hashimoto's disease, and poor exercise tolerance. It is recommended to support glutathione with other nutrients such as alpha lipoic acid, cordyceps, and milk thistle for better utilization.

Improve energy and exercise tolerance by supplementing with mitochondrial nutrients: CoQ10 (100–200 mg per day), l-carnitine (1–2 g daily), and a complex of B vitamins, including methyl folate and B12.

Electrolytes with additional minerals and vitamin C as well as 100–150 mg of sodium and 150 mg of potassium are optimal. These are ideal for low cortisol and insulin-resistance issues. We recommend hydrate + support by Better by Dr. Brooke or Optimal Electrolytes by Seeking Health.

Sleep Support

Utilize alone or in combination these calming herbs: lemon balm, valerian, passionflower, and chamomile, all in doses of 100–300 mg each. We recommend calm + sleep by Better by Dr. Brooke.

Glycine: Take 3 g per day, one hour before bedtime.

L-theanine: Take 200 mg at bedtime.

Magnesium glycinate: Take 300–600 mg at bedtime.

MAOA and COMT Support

If you suspect your sleep issues are due to sluggish MAOA or COMT enzymes, avoid supplements with quercetin, rhodiola, or ECGC (green tea) later in the day.

Increase riboflavin from lamb, liver, salmon, and eggs or consider taking 100 mg riboflavin 1 or 2 times per day.

Avoid calcium and iron supplements in the evening; instead, take them earlier in the day as they will slow COMT. Do take 100–400 mg magnesium in the evening to support metabolism of stimulating neurotransmitter such as epinephrine and to help you sleep and be less anxious. Magnesium glycinate is our favorite because the glycine in this form also supports calm and sleep.

Chapter 4

Digestive Support

Digestive Enzymes

digest + better from Better by Dr. Brooke: Take 1–2 per day with meals.

Enzymix Pro Apex Energetics: Take 1–2 per day with meals.

For low stomach acid you can supplement with HCL, whether in a digestive enzyme or alone. Start with 200 mg HCL and increase as necessary (up to 600 mg); stop if any burning occurs. If HCL does cause burning, you can instead try 1 to 2 teaspoons of apple cider vinegar diluted in water for five minutes before a meal for added digestive benefit. If this also causes burning, stop and see a functional medicine doctor for assistance or visit your primary care doctor for evaluation.

Hangry B*tch Gut-Healing Protocol

repair + calm from Better by Dr. Brooke: Take 2 teaspoons in water twice daily. These products will help heal your intestinal lining. If choosing other products, look for l-glutamine in doses of 3–10 g two times per day and ideally herbs such as slippery elm, DGL (deglycyrrhizinated licorice), or marshmallow root.

remove + rebalance from Better by Dr. Brooke: Take 1 packet 2 times per day with food.

replace + restore from Better by Dr. Brooke: Take 2 capsules twice daily. OR Strengtia by Apex Energetics: Take 2 caps twice daily.

After three weeks on this protocol, reduce the replace + restore or Strengtia to just 2 caps per day and add 2 capsules per day of a *Lactobacillus* and *Bifidobacterium* blend (we suggest Sibiotica from Apex Energetics or Probiotic Synergy from Designs for Health).

In general, rotate probiotic products every two to three months to get a variety of strains. Probiotics we love include Sibiotica (Apex Energetics), Probiotic Synergy (Designs for Health), and Therabiotic (Klaire Labs). If tolerated, spore-form or soil-based probiotics including Prescript Assist, Primal Defense (Garden of Life), or Megaspore are good choices as well. When choosing probiotics, look for products that give you 25–100 billion units per day.

Collagen is also great for gut healing, among many other things. We recommend Hangry B*tch Collagen and Vital Proteins Collagen Peptides.

Chapter 6

More Sleep Suggestions

To Boost GABA

GABA as "PharmaGABA": Take 100–200 mg per day.

Glycine: Take 3 g per day, one hour before bedtime. If this increases anxiety and sleeplessness, it means you have some issues likely converting the amino acid glutamate to GABA; this can be worth exploring with your functional medicine doctor.

To Raise Serotonin

Inositol: Take 1000 mg at bedtime.

5-HTP: Take 50–100 mg at bedtime.

St. John's wort: Take 300 mg at bedtime.

Serotonin-boosting supplements can give very vivid dreams, which can make you wake less rested the next day. If this occurs, take earlier in the day or avoid. Do not take supplements that boost serotonin if you are also taking MAO inhibitors or SSRIs (selective serotonin reuptake inhibitors).

Chapter 8

Low Cortisol, Low Thyroid, High Cortisol, and Insulin Resistance

Low Cortisol

Pantothenic acid: Take 500 mg per day.

Licorice root: Take 50–100 mg (standardized to 20 percent glycyrrhizic acid) in the morning and possibly again at lunch as well. Some people benefit from doses as high as 400 mg, but you should not exceed 600 mg per day or take it if you have hypertension.

hydrate + support electrolytes from Better by Dr. Brooke: Take 1 serving per day. OR Seeking Health Optimal Electrolytes: Take 1 serving per day.

Ideal adaptogens for low cortisol include *Panax ginseng* (aka Korean ginseng), which improves stamina and energy with exercise. Take up to 3 g per day. *Withania somnifera* (aka ashwagandha or Indian ginseng) is great for blood sugar issues. It appears to act in a similar way to cortisol, so it can be a bit stimulating for some, but it is usually great for low cortisol. This herb is also great for the thyroid. The dose is typically 200–500 mg 1 or 2 times per day of a standardized herb containing 1.5 percent with anolides.

Grain free, fruit and veggie fiber powder: cleanse + balance from Better by Dr. Brooke: Take 1–4 servings per day.

Low Thyroid

Be sure your multivitamin or other supplement contains at least 30 mg of zinc and 200 mcg of selenium.

Ashwagandha: Take 200–500 mg 1 or 2 times per day of a standardized herb containing 1.5 percent with anolides.

Commiphora wightii, aka guggul, increases conversion of T4 to active T3. The dose is typically 750 mg daily. Consider better + thyroid from Better by Dr. Brooke.

If you have Hashimoto's disease, using 1–3 g of turmeric per day can help lower inflammation and antibodies.

High Cortisol

Magnesium: Take 300–1200 mg per day in divided doses (i.e., 300 mg 1 to 4 times per day).

Omega-3 fatty acids: Take 2–6 g per day until inflammation or stress is resolved, ideally not longer than three months. We recommend Ultimate Omega (Nordic Naturals) or OmegAvail Ultra (Designs for Health).

Phosphatidyl serine: Take 400 mg 1 or 2 times per day. We recommend Designs for Health brand. This should not be taken with psychotropic medications.

For high cortisol–related sleep issues (wired at bedtime), try taking a tincture of passiflora (40 drops at bedtime; we recommend HerbPharm brand). Also try magnolia bark (*Magnolia officianalis*), which is typically taken at doses of 225 mg per day at bedtime. Consider Cortisol Manager from Integrative Therapeutics.

Adaptogens for High Cortisol

Rhodiola prevents stress-induced catecholamine (aka adrenaline) activity, improves cognitive function, and supports the immune system. The dose is 100–300 mg daily of a product with 3 percent total rosavins.

Holy basil (aka tulsi): A good starting place for most people is 300 mg per day spread over a few doses.

Eleutherococcus (aka Siberian ginseng) optimizes the HPA (brain to adrenals) axis functioning under stress. It can be taken in capsule form or try ⅛ teaspoon of solid extract 1 to 3 times daily. Capsule doses are typically 100–200 mg of a product standardized to 0.8 percent eleutherosides. Taking this too late in the day can affect your ability to fall asleep, so take at breakfast or lunch. Avoid this supplement if you have high blood pressure.

Adaptogens are typically best taken in a blended product. These are our favorites:

adapt + cope from Better by Dr. Brooke: Take 1–2 capsules with meals 2 to 3 times per day

Adrenotone from Designs for Health: Take 1–3 capsules with breakfast and lunch.

Insulin Resistance

Berberine: Take 200–500 mg per day with meals. Consider better + berberine from Better by Dr. Brooke.

Minerals such as vanadium (100–200 mg per day) and chromium (500–1000 mcg 1 or 2 times per day) are helpful, as is the antioxidant alpha lipoic acid (200–600 mg per day; must be R form). Our favorite multi for insulin-resistance issues is balanced + beautiful from Better by Dr. Brooke because it includes all of these nutrients. The dose is 2 capsules with meals 3 times per day.

As with elevated cortisol, a higher dose of omega-3 fatty acids (2–6 g per day) is helpful for a few months. Ultimate Omega (Nordic Naturals) or OmegAvail Ultra (Designs for Health) are our favorites.

If you have PCOS, inositol is a great addition and should include d-chiral and myo forms. Consider sensitize + support from Better by Dr. Brooke (take 2 capsules 1 or 2 times daily).

Also considedr cleanse + balance fiber powder from Better by Dr. Brooke: Take 1–4 servings per day.

For Both Low Cortisol and Insulin Resistance:

Ideally, you'll support both adrenals and insulin balance with adaptogens such as adapt + cope (take 1 or 2 capsules with breakfast and lunch) and balanced + beautiful (2 capsules with meals 3 times per day), both from Better by Dr. Brooke.

Chapter 9

Low Thyroid or Exercise Intolerance

CoQ10: Take 100–200 mg 1 or 2 times per day. (Our favorite product is Q-Evail 100 or 200 mg capsules from Designs for Health.)

L-carnitine tartrate: Take 1–2 g per day.

Creatine: Take 1000 mg 1 to 3 times per day. We recommend creatine magnesium chelate (rather than creatine monohydrate) for less digestive upset and ease of use. Our favorite brand is Seeking Health.

Resveratrol: Take 100–400 mg per day.

Turmeric: Take 1–3 g per day.

Electrolytes: hydrate + support from Better by Dr. Brooke: Take 1 serving per day.

BCAAs: Taking 100 mg/kg body weight per day can be helpful. During a workout BCAAs help with endurance while taking them post-workout helps with recovery. For most women, 5–8 g per day total is adequate with 3–5 g of that taken post-workout. (Note that if your insulin resistance is significant, BCAAs can up your cravings and appetite. Watch your ACES and blood work to monitor.) Our favorite products are recover + replete from Better by Dr. Brooke and NOW Brand BCAAs. It is difficult to get this high dose in capsules, and unflavored/unsweetened BCAA powders are very bitter (however, Pure Encapsulations does make one), but avoid products with aspartame or sucralose.

Glutathione support such as n-acetyl cysteine (300 mg 1 to 3 times per day; NAC doses typically range from 600–2400 mg) OR liposomal glutathione (100-500 mg per day). Liposomal glutathione brands we love include Designs for Health and Better by Dr Brooke (both liquid) and Pure Encapsulations (capsules).

And to adequately support glutathione recycling after it's been used as an antioxidant, be sure you're getting 200–600 mg alpha lipoic acid per day (found in the balanced + beautiful multi from Better by Dr. Brooke) or 200 mg milk thistle per day (try Vital Nutrients Milk Thistle Extract). For ease we recommend Glutathione Recycler from Apex Energetics. Cordyceps is also helpful to support glutathione balance and we love the cordyceps elixirs from Four Sigmatic. Save 15 percent at www.us.four sigmatic.com and use code BETTEREVERYDAY at checkout.

Chapter 10
Female Hormones and Testosterone

Low Testosterone

Zinc: Take 30 mg per day.

Vitamin D: Make sure you have adequate levels aiming for 50–80 ng/dL 25-OH vitamin D on lab testing

Maca boosts estrogen, testosterone, and DHEA. Take 75–100 mg per day.

Estrogen and Progesterone General Support

Zinc: Take 30 mg per day.

Magnesium: Take 300–1200 mg per day in divided doses. We prefer magnesium glycinate for its added calming effect; try Pure Encapsulations.

For all Estrogen, Progesterone, or Testosterone Issues

Utilize adrenal adaptogens and blood sugar support as needed. See pages 159–65 under chapter 8 for specifics.

Estrogen Dominance

DIM (di-indole-methane): Take 200 mg per day.

Glutathione or n-acetyl cysteine (300g 1 to 3 times per day; doses of NAC typically range from 600–2400 mg) OR liposomal glutathione (100–500 mg per day or more)

Vitamin B6: Take 50–100 mg per day.

Turmeric: Take 1–3 g per day.

Green tea, which you can drink (4–8 cups per day) or take in supplemental form at 200 mg per day.

If you tend toward constipation, you can utilize calcium d-glucarate 1000–1500 mg per day.

Low or Fluctuating Estrogen (i.e. Perimenopause and Menopause)

Phytoestrogen herbs such as black cohosh: Take 80–100 mg 1 or 2 times per day.

Hot flashes:

Rheum rhaponticum, extract called ER731 found in Estrovera from Metagenics (4 mg per day) or Herbpharm's Rhubarb extract is excellent for hot flashes.

Low Progesterone

Chaste tree (aka vitex) is typically given from ovulation (typically around day 14) until the start of the next period; doses range from 200 mg or more per day. We recommend Pure Encapsulations brand chaste tree/vitex or Progestaid (Apex Energetics) if you also have heavy bleeding (take 2 capsules 2 times per day from day 14 to day 1).

PCOS

Insulin support (see chapter 8) including the following:

balanced + beautiful from Better by Dr. Brooke: Take 2 capsules 3 times per day with meals.

better + berberine (if needed): Take 1–2 capsules with meals. (Watch your blood sugar with ACES and/or a glucometer.) Or other berberine capsules 200–500 mg per day.

sensitize + support (inositol blend from Better by Dr. Brooke): Take 2 capsules 1 to 2 times per day.

Address inflammation with turmeric (take 1–3 g per day) and omega-3 fatty acids (2–6 g per day for up to three months; try Designs for Health or Nordic Naturals brands).

High testosterone or other androgen symptoms can be addressed with 30 mg zinc 1 to 3 times per day or herbs such as nettle root or saw palmetto. Consider taking 2 clear + normalize capsules from Better by Dr. Brooke twice per day.

Address any estrogen, progesterone or testosterone issues with the suggestions above.

Inflammation

Include turmeric liberally in your food; however, if you have significant inflammation, a supplemental dose is warranted (1–3 g per day). Other potent herbal anti-inflammatories include boswellia, ginger, and resveratrol.

Antioxidants and bioflavonoids such as EGCG in green tea, 200 mg per day, and pycnogenol, 100–200 mg per day, are also amazing.

Systemic enzymes can help "munch up" inflammation in your system and reduce your symptoms. These are taken between meals. Consider Pure Encapsulations Systemic Enzymes or quell + quiet enzymes with anti-inflammatory herbs (such as turmeric, boswellia, or ginger), from Better by Dr. Brooke.

Glutathione support as n-acetyl cysteine (300 mg 1 to 3 times per day; doses of NAC typically range from 600–2400 mg per day) OR liposomal glutathione (100–500 mg per day or more) as well as nutrients that recycle this important antioxidant, such as milk thistle, alpha lipoic acid, and cordyceps, can be utilized.

Testing Resources

General Blood Work and Thyroid Testing

Email Dr. Brooke directly at
   drbrooke@betterbydrbrooke.com

Direct Labs
   www.directlabs.com/BetterByDrBrooke

Life Extension
   www.lifeextension.com

Thyroid testing at home
   www.canaryclub.org

Food Sensitivity Testing

Cyrex Labs
www.cyrexlabs.com

Hormone Testing

Precision Analytical
www.DUTCHtest.com

Genova Diagnostics
www.gdx.net

Diagnostechs
www.diagnostechs.com

Organic Acid Testing

Ideal for fatigue, exercise intolerance, or unresolving hormone issues.

Genova Diagnostics
www.gdx.net

Digestive Function Testing

Stool analysis (microbiome balance, infection, digestive capacity, inflammation, etc.)

Genova Diagnostics
www.gdx.net

Doctor's Data
www.doctorsdata.com

Diagnostic Solutions
www.diagnosticsolutionslab.com

SIBO Testing

Genova Diagnostics
www.gdx.net

Aerodiagnostics
http://aerodiagnostics.com/

References

Due to space constraints and our desire to bring you more content we had to limit the references provided herein. We've selected key references here, but this is in no way a complete list of scientific and medical literature on which we've based this book and our program. A complete list of references is available for free at www.sarahanddrbrooke.com. Thank you for your understanding!

Introduction

Dembe A. E. and X. Yao. "Chronic Disease Risks from Exposure to Long-Hour Work Schedules Over a 32-Year Period," *J Occup Environ Med* 58, no.9 (Sep 2016): 861–7. https://www. ncbi.nlm.nih.gov/pubmed/27305843.

Chapter 1: Too Tired to Be Happy

Aschbacher K., A. O'Donovan, O. M. Wolkowitz, F. S. Dhabhar, Y. Su, and E. Epel. "Good stress, bad stress and oxidative stress: insights from anticipatory cortisol reactivity," *Psychoneuroendocrinology* 38, no. 9 (Sep 2013): 1698–708. doi: 10.1016/j.psyneuen.2013 .02.004. Epub 2013 Mar 13. https://ncbi.nlm.nih.gov/pubmed/23490070.

Davis B. J., R. R. Maronpot, and J. J. Heindel. "Di-(2-ethylhexyl) phthalate suppresses estradiol and ovulation in cycling rats," *Toxicol Appl Pharmacol* 128, no. 2 (Oct 1994): 216–23. https://www.ncbi.nlm.nih.gov/pubmed/7940536.

Langer P. "The impacts of organochlorines and other persistent pollutants on thyroid and metabolic health," *Front Neuroendocrinol* 31, no. 4 (Oct 2010): 497–518. doi:10.1016/j .yfrne.2010.08.001. Epub 2010 Aug 24. https://www.ncbi.nlm.nih.gov/pubmed/20797403.

Lovekamp-Swan T. and B. J. Davis. "Mechanisms of phthalate ester toxicity in the female reproductive system," *Environ Health Perspect* 111, no. 2 (Feb 2003): 139–45. https://www.ncbi.nlm.nih.gov/pubmed/12573895.

Powell D. J., C. Liossi, R. Moss-Morris, and W. Schlotz. "Unstimulated cortisol secretory activity in everyday life and its relationship with fatigue and chronic fatigue syndrome: a systematic review and subset meta-analysis," *Psychoneuroendocrinology* 38, no. 11 (Nov 2013): 2405–22. doi: 10.1016/j.psyneuen.2013.07.004. Epub 2013 Aug 2. https://www .ncbi.nlm.nih.gov/pubmed/23916911.

Rodríguez A., J. Gómez-Ambrosi, V. Catalán, M. J. Gil, S. Becerril, N. Sáinz, C. Silva, J. Salvador, I. Colina, and G. Frühbeck. "Acylated and desacyl ghrelin stimulate lipid accumulation in human visceral adipocytes, *Int J Obes* Lond. 33, no. 5 (May 2009): 541–52. doi: 10.1038/ijo.2009.40. Epub 2009 Feb 24. https://www.ncbi.nlm.nih.gov/pub med/19238155.

Silverman M. N. and E. M. Sternberg. "Glucocorticoid regulation of inflammation and its functional correlates: from HPA axis to glucocorticoid receptor dysfunction," *Ann N Y Acad Sci.* 1261 (Jul 23 2012): 55–63. doi: 10.1111/j.1749-6632.2012.06633.x. https://www .ncbi.nlm.nih.gov/pubmed/22823394.

Chapter 2: Stressed-Out B*tches

Kalantaridou S. N., A. Makrigiannakis, E. Zoumakis, and G. P. Chrousos. "Stress and the female reproductive system," *J Reprod Immunol* 62, no. 1–2 (Jun 2004): 61–8.

Shewchuk B. M. "Prostaglandins and n-3 polyunsaturated fatty acids in the regulation of the hypothalamic-pituitary axis," *Prostaglandins Leukot Essent Fatty Acids* 91, no. 6 (Dec 2014): 277–87. doi: 10.1016/j.plefa.2014.09.005. Epub 2014 Sep 28. https://www.ncbi .nlm.nih.gov/pubmed/25287609.

Soenen S., E. A. Martens, A. Hochstenbach-Waelen, S. G. Lemmens, and M. S. Westerterp-Plantenga. "Normal protein intake is required for body weight loss and weight maintenance, and elevated protein intake for additional preservation of resting energy expenditure and fat free mass," *J Nutr* 143, no. 5 (May 2013): 591–6. doi: 10.3945/jn.112 .167593. Epub 2013 Feb 27. https://www.ncbi.nlm.nih.gov/pubmed/23446962.

Stratakis C. A. and G. P. Chrousos. "Neuroendocrinology and pathophysiology of the stress system," *Ann N Y Acad Sci* 771 (Dec 1995): 1–18. https://www.ncbi.nlm.nih.gov /pubmed/8597390.

Takahashi N., M. Harada, Y. Hirota, L. Zhao, J. M. Azhary, O. Yoshino, G. Izumi, T. Hirata, K. Koga, O. Wada-Hiraike , T. Fujii, and Y. Osuga. "A Potential Role for Endoplasmic Reticulum Stress in Progesterone Deficiency in Obese Women," *Endocrinology* 158, no. 1 (Jan 2017): 84–97.

Chapter 4: What a Hangry B*tch Should Eat

Adlercreutz, H., et al. "Studies on the role of intestinal bacteria in metabolism of synthetic and natural steroid hormones." *Journal of Steroid Biochemistry* 20, no. 1 (Jan 20 1984): 217–229.

Alexander, D. D., et al. "A review and meta-analysis of red and processed meat consumption and breast cancer," *Nutrition Research Reviews* 23, no. 2 (Dec 23 2010): 349–365.

Boas M., U. Feldt-Rasmussen, N. E. Skakkebaek, and K.M. Main. "Environmental chemicals and thyroid function," *Eur J Endocrinol* 154, no. 5 (May 2006): 599–611. https://www. ncbi.nlm.nih.gov/pubmed/16645005.

Fabricio G., A. Malta, A. Chango, and P. C. De Freitas Mathias. "Environmental Contaminants and Pancreatic Beta-Cells." *J Clin Res Pediatr Endocrinol* 8, no. 3 (Sept 1 2016): 257–63. doi: 10.4274/jcrpe.2812. Epub 2016 Apr 18. https://www.ncbi.nlm.nih.gov /pubmed/27087124.

Fasano A. "Zonulin and its regulation of intestinal barrier function: the biological door to inflammation, autoimmunity, and cancer," *Physiol Rev* 91, no. 1 (Jan 2011): 151–75. doi: 10.1152/physrev.00003.2008. https://www.ncbi.nlm.nih.gov/pubmed/21248165.

Freed D. L. "Do dietary lectins cause disease?" *BMJ* 318, no. 7190 (Apr 17 1999): 1023–4.

Shewry P. R. "Wheat," *J Exp Bot* 60, no. 6 (Apr 1 2009): 1537–53. doi: 10.1093/jxb/erp058. https://www.ncbi.nlm.nih.gov/pubmed/19386614.

Patrick L. "Thyroid disruption: mechanism and clinical implications in human health," *Altern Med Rev* 14, no. 4 (Dec 2009): 326–46. https://www.ncbi.nlm.nih.gov/pubmed /20030460.

Chapter 5: Getting It Right with Exercise

Menshikova E. V., V. B. Ritov, L. Fairfull, R. E. Ferrell, D. E. Kelley, and B. H. Goodpaster. "Effects of exercise on mitochondrial content and function in aging human skeletal muscle," *J Gerontol A Biol Sci Med Sci* 61, no. 6 (Jun 2006): 534–40. https://www.ncbi.nlm .nih.gov/pmc/articles/PMC1540458.

Godfrey R. J., G. P. Whyte, J. Buckley, et al. "The role of lactate in the exercise-induced human growth hormone response: evidence from McArdle disease," *Br J Sports Med* 43, no. 7 (Jul 2009): 521–525.

Kraemer W. J. and N. A. Ratamess. "Endocrine responses and adaptations to strength and power training," *Sports Med* 35, no. 4 (2005): 339–361.

Schoenfeld B. J., B. Contreras, G. Tiryaki-Sonmez, J. M. Wilson, M. J. Kolber, and M. D. Peterson. "Regional differences in muscle activation during hamstrings exercise," *J Strength Cond Res* 29, no. 1 (Jan 2015): 159–64. doi: 10.1519/JSC.0000000000000598. https://www.ncbi.nlm.nih.gov/pubmed/24978835.

Schoenfeld B. J., B. Contreras, J. Krieger, J. Grgic, K. Delcastillo, R. Belliard, and A. Alto. "Resistance Training Volume Enhances Muscle Hypertrophy but Not Strength in Trained Men," *Med Sci Sports Exerc* 51, no. 1 (Jan 2019): 94–103. doi: 10.1249/ MSS.0000000000001764. https://www.ncbi.nlm.nih.gov/pubmed/30153194.

Chapter 6: Week 1

Massoudi M. S., E. N. Meilahn, T. J. Orchard, T. P. Jr Foley, L. H. Kuller, J. P. Costantino, and A. M. Buhari. "Prevalence of thyroid antibodies among healthy middle-aged women. Findings from the thyroid study in healthy women," *Ann Epidemiol* 5, no. 3 (May 1995): 229–33. https://www.ncbi.nlm.nih.gov/pubmed/7606312.

McGrogan A., H. E. Seaman, J. W. Wright, and C. S. de Vries. "The incidence of auto-immune thyroid disease: a systematic review of the literature," *Clin Endocrinol* (Oxf). 69, no. 5 (Nov 2008): 687–96. doi: 10.1111/j.1365-2265.2008.03338.x. Epub 2008 Jul 31. https://www. ncbi.nlm.nih.gov/pubmed/18673466.

Purohit V. "Moderate alcohol consumption and estrogen levels in postmenopausal women: a review," *Alcohol Clin Exp Res* 22, no. 5 (Aug 1998): 994–7. https://www.ncbi .nlm.nih.gov/pubmed/9726268.

Chapter 7: The Hangry B*tch Hormone Quiz

D'Eon, T. and B. Braun. "The roles of estrogen and progesterone in regulating carbohydrate and fat utilization at rest and during exercise," *J Womens Health Gend Based Med* 11, no. 3 (Apr 2002): 225–37. https://www. ncbi.nlm.nih.gov/pubmed/11988133.

Diamanti-Kandarakis E., J. P. Bourguignon, L. C. Giudice, R. Hauser, G. S. Prins, A. M. Soto, R. T. Zoeller, and A. C. Gore. "Endocrine-disrupting chemicals: an Endocrine Society scientific statement," *Endocr Rev* 30, no. 4 (Jun 2009): 293–342. doi: 10.1210/er.2009-0002. https://www. ncbi.nlm.nih.gov/pubmed/19502515.

Dreon D. M., J. L. Slavin, and S. D. Phinney. "Oral contraceptive use and increased plasma concentration of C-reactive protein," *Life Sci* 73, no. 10 (Jul 25 2003): 1245–52. https://www.ncbi.nlm.nih.gov/pubmed/12850240.

Fasano A. "Leaky gut and autoimmune diseases," *Clin Rev Allergy Immunol* 42, no. 1 (Feb 2012): 71–8. doi: 10.1007/s12016-011-8291-x. https://www.ncbi.nlm.nih.gov/pubmed/22109896.

Fasano A. "Physiological, pathological, and therapeutic implications of zonulin-mediated intestinal barrier modulation: living life on the edge of the wall," *Am J Pathol* 173, no. 5 (Nov 2008): 1243–52. doi: 10.2353/ajpath.2008.080192. Epub 2008 Oct 2. https://www.ncbi.nlm.nih.gov/pubmed/18832585.

Kharrazian D. and A. Vojdani. "Correlation between antibodies to bisphenol A, its target enzyme protein disulfide isomerase and antibodies to neuron-specific antigens," *J Appl Toxicol* 37, no. 4 (Apr 2017): 479–84. doi: 10.1002/jat.3383. Epub 2016 Sep 9. https://www.ncbi.nlm.nih.gov/pubmed/27610592.

Chapter 8: Week 2

Byrnes S. E., J. C. Miller, and G. S. Denyer. "Amylopectin starch promotes the development of insulin resistance in rats," *J Nutr* 125, no. 6 (Jun 1995): 1430–7. https://www.ncbi.nlm.nih.gov/pubmed/7782895.

Davis, William. *Wheat Belly*. New York: Rodale Books, 2011.

Gärtner, R., B. C. Gasnier, J. W. Dietrich, B. Krebs, and M. W. Angstwurm. "Selenium supplementation in patients with autoimmune thyroiditis decreases thyroid peroxidase antibodies concentrations." *Journal of Clinical Endocrinology & Metabolism* 87, no. 4 (Apr 2002): 1687–91. https://www.ncbi.nlm.nih.gov/pubmed/11932302.

Soares F. L., R. de Oliveira Matoso, L. G. Teixeira, Z. Menezes, S. S. Pereira, A. C. Alves, N. V. Batista, A. M. de Faria, D. C. Cara, A. V. Ferreira, and J. I. Alvarez-Leite. "Gluten-free diet reduces adiposity, inflammation and insulin resistance associated with the induction of PPAR-alpha and PPAR-gamma expression," *J Nutr Biochem* 24, no. 6 (Jun 2013): 1105–11. doi: 10.1016/j.jnutbio.2012.08.009. Epub 2012 Dec 17. https://www.ncbi.nlm.nih.gov/pubmed/23253599.

Toulis, K. A., A. D. Anastasilakis, T. G. Tzellos, D. G. Goulis, and D. Kouvelas. "Selenium supplementation in the treatment of Hashimoto's thyroiditis: A systematic review and a meta- analysis," *Thyroid* 20, no. 10 (Oct 2010): 1163–73. doi: 10.1089/thy.2009.0351. https://www.ncbi.nlm.nih.gov/pubmed/20883174.

Chapter 10: Week 4

D'Eon T. and B. Braun. "The roles of estrogen and progesterone in regulating carbo-hydrate and fat utilization at rest and during exercise," *J Womens Health Gend Based Med* 11, no. 3 (Apr 2002): 225–37. doi: 10.1089/152460902753668439. https://www.ncbi.nlm.nih.gov/pubmed/11988133.

Index